Mission Statement

Future Medicine Publishing was created to help alleviate our present medical crisis by informing the public of effective and affordable alternatives in health care and promoting freedom of choice in medicine.

Responding to a growing consumer demand for alternatives to conventional medicine, we produced *Alternative Medicine: The Definitive Guide*, a landmark work resulting from a global effort spanning four years, a two million dollar budget, and involving over 400 leading alternative health professionals. *You Don't Have to Die: Unraveling the AIDS Myth* continues our tradition of investigating and reporting on crucial health issues in order to help save lives and reduce needless suffering.

As the "Voice of Alternative Medicine," our goal is to help bring about a rebirth of heath care in America. We seek to unite the most successful approaches to health maintenance, disease prevention, and the treatment of chronic illness from both conventional and alternative medicine. We envision this integration as the hallmark of future medicine and the catalyst for the dawning of a new Health Age in America.

You Don't Have to Die

Unraveling the AIDS Myth

Leon Chaitow, N.D., D.O.
and James Strohecker
with the Burton Goldberg Group

Scientific Appendix by
Robert Jacobs, N.M.D., D. Hom. (med)

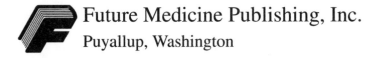

Future Medicine Publishing, Inc.
Puyallup, Washington

ISBN: 0-9636334-4-9

Library of Congress Catalogue Card Number: 94-72701

Publisher's Cataloging in Publication Data

Chaitow, Leon.
    You don't have to die : unraveling the AIDS myth / Leon
Chaitow, James Strohecker and the Burton Goldberg Group.
    p. cm.
    Includes bibliographical references and index.
    Preassigned LCCN: 94-72701.
    ISBN 0-9636334-4-9

    1. AIDS (Disease)—Alternative treatment.
I. Strohecker, James.   II. Burton Goldberg Group (Firm)
III. Title.
RC607.A26C53 1994   616.97'9206
                                     QBI94-1568

Cover design by 3DMARK, Inc.
Typesetting: Patti Zeman

Printed in the United States of America.

9 8 7 6 5 4 3 2 1

Future Medicine Publishing, Inc.
10124 18th Street, Court East
Puyallup, WA 98371
1-800-435-1221

Dedication

To all the courageous physicians and scientists who have flown in the face of conventional thinking in order to discover the underlying causes and effective treatments for AIDS. And to all those who have needlessly suffered and died due to the short-sightedness of conventional medicine.

Credits

Executive Editor: James Strohecker

Senior Contributing Editors: Celia Farber, Larry Trivieri

Contributing Editor: Mari Florence

Research: Denise Domb, Chris Breyer

Copy Editor: Robin Quinn

Production: John Coyle

Table of Contents

Message to the Reader   ix
Introduction   AIDS—A Reevaluation   xi

PART ONE   UNDERSTANDING AIDS
Chapter 1   Unraveling the Myths   3
Chapter 2   Major Risk Groups and the Many
             Causes of AIDS   25
Chapter 3   Lifestyle Influences and Immune
             Suppression   35
Chapter 4   Prognosis for the Future   45

PART TWO   ALTERNATIVE TREATMENTS
            FOR AIDS
Chapter 5   Diet and Nutritional Supplements   61
Chapter 6   Herbal Medicine   85
Chapter 7   Nutritional and Herbal Treatment of
             Illnesses Associated with AIDS   99
Chapter 8   Acupuncture and Traditional Chinese
             Medicine   113
Chapter 9   Naturopathic Medicine   123
Chapter 10   Mind/Body Medicine   137
Chapter 11   Oxygen Therapy   155
Chapter 12   Hyperthermia   169
Chapter 13   Massage and Touch Therapies   183

PART THREE LONG-TERM SURVIVORS
Chapter 14   Success Stories: The Physician-Patient
             Partnership   197
             Dr. Jon Kaiser   198
             Dr. Joan Priestley   205

	Dr. Laurence Badgley	211
	Dr. Gerhard Orth (Germany)	216
	Dr. Hulda Regehr Clark	220
	Dr. Stanislaw Burzynski and Antineoplaston AS2-1	221
	Dr. Robert Cathcart III and Vitamin C	224
	Dr. Ignacio Coronel and L-51 (Mexico)	225
	Gaston Naessens and Somatidian Orthobiology (Canada)	226
	Dr. Qingcai Zhang and Chinese Bitter Melon	235
Chapter 15	A Woman's Journey: Sharon Lund	241

RESOURCES

Where to Find Help

AIDS Organizations	255
Buyer's Clubs	259
Recommended Reading	260
Choosing an Alternative Health Professional	263
Appendix: Human Immunodeficiency Virus	267
Glossary	279
Endnotes	291
Index	305

Message to the Reader

The message that "HIV=AIDS=Death" has been so widely disseminated that to challenge it seems heretical. We will doubtless be accused of heresy and of putting lives at risk due to our questioning the emphasis placed on HIV by government agencies, research institutions, and the media. But the truth is that while HIV may be a part of the process in many individuals, it is almost certainly never sufficient to cause AIDS on its own.

The excessive emphasis on HIV as "the cause" of AIDS, and the lack of attention to methods of encouraging and modulating the immune system, have led to the present crisis. This is the single most important reason for the writing of this book. The propaganda relating to HIV has been so intense, in fact, that many of the researchers and clinicians quoted in later sections of the book are still working within, or are largely influenced by, the mind-set in which HIV is the key element.

Lest we be accused of inconsistency because some of the research and clinical evidence which we will present has a focus on HIV, we wish to make our position clear from the outset. We do not believe, based on the evidence we have seen and which we will outline, that HIV is a sufficient single cause of AIDS. Nor do we believe that being HIV positive leads inevitably to AIDS, or that AIDS is necessarily irreversible.

We do believe that attention to enhancement and modulation of immune function presents an opportunity for recovery of health. We sincerely believe that this approach will be increasingly adopted as the HIV myth is discredited, and that we will look back and wonder why billions of dollars have been wasted in HIV-oriented research.

An Important Message:
This book is intended as an educational tool to acquaint the reader with alternative methods for the treatment of AIDS and HIV infection. The publisher hopes the book will enable the reader to improve his or her well-being and to better understand, assess, and choose the appropriate course of treatment for an illness or health condition.

Because the methods described in this book are, by definition, alternative methods, many of them have not been investigated and/or approved by any government or regulatory agency. National, state, and local laws vary regarding the use and application of many of the treatments that are discussed. Accordingly, this book should not be substituted for the advice and treatment of a physician or other licensed health professional, but rather should be used in conjunction with professional care. Pregnant women in particular are especially urged to consult with their physician before using any therapy.

Your health is important. Use this book wisely. Discuss the alternative treatment options described herein with your doctor. Ultimately, you, the reader, must take full responsibility for your health and how you use this book. The publisher expressly disclaims responsibility for any adverse effects resulting from your use of the information contained herein.

Introduction:
AIDS—A Reevaluation

W hen we think of AIDS (Acquired Immune Deficiency Syndrome), we think of a virus called HIV (human immunodeficiency virus). This association has existed ever since 1984, when Robert Gallo, M.D., announced that it was the HIV virus (then referred to as HTLV-111, or human T-cell lymphotropic virus) that was the cause of AIDS. From that time on, it has been the popular belief that this single factor alone, namely exposure to this virus, determines whether or not a person will contract AIDS and therefore live or die. And this has been compounded by the mainstream media, which for the most part has relentlessly perpetuated this theory, thereby assuring that millions of Americans will live in fear of "catching" what is now known as "the AIDS virus." Though it makes a good, simple story, the HIV/AIDS hypothesis is far from being conclusively substantiated scientifically.

Research has shown quite clearly that AIDS is a complex disease, and is determined by many more factors than whether or not a person has been exposed to HIV. Worldwide, more than four thousand known cases of AIDS exist without any trace of HIV, and these cases have been documented in the medical literature.[1] And, while as many as one million Americans have tested positive for HIV, many have remained healthy and asymptomatic for upwards of fourteen years after their diagnoses.[2] This does not discount the sad fact that thousands of people who were also HIV positive became sick and died. But it does strongly suggest that this correlation between AIDS and HIV is not sufficient proof of causation, particularly since no research has focused on what other factors may have contributed toward the disease progression. In other words, almost fourteen years into the AIDS crisis, a realization is now emerging that HIV, the presumed cause of AIDS, may have less to do with AIDS than is widely believed, and may in fact be but one piece in a very complex puzzle, the other pieces of which must be addressed in order to bring AIDS under control.

xii

Unanswered Questions

There are many unresolved issues surrounding AIDS. Despite years of our being warned otherwise, AIDS has not spread significantly outside of the original risk groups associated with it when the syndrome was first identified.[3] And, perhaps even more curiously, repeated studies have shown that prostitutes, unless they are also IV drug users, face no greater risk for contracting AIDS than does anyone else.[4] It has also been observed that AIDS patients tend to have a host of other immunosuppressive factors in their background, beyond infection with HIV alone. These facts raise a number of serious questions. Is AIDS really caused by a single virus that is spread primarily through sex? If not, then what is it that really determines who gets AIDS and who doesn't? And why do some people infected with HIV get sick while others with the same infection remain healthy?

Ever since Dr. Gallo's pronouncement, virtually all research has focused on HIV and little or no attention has been paid to alternative causes. For this reason, it may take decades before we have the answers to these questions. It is a shame that so much time, research, and funds have been wasted looking for answers in the wrong direction. In the meantime, it is important that people with AIDS or other forms of immune suppression learn how to stay well and survive. That is the focus of this book.

We have found that the most successful approaches to AIDS have been taken by those within the field of alternative medicine, outside the mainstream of conventional approaches. The people who are recovering and surviving are those who have eliminated immunosuppressive activities from their lives and improved their nutrition and overall health. They have chosen not to accept an AIDS diagnosis as a death sentence, and instead have adopted a personal and realistic vision of health.

This book will present the inspiring stories of some of these survivors, as well as treatments which we feel offer the best hope for those who suffer from immune deficiency. With the brunt of AIDS research funds still being funnelled into the development of toxic drugs and therapies that have yielded only dismal results thus far, it is obvious that the time has come to consider other approaches (that are proving to be successful) as well. And as more people begin to take their health into their own hands, it is likely that they will begin utilizing these alternative therapies.

Alternative Medicine and AIDS: Success Stories

A basic premise of alternative medicine is that virtually all diseases, if properly approached and treated in time, are reversible. This includes AIDS, as the following stories illustrate.

Mark,* a man suffering from AIDS for five years, came to Joan Priestley, M.D., of Anchorage, Alaska. His doctors had told him that his case was terminal and had given him five months to live. He was suffering from severe weight loss and diarrhea, and was ravaged by opportunistic infections and Crohn's disease. Today, over one year after beginning aggressive treatment with Dr. Priestley, Mark is symptom-free, has regained forty pounds, and is living a productive, engaging life. This is despite a continued low T-cell count (which is considered a marker for AIDS and HIV infection).

A patient suffering from night sweats and fever, and diagnosed as HIV positive, was weak and faint all of the time as his T-cell count continued dropping. He sought out Robert Cathcart III, M.D., of Los Altos, California, a pioneer in the use of vitamin C therapy as a treatment for illness. Fifteen months after beginning intravenous vitamin C treatments, the patient's T-cell count had risen from under 300 to 600. Not only did he feel healthy, for the first time in his life he went over a year without experiencing a cold or flu.

In 1984, Jon was diagnosed with Kaposi's sarcoma, a form of skin cancer common to gay men with AIDS. He had also been suffering from hepatitis for a year. After adopting a protocol of nutritional supplementation, herbs, and diet under the supervision of Laurence Badgley, M.D., of Foster City, California, his symptoms began to improve. Today, over nine years later, Jon is healthy and working two full-time jobs.

These are just three cases of people with AIDS who have turned their illness around and are now on the road to health. Other cases in Part Two, "Alternative Treatments for AIDS,"

* Note: To protect patient confidentiality, the names of patients presented in this book have been changed.

and Part Three, "Long Term Survivors," further illustrate the various alternative methods that are being used outside of the framework of conventional medicine to keep people with AIDS alive and healthy. To understand how and why such treatments work, though, it is important to examine what AIDS is and what it is not.

Smoke and Mirrors: The Continuing Debate

When we say "AIDS," the common assumption is that we are referring to something specific and definable, as is the case with all other diseases. But the fact is that AIDS has a constantly evolving definition which differs from risk group to risk group, and from country to country. In part, AIDS is a media construct, a patchwork of sound bites. That is not to say that it is a mere phantom created by the mass media, only that the rigid and simplified version of AIDS which we get through the media has very little to do with the reality. And beyond the media distortion is the problem that even the experts do not agree on what that reality is.

As we approach the mid-nineties, the AIDS discourse is increasingly becoming more defined by bewilderment and reassessment, and less by dogma. Gradually, AIDS experts are peeling away the layers of what they thought they knew. What will remain when all the old dogmas are dissolved will be the new definition of AIDS.

Perhaps we will find that it is not a single syndrome, but a grouping of several. Perhaps we will find that it is not even a new syndrome at all, but an old one newly named. The answers are yet to be found. Meanwhile, the more pressing task remains of attempting to make some sense out of what we do know.

That is the aim of this book. We hope to provide you with the most sensible approaches to avoiding and surviving AIDS that can be determined at this time, in a manner that enables you to make informed decisions, and that quite possibly saves lives. In addition, we hope to make sure the debate about the true cause or causes of AIDS remains open, rigorous, undistorted, and apolitical. Otherwise we may never have the answers we need to conquer AIDS once and for all.

Part One: Understanding AIDS

"My dear Kepler, what do you say of the leading philosophers here, to whom I have offered a thousand times of my own accord to show my studies, but who, with the lazy obstinacy of a serpent who has eaten his fill, have never consented to look at the planets or moon, or telescope? Verily, just as serpents close their ears, so do men close their eyes to the light of truth."

—Galileo in a letter to Johannes Kepler ca. 1630

1   Unraveling the Myths

AIDS has proven to be a perplexing phenomenon fraught with paradoxes which cloud our understanding of the cause and nature of the disease. Over four thousand cases of AIDS with no trace of HIV infection, the virus thought by most scientists to cause the illness, have been medically documented worldwide.[1] And there are many people with HIV infection who, if their HIV test results can be trusted (see Chapter Four), have remained healthy for at least ten years after becoming infected. There are also a number of people who were at one time HIV positive and who are now HIV negative,[2] and growing numbers of people who have suffered from full-blown AIDS symptoms, but have since completely recovered from the disease, establishing that AIDS is reversible. Finally, there is increasing evidence that AIDS may not even be a new disease syndrome at all.

Although AIDS was recognized and named only fifteen years ago, some doctors insist it has been around for decades and perhaps even longer. And their arguments are not simply based on speculation. There are recorded cases of patients who not only displayed clusters of symptoms virtually identical to those defining our current picture of AIDS, but who were also actually infected with HIV, as identified from frozen specimens kept since the 1950s and 1960s.[3] Even more puzzling is the possibility of other cases which meet all of the symptomatic definitions of AIDS, but without any possibility of knowing whether or not HIV was also present, dating back to 1872.[4]

These are some of the most obvious areas of confusion, because the statements above contradict the commonly-held beliefs that AIDS is new, that HIV, on its own, causes AIDS, and that a test showing someone to be HIV positive means that the onset of AIDS is inevitable. In light of these issues, the debate about what AIDS is and how it is caused is widening, as an increasing number of scientists come to the view that we have been presented with a greatly simplified picture of AIDS and that the answers to reversing the condition lie in unraveling the truth.

Examining AIDS, we find that it is defined primarily by what appears to be a breakdown of the body's defense systems, resulting in severe immune deficiency. But it is distinguished from virtually every other disease in history by the fact that it has no constant, specific symptoms. Once the immune system has begun to malfunction, a broad spectrum of health complications can set in, and "AIDS" has now become an umbrella term for any or all of twenty-eight previously known diseases and symptoms. According to the Centers for Disease Control (CDC), when a person has any of these microbial diseases or opportunistic infections, and also tests positive for antibodies to HIV, a diagnosis of AIDS is warranted.[5]

Differences in AIDS Cases Worldwide

The diseases that define AIDS differ widely from country to country, and even from risk group to risk group. In the United States and Europe, some of the most common diseases associated with AIDS are Kaposi's sarcoma (a form of cancer), pneumocystis carinii pneumonia (PCP), candidiasis, and mycobacterial infections such as tuberculosis, toxoplasmosis (a disease caused by protozoa that damages the central nervous system, eyes, and the body's internal organs), cytomegalovirus (an infectious agent which is often considered a prime suspect as a co-factor for AIDS), and the herpes virus. Other more general conditions not included in the twenty-eight indicator diseases, but often associated with the disease, include diarrhea, weight loss, night sweats, fevers, rashes, and swollen lymph glands.

There are some striking differences between the various "risk groups," or groups of people within which AIDS has remained concentrated since it was first discovered. Kaposi's sarcoma, for instance, one of the earliest symptoms by which AIDS was diagnosed, is twenty times more common in gay men with AIDS than in all other American AIDS patients.[6] Tuberculosis, meanwhile, is mainly seen in intravenous drug users. AIDS in Africa, by contrast, lacks the distinction of "risk groups," but is said to be distributed evenly among the population and between the sexes. There, AIDS is defined primarily by diarrhea, wasting, fever, and a persistent cough. All these symptoms, which are factors in most tropical diseases, have been reported in Africa for over one hundred years and are still quite common there independent of an AIDS diagnosis.

A 1993 report by the eleven member U.S. National Research Council concluded that AIDS hardly exists in many geographical areas and population groups. The disease syndrome seems to be localized in areas in which there are concentrations of "socially disadvantaged" groups, such as drug-users, the poor and under-educated, and homosexuals. A virus alone is unlikely to discriminate in this way. The evidence points, rather, to social and behavioral factors as key elements in AIDS causation.[7]

Because of these and other discrepancies, there is much confusion and dissent about what AIDS really is, and even if it is accurate to classify it as a disease entity. The common factor that all these disconnected symptoms and diseases revolve around is HIV. If HIV antibodies are detected, these diseases converge as AIDS; if not, then an AIDS diagnosis is not given. In other words, any degree of immune suppression, in the presence of HIV, is classified as AIDS. But the same degree of immune suppression, in the absence of HIV, is by conventional definition not AIDS.

This has led to a kind of diagnostic chaos never before seen in modern medicine. The answer as to who has AIDS and who doesn't may depend on which doctor a person questions. Further confusing the issue, there is also, as we have already mentioned, tremendous dispute about whether, in fact, HIV is the cause of AIDS. This question has been argued in the media, the AIDS community, and in the scientific literature—and it remains unresolved.

Today, the scientific community researching AIDS is dividing into two camps. One camp, and by far still comprising the majority viewpoint, believes that HIV causes, or triggers, the immune suppression that leads to AIDS. The other camp argues that various environmental risk factors, such as recreational and pharmaceutical drugs, sexually transmitted diseases, and bacterial infections, are the real causes of the immune suppression, and that HIV is just a by-product of an already suppressed immune system. The debate between the two camps also raises questions about how people contract AIDS. Do they "catch" it all at once, or do they acquire it over a period of several years due to the continual stress placed upon their immune systems because of the co-factors outlined above? Questions like this one are what need to be resolved before the true nature of the relationship between AIDS and HIV can be fully understood.

The Trouble with Defining AIDS

By January 1, 1993, the original definition of AIDS was radically altered and expanded. Previously, in order to be diagnosed as having AIDS, it was necessary to have one or more of twenty-five symptoms listed by the Centers for Disease Control (CDC), as well as being HIV positive. Beginning that January, however, the CDC added three new conditions—cancer of the cervix, bacterial pneumonia, and tuberculosis—which, when found in combination with the HIV virus, would also constitute AIDS.

The effect of this decision will be to dramatically and artificially inflate the statistics of people who have AIDS. In the United States alone, the figures will show a rise from 250,000 to 400,000 (from 1982 to date), in part due to a huge increase in the number of women with a sudden AIDS diagnosis as a result of having cervical cancer. This figure increase has caused famed British epidemiologist, Professor Gordon Stewart, to ask the pertinent question: "Will any woman with cervicitis, any man with urethritis, or prostatitis, or genitourinary cancer, or any cancer, or perhaps severe infection, or any other unspecified, wasting, or multiple disease, who happens to be HIV positive, be diagnosed and registered as having AIDS and treated for HIV disease, because those in the business can expand their domain across any diagnostic code and scruple?"[8] Thus far, Professor Stewart's query has received no satisfactory answer.

The HIV Debate

Most AIDS scientists freely refer to HIV as "the causative agent of AIDS," or the "primary cause of AIDS," but when asked just exactly what body of scientific evidence supports their view, they are less certain. Although there definitely is a strong correlation between HIV and AIDS, meaning that most people with AIDS also test positive for HIV, it is not a total correlation, and certainly not proof of causation. Despite some 60,000 papers written on HIV,[9] the evidence that the virus causes AIDS still remains tenuous and, in the minds of some at least, can best be described as circumstantial; the damage is done, the cells are depleted, and HIV is present at the scene of the crime.[10]

The truth is that despite billions of dollars and years of research from around the world, no definitive answer has been found which actually shows *how* HIV causes AIDS. Even those in the mainstream who assert that there is no question as to *whether* HIV causes AIDS admit the precise mechanism by which the virus does its work has yet to be clearly found. Meanwhile, those who hold to the dissident view insist that we do not yet know whether HIV is the cause of AIDS in the first place.

The HIV/AIDS hypothesis was first revealed at a press conference on April 23, 1984, when Robert Gallo, M.D., of the National Cancer Institute, stepped up to a podium before a packed press conference in Washington, D.C. and announced that the cause of AIDS had been found.* It was, he claimed, a

* **Note:** *Dr. Gallo has been the subject of extreme controversy following his pronouncement. Most of it has focused on the question of whether he "discovered" HIV, or merely held up, as his own discovery, a year-old viral sample that had been sent to him by his colleague, Dr. Luc Montagnier of the Pasteur Institute in Paris. In 1993, a government-appointed panel officially exonerated Dr. Gallo from the charges. However, in July 1994, the National Institutes of Health acknowledged that Dr. Gallo used a French-provided virus in inventing the American HIV test kit.[11] Despite the continuing controversy, Dr. Gallo remains a leading force in conventional AIDS research.*

new retrovirus (RNA virus with tumor-causing properties), supposedly isolated in his own lab, that he named HTLV-lll (human T-cell lymphotropic virus), and which was later renamed as HIV. At the time of the announcement, this hypothesis was based on nothing more than a strong correlation between AIDS cases and HIV. Most, though not all, of the AIDS patients studied showed antibodies to HIV, and half of them also had detectable levels of the live virus. With the help of the world media, Dr. Gallo's hypothesis soon became accepted as fact. The first reports stated that the "probable" cause of AIDS had been found, but very soon the word "probable" was dropped as HIV found its new identity as "the AIDS virus."

"Nobody in their right mind would jump into this thing like they did," says Kary Mullis, Ph.D., of La Jolla, California, recipient of the 1993 Nobel Prize in Chemistry, and inventor of the Polymerase Chain Reaction (PCR), one of the mainstays of AIDS viral technology. "It had nothing to do with any well-considered science. There were some people who had AIDS and some of them had HIV—not even all of them. So they had a correlation. So what?"[12]

In 1987, molecular biologist Peter Duesberg, Ph.D., Professor of Molecular and Cell Biology at the University of California at Berkeley, launched a frontal attack on the HIV/AIDS hypothesis in the journal *Cancer Research*. Dr. Duesberg, a world-renowned scientist and long-standing member of the National Academy of Sciences, is known as one of the world's leading experts on retroviruses and helped map their genetic structure. After examining the scientific literature on HIV and AIDS, Dr. Duesberg concluded that the virus was "harmless," pointing out, among other things, that HIV was a latent, inactive virus, which infected very few cells. Dr. Duesberg stated flatly that he "wouldn't mind being injected with it."[13]

Perhaps the most striking point of Dr. Duesberg's critique of the HIV-AIDS hypothesis was that HIV showed very little direct cell-killing activity. In fact, when he viewed HIV (using a microscope) amidst lymphocytes (cells important in the creation of antibodies), the virus didn't move at all while the cells remained perfectly intact. According to Dr. Duesberg, this is

AIDS Without HIV

Growing numbers of cases of severe immune suppression have been reported that appear to be clinically identical to AIDS, but which do not test positive for HIV. Patients who are HIV negative yet fulfill all the criteria for AIDS as defined by the Centers for Disease Control (CDC) and the World Health Organization, including Kaposi's sarcoma (KS) and pneumocystis carinii pneumonia (PCP), are now a well-established phenomenon.[14] For example, CDC records cite dozens of cases of HIV negative homosexual males with Kaposi's sarcoma and associated opportunistic infections, and around fifteen cases have been recorded of HIV negative patients with another diagnostic disease for AIDS—MAI (Mycobacterium avium intracellulare). CDC reports also exist of PCP among HIV negative patients.[15]

According to Robert Root-Bernstein,Ph.D., Associate Professor of Physiology at Michigan State University, "There is no longer any doubt that HIV is not necessary to cause immune deficiency. The question is whether the causes of HIV-free AIDS are also at work in people with HIV, and therefore what role HIV plays in causing AIDS in anyone."[16] The CDC now reports that as many as 5 percent of people who develop opportunistic diseases diagnostic of AIDS remain HIV-free in the United States.[17]

According to Peter Duesberg, Ph.D., a professor at the University of California at Berkeley, and one of the world's leading experts on retroviruses, there are over four thousand such cases documented in the medical literature, including cases in Africa and Europe.[18] Because HIV is not present, these cases are not registered as AIDS. The CDC's rationale for this has been oversimplified: AIDS is caused by HIV. Therefore, if HIV is not present, the cases cannot be AIDS.

Despite many cases of HIV-free AIDS having been documented in the literature for several years, it was not until the International AIDS Conference in Amsterdam in July of 1992, that the world media reacted, writing front page stories about the "new disease," and criticizing CDC officials for not taking the "handful" of cases more seriously. A single abstract sparked the uproar, written by an American doctor who reported on six cases of AIDS with no HIV. Upon hearing the doctor's presentation, several more doctors started to volunteer cases of their own that fit the same description.

As scientific opinion has slowly begun to recognize that there can be AIDS without HIV, the task remained to re-educate the public, which has been well indoctrinated with the message that "HIV=AIDS=Death." The time had come to alter the name of the disease.

The World Health Organization has announced that the condition previously called AIDS would henceforth be referred to as "HIV Disease."[19] Quite obviously it is impossible to have HIV Disease without HIV, so the new name becomes a self-fulfilling definition. But what happens to the people with "non-HIV AIDS"? What disease do they have?

Seeking to calm the ensuing chaos, the CDC quickly settled on a new name for the "mysterious new disease." Cases of what look like clinical AIDS, where no HIV is present, are now called "ICL," which stands for idiopathic CD-4 lymphocytopenia. "Idiopathic" refers to a disease for which the cause is not known. "That's what they should call AIDS," says Harvey Bialy, Ph.D, scientific editor of the journal *BioTechnology*, and an outspoken critic of the HIV causation theory of AIDS. "ICL," he says, "it's perfect!"[20]

The choice seems simple—either the diagnostic criteria being used for AIDS are accurate or they are not. If someone can have all the symptoms of AIDS and not be HIV positive, it may be possible that people with the same symptoms, who do have HIV, have the symptoms for reasons other than the presence of that virus. If such is the case, we need to be looking at what those other reasons might be. It may be that HIV is largely involved, but it is becoming clear that it requires co-factors before it can develop into AIDS.

to be expected. "Retroviruses are not typically cytocidal, that is, they do not kill cells," he states.[21]

The mainstream AIDS research community, for its part, contends that direct cell killing is not necessary in order to implicate HIV as the disease's cause, believing that the virus kills cells by one of several highly-complex indirect mechanisms. One of these is *apoptosis*, a mechanism by which HIV is said to program cells to kill themselves in the future. Dr. Duesberg counters that there is no evidence for any of these elaborate mechanisms, and that HIV is far too simple in its genetic structure to be able to perform all these feats.

Harvey Bialy, Ph.D., scientific editor of the journal *BioTechnology*, agrees. "HIV is an ordinary retrovirus," he says. "It only contains a very small piece of genetic information. There's no way it can do all these elaborate things they say it does."[22]

Dr. Duesberg further argues that the HIV-AIDS theory fails to fulfill the standard set of rules used to determine whether a particular organism causes a particular disease. These rules, known as "Koch's Postulates," were established by German bacteriologist Robert Koch, who determined the causes of tuberculosis, anthrax, and several other infectious diseases using the following rules:

- The suspected organism has to be present in each and every case of the disease, and in sufficient quantities to cause disease.
- The agent is not found in other diseases.
- After isolation and propagation, the agent can induce the disease when transmitted to another host.

Dr. Duesberg concedes that there are limitations to Koch's Postulates, especially since most pathogens (disease-causing agents) are pathogenic only when the immune system is already below par. However, he argues, HIV has been shown to fail all three postulates:

- It has already been established that the virus is not present in every case of AIDS-like disease.
- It is found not in one, but in twenty-eight distinct diseases.
- Chimpanzees inoculated with HIV have consistently failed to develop AIDS. (There are, at present, 125 to 150 chimpanzees around the world in captivity who have been injected with HIV, some as long as ten years ago. None of the chimps has developed any symptoms of AIDS.[23])

A British study conducted in 1987 also looked at accidental exposure to HIV by medical personnel (scratched with a needle previously used on infected individuals, for example). The study noted, "One surprising and mildly reassuring fact is that when health workers were examined after needlestick wounds only one out of fifteen hundred in the United Kingdom and the United States became infected."[24]

Another mystery is why, if HIV is an infectious, deadly virus, it does not spread equally between the sexes. According to the CDC, 85 percent of those diagnosed with AIDS in the United States have been men. But if HIV were the cause, it would spread equally between men and women; viruses are not gender specific.

Meanwhile, in Africa, AIDS has been diagnosed equally in men and women. A virus does not overwhelmingly choose men on one continent, and men and women on another. Although there is a distinct form of the virus, HIV-2, in Africa, the end result of HIV-1 and HIV-2 are thought to be the same. And there are other reasons why Africa has a different pattern of AIDS. For example, there is mounting evidence of different criteria being used in making an AIDS diagnosis in Africa. In addition, false positive HIV tests have been linked to malaria, a disease that is endemic in Africa, as is tuberculosis, malnutrition, and the use of many immune-supressive drugs.[25]

Dr. Duesberg's paper catalyzed the long and bitter battle that was to come. At this writing, it still hasn't been resolved. The AIDS establishment stands firmly by its conviction that HIV is the cause, or at least the primary cause of AIDS, although they are moving closer to Dr. Duesberg's position by conceding, finally, that HIV may not be able to do the job alone, without the help of one or several co-factors.

A Shift in Focus in the HIV Debate
For several years following Dr. Duesberg's published critique of the AIDS/HIV hypothesis, the HIV orthodoxy stuck to their guns, greeting Dr. Duesberg with scorn and retribution, yet no real scientific rebuttal, as they continued to insist that HIV could kill and that it did cause AIDS by directly wiping out the CD4 cells of the immune system. Gradually, however, their certainty started to wane. At the Sixth International Conference on AIDS in San Francisco in 1990, the French discoverer of HIV, Dr. Luc Montagnier, former chief of the

Pasteur Institute's Viral Oncology Unit and now head of its Department of Retroviral AIDS Research, made a stunning announcement. To the astonishment of his colleagues, he reported that he no longer believed HIV could cause AIDS "by itself," without the help of one or several co-factors.[26]

Dr. Montagnier proposed that an organism called a mycoplasma was working in conjunction with HIV to cause the disease. He noted that when HIV isolates contaminated with mycoplasma were exposed to antibiotics, the damage to the CD4 cells stopped. This led him to theorize that the antibiotics had eliminated the mycoplasma infection, and that it was this infection, not HIV, which was the source of the damage to the cells, since HIV by itself, as he had already observed, barely killed any cells.

Dr. Montagnier was soundly criticized by his colleagues who were present at the conference. HIV scientist Jay Levy, of the University of California at San Francisco, for example, rushed to the microphone after Dr. Montagnier's presentation and dismissed the findings. And James Curran, head of the AIDS program at the Centers for Disease Control, called Dr. Montagnier's mycoplasma theory "nonsense." Other AIDS researchers were similarly upset and dismissive.[27] Nonetheless, as a result of his and Dr. Duesberg's assertions, eventually a new camp of scientists started to emerge, those who believed that HIV plus co-factors caused AIDS.

Three years following Dr. Montagnier's statements, in September of 1993, Dr. Gallo convened an eight-day meeting of five hundred AIDS scientists in Bethesda, Maryland. Among those invited, surprisingly, was one of his long-standing opponents, Joseph Sonnabend, M.D., a New York City AIDS physician and researcher and Director of the Community Research Initiative on AIDS. It was Sonnabend who had pioneered the notion of a multifactorial cause of AIDS. "Strange as it may seem," Dr. Gallo told *Science* magazine,[28] "I have a linkage to Sonnabend's early notions." At the close of the meeting, the press was informed that there had been a radical "shift in focus," in AIDS research, away from emphasizing HIV, and toward co-factors and alternative, new theories about what causes AIDS. Particular emphasis was placed on the theory that AIDS is an "autoimmune" disease, meaning that the damage is not caused directly by the virus, but results from "an immune system that goes haywire, attacking itself and other parts of the body."

This is only the latest change in the constantly shifting and often contradictory debate about what really causes the disease syndrome we call AIDS. But this latest concession, with its de-emphasizing of HIV's central role in AIDS, represents a critical turning point in a long-standing scientific battle. However, the public is not yet aware of this shift in focus and must be educated on these matters in order to create the demand for funding for serious research into new alternative treatments for AIDS which are based on this more complex understanding of the AIDS disease process.

Co-factors

The co-factors which the AIDS establishment are now finally conceding may be involved along with HIV in causing AIDS include recreational and pharmaceutical drug use, recurrent infections, chronic use of antibiotics, poor nutrition, and pollution, as well as many psychoneuroimmunological factors, such as stress, fear, and despair.

When AIDS was first recognized in 1980-81, the syndrome was called GRID, for Gay Related Immune Deficiency, since it was initially only found in gay men. The first few hundred cases were seen in male homosexuals who lived in major cities, particularly New York and San Francisco. Those in this group had frequently used both recreational and pharmaceutical drugs, and had been exposed to numerous bacterial infections and sexually transmitted diseases.[29] In fact, the CDC's initial supposition was that AIDS is caused by drugs, most specifically amyl nitrates, or "poppers," a drug that was prevalent in gay circles of that era, and which is known to be carcinogenic in laboratory animals.[30]

Other groups, however, soon started showing up as targets for the host of opportunistic diseases characteristic of AIDS. They included hemophiliacs, intravenous drug users, and the third world poor. As with gay men, all these risk groups shared similar symptoms of immune suppression caused by a number of possible factors, including drug use, frequent exposure to various bacteria and germs (as from a blood transfusion or a dirty needle), unsafe sexual practices, malnutrition, unsanitary eating and living conditions, or a combination of all or some of the above.

Before HIV was declared to be the single cause of AIDS, many of these various immunosuppressive factors were being investigated for their possible roles in causing the disease. In 1984, however, with the discovery of HIV, these other investigations stopped cold. Now, ten years later, there is a vast amount of research on HIV, and very little on any of the possible co-factors. "We were all forced into a very dogmatic and simplistic view of what caused AIDS," says Michael Lange, M.D., an infectious disease specialist at St. Luke's Roosevelt Hospital in New York City. "Today I think even the greatest proponents of HIV no longer believe that it does all that damage to the immune system by itself. There have to be other factors involved. And because of the HIV hypothesis, there's been little or no research done on what those other factors may be."[31]

AIDS and the Immune System

Aside from the presence of HIV antibodies, another marker for AIDS is a steady decline in CD4 (also called T4) immune cells. A deficiency of CD4 cells makes it difficult to fight off infections. In a healthy person, the CD4 count should hover between 900 and 1,600 per cubic millimeter of blood, but in a person with AIDS it can decline to as low as zero. In 1993, the CDC announced that a diagnosis of AIDS was permissible when CD4 cells dropped below 200, together with a positive HIV test, even in the absence of an AIDS indicator disease.

Virtually all AIDS therapies, both mainstream and alternative, have used the CD4 count as a marker for immune suppression. For example, in 1989, a CD4 cell count of less than 500 was determined to be the cutoff point after which AZT therapy was advised.[32] More recently, however, studies have shown that the "normal" range of CD4 counts is lower than previously thought in the general population.[33]

But just as the role of HIV in causing AIDS is being debated, the issue of whether or not CD4 counts are a valid means of assessing decline in immune function has also been called into question. New research shows that CD4 helper T cells

Immune System Cells

CD4: A protein marker embedded on the surface of helper T-lymphocytes (T4 cells); also found to a lesser degree on the surface of monocyte/macrophage and other immune cells. HIV invades cells by first attaching to the CD4 molecule (CD4 receptor).

CD8: A protein marker embedded in the cell surface of suppressor T-lymphocytes (T8 cells).

Lymphocytes: Cells produced chiefly by lymphoid tissue which are the cellular mediators of immunity. See T cells and B cells.

T cells (T-lymphocytes): A thymus-derived white blood cell that participates in a variety of cell-mediated immune reactions. Three fundamentally different types of T cells are recognized: helper (T4), natural killer (NK), and suppressor (T8). The ratio of T4 (helper) to T8 (suppressor) cells should be 2:1. In AIDS, this ratio is usually reverse (1:2 or less).

- **T4 cells (T-helper lymphocytes):** Immune cells called helper cells which activate themselves (cloning to produce large numbers) in response to an antigen (a substance which, when introduced into the body, is capable of inducing the production of a specific antibody), and bring into action B cells. Derived from the thymus gland (hence "T" cells), T4 cells produce lymphokines (proteins) which stimulate the macrophages (see below) to attack the invading organism.
- **T8 cells (T-suppressor lymphocytes):** Immune cells called T-suppressor cells that halt antibody production and other immune responses. T8 cells modulate activity of T4 and B cells and prevent over-reaction by the immune system. When the ratio of T4 to T8 cells alters in dominance of the latter, as in AIDS, the ability to neutralize invading organisms diminishes dramatically, or vanishes altogether.

• **Natural killer cells (NK cells):** Large granular lymphocytes that attack and destroy tumor cells and infected body cells. They are known as "natural" killers because they attack without first having to recognize specific antigens.

B cells (B-lymphocytes): One of two major classes of lymphocytes. Derived from the bone marrow (hence "B" cells). During infections, these cells are transformed into plasma cells which produce large quantities of antibodies directed at a specific pathogen. This transformation occurs through interactions with various types of T cells and other components of the immune system.

Macrophage: Scavenger cells that have the ability to recognize and ingest all foreign antigens, especially harmful bacteria, as well as cell debris and other waste in the blood. The macrophage may be a reservoir for HIV.

Monocyte: A large white blood cell which acts as a scavenger capable of destroying invading bacteria or other foreign material. Precursor to the macrophage.

---

target extracellular infections, whereas most damage in AIDS and other viral infections occurs intracellularly, where the CD8 suppressor T cells (also called T8 and vital for proper immune function) are the dominant factors.[34]

The controversial suggestion coming from some well-informed quarters is that the focus by researchers on the CD4 cell status and its decline during AIDS might be diverting attention from the more important factor of trying to enhance the potential of CD8 cells, since their task is to act intracellularly against invading organisms such as HIV.

This leads to the question as to whether HIV/AIDS research has been wrongly directed, since much of the current research effort involves suppressing the immune system's ability to destroy the HIV-infected CD4 cells. Allowing a transient increase in the total number of CD4 cells may actually result in increasing the number of HIV-infected CD4 cells.[35]

A more appropriate goal could therefore be the boosting of CD8 status with acceptance that the decline in CD4 cells numbers represents a natural process during intracellular infection.

T4 and T8 Cells

According to official doctrine, HIV also destroys T4 cells, another critical part of the immune system. (The terms CD4 and T4 cells are virtually interchangeable.) T4 cells scout out and identify invading pathogens, and trigger other immune system cells to attack these invaders. With a drastic reduction in T4 cells, the ability to respond against potential disease is reduced. As a result, pathogens which ordinarily would have no effect on the body become potent enemies.

Another phenomenon in people with AIDS is a curious reversal of the ratio between T4 and T8 cells. While a healthy person has a high T4 cell count and a low count of T8 cells, a person with AIDS has the opposite ratio.

This drop in T-helper cell levels (as evidenced by lower levels of their protein marker CD4) may show a self-preservation tactic on the part of the body as infected cells are eliminated. This is supported by the fact that many scientists have observed that ill-health does not necessarily follow a low CD4 (and therefore T-helper cell) count, at least not in the short term. Researchers have found people whose T4 counts are almost non-existent (under 10) who show no signs of disease.[36]

Prior to AIDS, T-cell counts were rarely performed, and scientific understanding of their significance remains unresolved. At the AIDS Conference in Berlin in 1993, researchers stressed that they no longer believed that CD4 counts were a particularly valuable marker for clinical disease progression, because certain drugs had raised CD4s with no improvement in health.

This is another indication that our understanding of AIDS has been oversimplified by the media, to mean, in part, nothing more than a deficiency of these immune system cells. While T-cell loss is certainly one of the markers for AIDS, blood tests of a typical patient reveal a far more complicated picture, a kind of immunological chaos that is commonly referred to as "immune collapse." As mentioned earlier, some scientists feel it is even more complex than that, and that AIDS is a problem of an immune system gone haywire, perhaps even attacking itself in a process known as "autoimmunity." While these and other theories continue to be debated, the only thing absolutely clear at present is that the immune systems of people with AIDS are damaged. Therefore, it is vital that attention be directed at those treatments which offer the best hope of restoring the immune system, thereby restoring health, as well.

A Move Away from Pharmaceutical Drugs

Because for so long it has been believed that AIDS is caused by the single virus, HIV, all mainstream medical approaches have been drug-based, as the major pharmaceutical companies joined the race to find the drug that would act as a "magic bullet" to cure AIDS. The results of this focus, however, have often verged on being disastrous.

Despite the investment of millions of dollars, and over a decade of research, the only drugs currently approved by the FDA to treat AIDS have proven so toxic and ineffective that there is concern that they might even be exacerbating the disease. These drugs—AZT, ddI, and ddC—are all antiviral agents designed to stop viral replication. But in the process they also destroy healthy cells, and cause complications ranging from bone marrow toxicity to acute pancreatitis, yielding only marginal and transitory beneficial effects as justification for the damage they cause.

The main drug which has been used in the treatment of AIDS, AZT, on which some 80 percent of all federal drug trials have focused, is actually an old chemotherapeutic drug from the 1960s.[37] Paradoxically, because of its effect on the white cells of the bone marrow, it causes severe immune suppression—the very condition it is supposed to correct.

Over the years, a great resistance has developed in the AIDS community toward these drugs, due to their high degree of toxicity and the fact that they are very expensive.[38] And it is now clear that the drugs, instead of prolonging life, may in fact be shortening it. "AZT itself causes T-cell mediated immune suppression[39] as well as drug associated anemia or leucopenia (loss of white cells) in at least half the patients treated with it," according to Robert Root-Bernstein, Ph.D., Associate Professor of Physiology at Michigan State University.[40] And the United Kingdom National AIDS Manual lists "peripheral neuropathy, malabsorption, bone marrow destruction, dementia, anemia, leucopenia, fatigue, rashes, nausea, insomnia, weight loss, muscle degeneration, and hair loss" as other toxic side-effects of AZT.[41]

The Questionable Benefits of AZT

There is a growing consensus among AIDS researchers that the benefits of AZT are at best minor and transitory. For instance, although AZT has been shown to produce a short term (months rather than years) increase in T-cell population, this is invariably followed by a rapid decline in their number to a point actually lower than that before treatment with the drug. And while, anecdotally, some physicians have reported that AZT seems to have helped some of their patients, some researchers have suggested that this may simply be due to AZT's anti-inflammatory effect, which, they say, could better be achieved with common aspirin.[42]

Nonetheless, from the time that AZT was approved by the FDA in 1987, up until the spring of 1993, it was the premier drug of mainstream AIDS treatment, filling up some 80 percent of all federal drug trials. When AZT was first approved, the FDA promised that it would only be prescribed to people in the late stages of AIDS, but those original parameters were quickly cast aside, and AZT became widely prescribed in all patient categories. By 1989, the National Institutes of Health (NIH) recommended that AZT be taken by people who were HIV positive yet still healthy, because studies had allegedly "proven" that AZT could stave off the onset of AIDS and, as the drug company's ads euphemistically phrased it, "put time on your side."

This notion proved to be sheer pharmaceutical industry propaganda. In 1991, the first major independent study that took a critical look at AZT was published by the Veterans Administration. The VA study, headed by Dr. John Hamilton, sought to demonstrate that AZT could prolong life, as claimed, in HIV positive, healthy individuals. Instead, the researchers found that there was "no statistical difference in progression to AIDS" between the AZT group and the placebo group. The VA study signaled the beginning of the end of AZT's supremacy over AIDS research.[43]

What little credibility the drug had left was shattered in one blow in the spring of 1993, with the release of the results of the Anglo-French study called "Concorde." This vast, four-year study examined AZT in more depth and for a longer period of time than any study conducted previously. For those who had placed their faith in AZT, the results were devastating.

Contrary to popular wisdom, the Concorde study showed that AZT did not forestall AIDS in people who were HIV positive but symptom-free. In fact, it was found that those who began taking AZT while symptom-free died sooner than those who were healthy yet HIV positive and received no treatment at all. This was a real blow to the drug's manufacturer, Burroughs Wellcome, particularly since HIV positive asymptomatics comprised 38 percent of their market for AZT. Their attempts at damage control included a four-page press release entitled "Wellcome's View On Concorde," which criticized the trial's conclusions as being faulty. However, the April 8, 1994 issue of the prestigious medical journal, *The Lancet*, published the final findings of the Concorde study, and confirms the verdict that "the results of Concorde do not encourage the early use of zidovudine (AZT) in symptom-free, HIV-infected adults."[44] Even though some doctors continue to prescribe AZT for individuals who are HIV positive, yet symptom-free, the Concorde study has essentially signaled at least the beginning of the end of AZT's reign as the primary drug of choice in the treatment of HIV and AIDS.

AZT Compared with Natural Methods

The Healing AIDS Research Project (HARP) at Bastyr University in Seattle, Washington treated sixteen male patients diagnosed with ARC (AIDS-Related Complex)[45] with nutrition, herbs, psychological counseling, and hyperthermia. None of the patients progressed to AIDS or died in the one-year period of the study (1988-1989). In contrast, we find that in standard AZT studies involving similar patient groups the progression (decline) rate was between 3 percent and 7 percent.[46]

The results of the HARP study indicate that natural methods of treating AIDS-related illness, which are much cheaper and have no toxicity, can produce better results over a one year period than do protocols based on the drugs of choice currently being used by conventional medicine. A longer HARP study is currently in progress as a follow-up to these findings. (For a more in-depth description of the study see Chapter Nine.)

Other Conventional AIDS Drugs: ddI and ddC

The other main drugs used to treat AIDS—ddI (dideoxynosine) and ddC (dideoxycytidine)—are also reverse transcriptase inhibitors, meaning that they inhibit the reverse transcriptase enzyme thought to be used by the HIV virus to enter the genetic material of a healthy T cell in order to convert its RNA into DNA. Both of these drugs also have potential side effects, although they differ from those posed by AZT. Among them are pancreatitis (mainly from use of ddI), hepatitis, irritability, abdominal pains, headaches, severe peripheral neuropathy, rashes, chest pain, fever, and nausea, with some of the effects being temporary while others are more severe and permanent.

Summary

Although many issues surrounding AIDS remain unresolved, a close look at the available evidence leads to the following conclusions:

- AIDS represents a generalized collapse of immune function. Although the HIV virus seems to be linked to the vast majority of AIDS cases, other cases of AIDS exist where the virus is not present, indicating that HIV, of itself, may not be enough to trigger the disease.
- Being HIV positive need not necessarily result in AIDS.
- The many co-factors which make an individual more susceptible to AIDS can be controlled.
- Having AIDS need not be fatal. A person with AIDS may recover if proper treatment is initiated before the damage associated with the disease becomes too advanced.
- AZT and other conventional AIDS drugs do not prolong life, are of limited benefit, and may even prove to be harmful.

Recommended Reading

AIDS and Syphilis—The Hidden Link. Coulter, H. Berkeley, California: North Atlantic Books, and Washington, DC: Wehawken Book Company, 1987.

According to Dr. Coulter, "The AIDS virus is probably another 'opportunistic' infection of an already destroyed immune system . . . the search should be for factors which undermine the immune system and thus predispose to infection with the AIDS virus and others which may otherwise be quite innocuous."

AIDS: The HIV Myth. Adams, Jad. New York: St. Martin's Press, 1989.

An exploration of Peter Duesberg's HIV hypothesis that debunks the theory that the virus causes AIDS.

AIDS INC.: Scandal of the Century. Rappoport, Jon. Foster City, California: Human Energy Press, 1988.

Investigative reporter Jon Rappoport uncovers the shocking truth about AIDS: Thousands are dying needlessly as the medical world and media pull off one of the biggest scandals of our time—all for the love of power and money. AIDS INC. takes you on a behind-the-scenes tour of laboratories, newsrooms, and even the White House to expose the real killers behind the disease and to propose a multifactorial model for the causation of AIDS. The author proposes that AIDS represents the confluence of many different factors within the "modern" lifestyle such as historically unprecedented sexual promiscuity, drug abuse, promiscuous use of pharmaceuticals, rampant sexually transmitted diseases, widespread malnutrition (even in the U.S where processed foods are common), and massive vaccination campaigns.

The AIDS War: Propaganda, Profiteering, and Genocide from the Medical-Industrial Complex. Lauritson, John. New York: Asklepios, 1993.

A leading AIDS dissident journalist debunks the HIV-AIDS hypotheses and AZT therapy. Contains the latest information regarding the dangers of using AZT to treat AIDS, as well as the censure Peter Duesberg received from the conventional medical establishment for his theory that HIV does not cause AIDS. (Available from Asklepios, 26 Saint Marks Place, New York City 10003.)

Alternative Medicine: The Definitive Guide. The Burton
Goldberg Group. Puyallup, WA: Future Medicine Publishing,
Inc., 1993.
*The most comprehensive reference on alternative medicine ever
compiled. Provides in-depth, easily understandable coverage of 43
alternative therapies and over 200 health conditions, with advice
from nearly 400 alternative physicians worldwide. See chapter on
"AIDS."*

Poison By Prescription: The AZT Story. Lauritson, John.
New York: Asklepios, 1990.
*An expose of the politics involved in AIDS research and how AZT, a
known toxic substance, became the conventional medical establishment's drug of choice for dealing with AIDS and HIV. (Available
from Asklepios, 26 Saint Marks Place, New York City 10003.)*

Rethinking AIDS. Root-Bernstein, Robert. New York: The
Free Press, 1993.
*A thorough investigation which indicates that HIV alone does not
cause AIDS.*

Surviving AIDS. Callen, Michael. New York: Harper Collins,
1990.
*Outlines the alternative medicine approach to health taken by the
author, one of the longest survivors of AIDS.*

A World Without AIDS. Chaitow, Leon, D.O., N.D.; and
Martin, Simon. London, England: Thorsons Publishing
Group, 1988. [Available only from Nutri Centre, 7 Park
Crescent, London W1   (FAX 011-4471-436-5171)]
*A convincing argument that conventional medicine approaches do
not "cure" disease, which outlines how AIDS can be treated using
methods of naturopathic medicine. Also includes an appendix
outlining twenty-one ways to strengthen the immune system.*

Newsletters

Rethinking AIDS
2040 Polk Street, Suite 321
San Francisco, CA 94109
FAX (415) 775-1984
*A monthly newsletter published by the Group for the Scientific
Reappraisal of the HIV Hypothesis. Comprised of over four hundred
scientists and physicians worldwide.*

2 Major Risk Groups and the Many Causes of AIDS

Before we can address the question of how best to treat the syndrome called AIDS, we must first examine the various factors that may be causing it, as our beliefs about the cause of a condition will have the most impact on our choice of treatment. This is particularly true for health professionals who base their treatment strategies on their own personal conclusions about causation. Physicians, for the most part, currently accept the hypothesis that the HIV virus alone is responsible for the onset of AIDS; consequently, few of them are presently willing to look beyond a strategy of attacking HIV, even though damage may be done to the patient's immune system as a result of these treatment methods.

There are health practitioners, however, particularly within the field of alternative medicine, who have a multifactorial approach to treating AIDS. Such practitioners do not believe that HIV alone is causing all the damage, and they look instead to other multiple immune-suppressive elements which may be present in a person's life. They are of the belief that these other factors can play as significant a role in causing AIDS, and perhaps even a greater one, than can the HIV virus of itself. And their view would seem to be borne out by the fact that for each of the major risk-groups for AIDS—the third world poor, gay men, IV drug users, blood transfusion recipients, and hemophiliacs—there tends to be characteristic immunosuppressive factors. An examination of these factors can go a long way in adopting a successful protocol for treating the disease.

The Third World Poor

The underclasses in non-industrial nations suffer from a variety of non-HIV immunosuppressive factors, all of which can produce the various symptoms associated with AIDS, including a lowered T-cell count.[1] For example, as long ago as November, 1984, researcher Maxime Seligmann, writing in

the *New England Journal of Medicine*, stated: "The common-
est cause of T-cell immunodeficiency worldwide is protein-
calorie malnutrition. Malnourished children have defects in . . .
T-cell function accompanied by . . . an increased susceptibility
to infections." Seligmann is describing the exact pattern of
AIDS, and concludes, "Bacterial superinfection in these children [suffering from malnutrition] is a major cause of serious
disease and death."[2]

This is only one of a number of studies which link serious
malnutrition to immune-system collapse and subsequent
opportunistic infection and disease, without the HIV virus
being present.[3] In countries like Uganda, where the public
health system is very deficient, malnourishment, typhoid
fever, endemic tuberculosis, worms, other intestinal parasites,
and malaria can all severely undermine people's health and
immune functioning. Another contributing factor is the use of
immunosuppressive drugs to combat malaria and other tropical diseases. These include antiparasitic drugs such as
Clotramizole and Ketoconazole, and antimalarial drugs such
as Chloroquine.[4] These conditions on their own, with no help
from HIV, can bring about the African AIDS profile.[5]

It should also be noted that malnutrition and various intestinal parasites have been on the rise in America's inner cities.[6]
These severe immunosuppressive factors are not byproducts
of the HIV virus; they are extremely debilitating on their own,
and can lead to opportunistic infections, presenting an exact
match of the AIDS profile.

Independent research scientist Hulda Regehr Clark, Ph.D.,
N.D., of San Diego, California, reports that a particular parasite, the human intestinal fluke *(Fasciolopsis buskii)*, is a key
co-factor in the progression of AIDS. According to Dr. Clark,
the presence of this parasite in the thymus gland sets the stage
for HIV to gain a foothold in the body. She has found that this
parasite becomes established in the thymus only when the solvent benzene has first accumulated there. If Dr. Clark's findings are accurate, we feel that a full-scale and intensive
research effort into the role of parasites as a co-factor in AIDS
and AIDS-related conditions should be undertaken immediately. (See Chapter Fourteen for a more in-depth explanation
of Dr. Clark's research.)

Gay Men

Gay men were the first people to be diagnosed with AIDS and have remained a major risk group ever since. Several health surveys have shown that those in this group who have come down with AIDS have shared certain immunosuppressive problems. In *Rethinking AIDS*, Robert Root-Bernstein, Ph.D., Associate Professor of Physiology at Michigan State University, writes, ". . . Investigators have confirmed that the presence of diverse antiviral antibodies, active infections, a history of syphilis, sexual promiscuity, unprotected anal intercourse, and use of multiple street drugs are all risks associated with the development of AIDS in gay men."[7] Conversely, he points out, gay men who have no such immunosuppressive factors in their history are at low risk for both immune suppression and AIDS.

Overuse of antibiotics is another serious problem, as it can upset the healthy balance of intestinal flora and other bacteria in the body.[8] In addition, a whole host of germs can become antibiotic-resistant. A landscape like this presents a strange picture to unknowing doctors who discover germs and infection running unchecked through their patient's body. The doctor may note that the patient's immune system is not stopping this onslaught, not realizing that too many antibiotics may have killed off *friendly* germs whose role it is to deplete the ranks of potentially harmful bacteria in the body, thereby keeping them under control. With this massive imbalance of bacteria, AIDS indicator-diseases have a much easier time blossoming.

In one of the only formal surveys done on gay men and their use of antibiotics, a research team interviewed the patrons of a gay bar in Memphis, Tennessee. Dr. Root-Bernstein reports, "Over 40 percent of the men surveyed responded that they 'routinely' treated themselves with prescription antibiotics. Chronic and high-dose antibiotic abuse can lead to significant immune suppression."[9]

Another factor common to some gay men, particularly those with multiple sex partners, is that they have contracted sexually transmitted diseases (STDs) a number of times, such as gonorrhea and syphilis. Steven Bailey, N.D., Assistant Professor of Pharmacognosy at National College of Naturopathic

Medicine in Portland, Oregon, states that approximately 97 percent of his HIV-infected patients report a history of gonorrhea. Such diseases are themselves immunosuppressive. "Syphilis, in particular," reports Joan McKenna, a research physiologist in San Francisco, "when undiagnosed or poorly treated, can eventually present as pneumocystis pneumonia, the number one disease symptom of AIDS. Certainly, repeated antibiotic treatment for these sexually transmitted diseases is also harmful to the immune system."[10]

The first five known AIDS cases in the United States, listed and described by the CDC (Centers for Disease Control), were gay men who had used inhalant drugs, at one time another common factor among homosexuals.[11] These inhalant nitrites (called poppers), taken as sexual stimulants, are extremely toxic. As Dr. Harry Haverkos, a researcher at the National Institute on Drug Abuse, states, "The proven potential for cancer-causing nitrosamine in bacon . . . is probably one-millionth of the dose from inhalation of poppers." Dr. Haverkos also indicates that Kaposi's sarcoma, one of the principal AIDS diseases in gay men, "is correlated to a degree with popper use."[12]

Combinations of the above pharmaceutical and recreational drugs,[13] and traditional sexually transmitted diseases, without the presence of HIV, are still enough to cause great damage to the immune system and thus open the door for those opportunistic infections which are generally assumed to be symptoms of AIDS and HIV. Immunosuppressive activities associated with anal intercourse can also result in such an outcome, due to the immunosupressive action of sperm as well as infections entering the bloodstream via abrasions or lesions in the rectum. (See Chapter Three.)

IV Drug Users

Studies now show that heroin users can present a complete AIDS profile without the presence of HIV. For example, of fifty IV heroin users who died from pneumonia (an AIDS indicator disease), twenty-six showed no sign of HIV. Likewise, in fifteen out of twenty-two deaths from endocarditis (inflammation of the lining membrane of the heart), and in five out of sixteen deaths from tuberculosis (both AIDS indicators), HIV could not be found.[14]

Many elements of this lifestyle contribute to a downward spiral of immune suppression which can lead to AIDS-like symptoms and diseases, with or without HIV. Among these factors is severe malnutrition, which should be another concern to drug users since many of them eat very poorly, using their money to buy drugs instead. "Nutritional studies have found that addicts as a group tend to be generally malnourished, to have anemia, decreased appetite, gastrointestinal distress, and emaciation, as well as key nutrient intake below two thirds the normal levels recommended," according to Dr. Root-Bernstein.[15] Dr. Bailey tells of one patient, age thirty, who was a heroin/cocaine addict. The patient had no body hair and reported only two bowel movements per month, noting an extreme absence of food intake.

Multiple infections are another immunosuppressive factor which drugs users run the risk of encountering, as sharing contaminated needles can result in a variety of needle-transmitted infections. Heroin itself is another factor, as a number of researchers identify heroin as being immunosuppressive.[16]

Further compounding the problem is the fact that many IV drug users turn to prostitution to support their drug habits. This, in turn, leads to a higher frequency of sexually transmitted diseases, abuse of antibiotics, and the resulting damage to the immune system.

Blood Transfusion Recipients

Those who insist that HIV is the sole and sufficient cause of AIDS typically cite a handful of highly publicized cases in which a person was exposed to HIV-tainted blood via a blood transfusion and then went on to die of AIDS some years later. The reality of the situation is far more complex, however. Transfusion patients are "far from free of immunosuppressive risks," notes Dr. Root-Bernstein, adding that 12,000 transfusion recipients were exposed to HIV through a contaminated blood supply between 1980 and 1985, yet only about 60 percent of those exposed to HIV-tainted blood became HIV positive.[17]

One study cited by him, conducted at the AIDS program of the Centers for Disease Control (CDC), reports that ". . . of 765 people who received HIV-tainted blood, HIV tests for 257 were performed; 113 (45 percent) were found to be HIV-seropositive within an average of five years following exposure to HIV; only 16 (6 percent) had developed AIDS."[18] Dr. Root-Bernstein concludes, "Only about half of patients transfused with blood from an HIV-seropositive donor develop antibodies to HIV. Even among these, the risk of subsequent AIDS seems to be quite varied."[19] Factors which may influence the subsequent development of AIDS include the immunosuppressive effects of blood transfusion, as well as the amount of blood transfused, he adds.

Immunosuppressive Effects of Blood Transfusion
A blood transfusion constitutes a rather severe assault to the immune system, especially if the blood itself contains other transmissible immunosuppressive viruses, such as cytomegalovirus, Epstein-Barr virus, and various hepatitis viruses. Since most people who have been accidentally infused with HIV have been exposed, at the same time, to all these other viruses as well, it's impossible to prove what really caused the immune suppression. All of the above mentioned viruses can be debilitating in and of themselves, and particularly so in combination with each other.

One of the most startling statistics regarding transfusion AIDS cases comes from a CDC study in which 331 out of 694 transfusion recipients of HIV-tainted blood had died within one year of transfusion. This represents 48 percent of the recipients. For comparison, however, in a study of HIV negative transfusion, 50 percent (73 out of 146) of recipients of blood that was not HIV infected died in the year after transfusion.[20] That is 2 percent *more* than in the HIV-infected group.

"All of the data," Dr. Root-Bernstein concludes, ". . . suggest that HIV has no influence on mortality and may or may not have any on morbidity. Statements such as those by James Curran and other AIDS researchers to the effect that transfusion patients prove the necessity and sufficiency of HIV as the cause of AIDS are wishful thinking."[21]

Effects of the Amount of Blood Transfused
According to the CDC, "persons receiving large volumes of blood may be more susceptible to infections because of [the]

severity of [the] underlying disease and other host factors or because they have an increased chance of exposure to other co-factors that modulate the clinical expression of infection with the virus [believed to be] causing AIDS (HIV)."[22]

The average blood transfusion involves less than 5 units of blood or plasma.[23] Among those who have received HIV-contaminated blood, the disease rate is thirty times higher in patients who received more than 10 units of blood compared to those receiving less than 10 units.[24] Blood transfusion recipients who were HIV positive and then developed AIDS received an average of 21 units of blood plasma during their hospitalization, whereas those who received an average of 7 units did not develop AIDS.[25]

Hemophiliacs

Hemophilia is a very serious disease in which the body's natural blood clotting capacity is impaired. Hemophiliacs, despite the usage of blood clotting factors, have an average life expectancy of only about fifty-five years.[26] During the 1970s, half of all hemophilia deaths were caused by uncontrolled bleeding.[27] As with heroin addicts, there are now studies which show that people in this group can present the complete immune-suppressed profile of AIDS without having HIV. One study reports severe immunodeficiency in six out of fourteen hemophiliacs who have no HIV.[28]

Non-HIV immunosuppressive elements among hemophiliacs include Factor VIII, the blood clotting element they receive for their deficiency condition. Some Factor VIII concentrates can expose a patient to the blood of over 100,000 donors per year. Various toxins and germs can be transmitted in this way, including hepatitis and cytomegalovirus.[29] Both of these infections are immunosuppressive, as are hemolytic anemia, and ITP, a blood platelet condition. Many hemophiliacs have these latter two blood problems, which can give rise to opportunistic infections characteristic of AIDS even if HIV is not present—making an AIDS diagnosis more likely. Therefore, HIV is clearly not necessary to produce this immune-suppressed profile, and if HIV happens to also be a part of the picture, it is not necessarily the cause of the immune suppression.

About 15,000 of the 17,000 to 18,000 hemophiliacs in the United States are HIV positive, and all were exposed before 1985. The mainstream AIDS model would predict that half of them would have AIDS or would have died by now, since the official latency period between HIV infection and AIDS is ten to fifteen years.[30] As of June 1991, however, only 1,535 cases of AIDS had occurred among hemophiliacs in the United States, or only 10 percent of all HIV positive hemophiliacs. The overwhelming majority who have been infected with HIV for eight or more years are apparently still free of AIDS.[31]

Most strikingly, new research from the United States and Italy has shown that HIV positive hemophiliacs who receive purified Factor VIII products demonstrate no decline in immune function and do not go on to develop AIDS.[32] This research, carried out over a four year period, has established that the "impure" Factor VIII blood products given to most hemophiliacs is the real trigger of immune decline, not HIV. When the old Factor VIII was used, T-cell counts fell steadily over the years, from a starting point around 400, to under 200 when AIDS-like symptoms began to appear. In those receiving the purified Factor VIII, T-cell counts stayed at 400 and showed no decline, and the patients developed no AIDS-like symptoms.

Former World Health Organization (WHO) advisor on AIDS, Professor Gordon Stewart of Glasglow University, calls these findings "immensely important," and says that the cause of the decline towards AIDS in HIV positive hemophiliacs can be laid at the door of the impure blood products (containing only 5 units of Factor VIII per milligram of blood versus up to 4,000 units in purified products). "If hemophiliacs with HIV are given ultra-purified Factor VIII, their immune system stays stable. If hemophiliacs are infused with impure blood concentrates they get changes that resemble AIDS, and if they get the high-purity product they don't get the changes. So the probability is that the hemophiliac's response is to foreign protein and not to HIV."[33]

This proves that the quality and purity of the blood clotting factor, not one's HIV status, is what determines whether a hemophiliac will suffer advanced immune suppression. This is one of the clearest examples we have thus far of how, by controlling the patient's co-factors, we can control the immune suppression associated with AIDS.

Conclusion

Whether we look at malnourished and disadvantaged people living in third world poverty, gay lifestyles which encourage multiple infections, drug use practices which produce massive immune suppression, historical blood transfusion methods (now hopefully safer), or the medical care of hemophiliacs, we can clearly see that factors other than HIV infections massively influence and modify co-factor infections and progression to AIDS. The conclusion can only be then that AIDS is multicausal and requires a therapeutic focus which addresses its varied causes and co-factors, rather than focusing simply on treating HIV alone.

"The primary cause of our disease is in us, always in us."

—*Antoine Bechamp (1883)*

3 Lifestyle Influences and Immune Suppression

The word "Lifestyle" has taken on explosive political implications in the AIDS debate, but in fact it is a neutral term, referring to just about everything we do, think, and feel daily. Lifestyle encompasses behavior (amount of exercise, sleep, sexual practices), nutrition, the use of both recreational and pharmaceutical drugs, and the far more difficult to identify emotional and spiritual traits comprised by our positive and negative attitudes, beliefs, prejudices, fears, and anxieties.

Many lifestyle factors over which we can exercise a degree of influence and control interact to decide just how well we are able to defend ourselves against illness and infection.

Cultivating the Environment for Health or Illness

The outcome of any infection depends on two factors—the degree of virulence and activity of the invading pathogen (be it virus, bacteria, yeast, parasite, etc.), and the degree of resistance offered by the environment in which that microorganism is acting.

Apart from our inherited characteristics, the body's ability to defend itself from illness depends upon the quality of our nutritional status (which profoundly affects immune/defense capabilities); the amount of acquired toxicity present in the body due to environmental pollution; drugs (whether medical or recreational); current or past medical problems or infections and how these were or are being handled;[1] and, most fundamentally, the host of mental and emotional factors which interact with our defense capacity via what is now called psychoneuroimmunology (the direct link between the mind, the nervous system, and the many facets of the immune system).

What we choose to eat, how we choose to live our lives, and how well we learn to avoid (when we can) or to handle stress in all its many forms certainly influences how well we handle infection and disease. We are largely in control of cultivating the environment in which invading pathogens find themselves, and the conscious step of accepting responsibility for this by living our lives for well-being can go a long way towards maintaining or restoring health.

Responsibility

One message shines through the hundreds of success stories of people who actively involved themselves in their own recovery after being severely ill with AIDS, cancer, and other supposedly "terminal" illnesses. In each case, the person involved showed a determination to be well and *accepted responsibility* for their lives and what they intended to do about their health.[2] In their effort to recover health, they were active players, not passive bystanders.

One argument used against such an active approach is that it can create feelings of guilt if it fails. And admittedly there will be times when the damage is too severe and the odds are too far weighted against complete recovery. Yet in such cases the effort to be well is itself a victory, as the person involved becomes empowered to take responsibility for his or her health.

Cumulative Effects of Stressors

If a person has multiple serious infections and has already been compromised by past or current illness, recreational drug use, overuse of immunosuppressive pharmaceutical drugs, poor diet, exposure to environmental toxins, emotional stress and spiritual emptiness, and lack of exercise or adequate rest, the chances of *any* treatment succeeding will be limited.[3]

Hans Selye, a top Canadian researcher, has shown that single stress factors are reasonably easy for an intact defense system to handle. But when two or more stress factors come to bear, the cumulative effect can be overwhelming, reducing the potential for recovery.

These stress factors need to be dealt with individually to improve the chance for successful recovery. This can be facilitated by getting enough sleep and rest, practicing relaxation and stress-coping techniques, improving the diet, encouraging detoxification, and doing whatever can be done by utilizing the best of conventional and/or alternative methods to deal with infections and other health problems.[4]

Common Lifestyle Influences on AIDS

Everyone on the planet has been affected by the toxic pollution of our air, water, soil, and food. Those of us in the faster-changing parts of this world suffer also from the decay of social mores. As if that were not enough, an increasing number of us have adopted negligently self-destructive lifestyles: eating poorly, smoking, abusing drugs, and draining ourselves emotionally, psychologically, physically, and spiritually. All of this strikes right at our most basic defense mechanism—our immune system.

Several of the worst stresses to the immune system come from excessive consumption of alcohol, tobacco, caffeine, and recreational use of marijuana, cocaine, heroin, opioides, amyl nitrites, and stimulant drugs. In addition, certain sexual practices can, in themselves, be immunosuppressive, as well as encouraging the acquisition of HIV. Immunosuppressive pharmaceutical drugs such as antibiotics and steroids, often used in treating co-factor illnesses, and AZT, the most widely sanctioned conventional medical treatment of AIDS, can also add to the deterioration of the immune system.

There is little doubt that these factors underlie the emergence of ever more virulent organisms which our increasingly weak immune systems struggle to control. As evidence of this, we see a dramatic and continuing rise in allergies, such as asthma in children, which are directly related to environmental pollution and immunological dysfunction, as well as the emergence of a host of "new" ailments such as Toxic Shock Syndrome and Chronic Fatigue Syndrome (CFS), and the explosive re-emergence of some older infections which had been thought to be controlled, such as tuberculosis. Tragically, such diseases are now also affecting huge wild animal populations and fish or crustacea that may also carry toxic metals and chemicals as well as disease organisms, thus entering our own food chain.

Alcohol

Alcohol consumption causes vitamin deficiency, specifically of folic acid, thiamine, vitamin B6, vitamin A, vitamin C, zinc, magnesium, and potassium.[5] Immune function is depressed (T and B lymphocytes and natural killer cells all decline) and infection is made more likely when alcohol is consumed in anything but extremely small quantities.[6]

Absolute avoidance of alcohol intake is suggested for anyone with AIDS/ARC, and moderate use, at most, is recommended for anyone who may be at risk for these conditions.[7]

Tobacco

Tobacco is a known depressant of immune function and anyone at risk should completely avoid smoking and the company of people who smoke.

Caffeine

Caffeine, found in black teas, coffee, chocolate, cocoa, soft drinks, and many pain-killing medications, belongs to a group of chemicals called *methylxanthines*. Other members of this group include *theophyllin*, found in black teas, and *theobromine*, found in chocolate. Among caffeine's many pharmacological effects is its action on serum adrenaline levels, according to Steven Bailey, N.D., Assistant Professor of Pharmacognosy at National College of Naturopathic Medicine in Portland, Oregon. Caffeine interferes with the body's natural metabolism in breaking down of adrenaline (or epinephrine), which is our stress hormone.[8]

"As a result, we run on an elevated adrenaline level, which is analogous to 'burning the candle at both ends,'" Dr. Bailey notes. "We may have more energy for a while, but we inevitably use up our reserves."

Negative effects of excess caffeine intake include stress on the digestive tract, inhibiting nutrient uptake from food; stress on the urinary tract, as well as on circulatory and possibly immune function;[9] and increased anxiety, depression, insomnia, and aggravation of pre-existing psychiatric states. Caffeine also artificially elevates serum insulin levels which is known to be destructive to white blood cells, adds Dr. Bailey.

"Recreational" Drugs[10]

There is overwhelming evidence that many of the symptoms of AIDS (including fever, extreme weight loss, swollen lymph glands, increased risk of infection, and septicemia, as well as many nervous system abnormalities) can also be produced by regular use of "street" drugs.[11]

A survey of just under four thousand self-identified American male homosexuals showed that in this high risk group for AIDS, during the previous six months, 83 percent had used one, and approximately 60 percent had used two or more, drugs during sexual activity,[12] ranging from amyl nitrite to cocaine, amphetamines, LSD, and phenylcyclidine.

Another study of three hundred and fifty male homosexuals showed that over 80 percent had used cocaine and/or amyl nitrites, and approximately 60 percent had used amphetamines.[13] Of all of these drugs, the negative properties of the aphrodisiac nitrites seem most dangerous as a risk factor for both AIDS and Kaposi's sarcoma, according to a detailed review by Peter Duesberg, Ph.D., of the University of California, Berkeley.[14] He reports (and gives extensive supporting evidence) that the drugs commonly used in high risk groups for AIDS are frequently toxic in themselves (and most are chemically contaminated or are not sterile, leading frequently to septicemia when used intravenously). Furthermore, Dr. Duesberg states, they promote malnutrition; have specific and profound immune suppressive effects; produce neurological and brain damage; and are in themselves responsible for many of the symptoms of the disease complex we call AIDS.

These, and the milder social drugs such as tobacco, should be avoided totally in any determined effort towards recovery from any aspect of immune suppression.

Marijuana: Marijuana is immunodepressive and encourages opportunistic infections by suppressing natural killer cell activity, as well as by slowing down many other aspects of immune function. It also plays a role in the reactivation of dormant infections such as herpes.[15]

Opioides: A combination of increased risk factors derive from the use of heroin, morphine, and other opioid drugs, including a massive increase in the likelihood of malnutrition developing, an enormous risk of acquiring HIV and other infections if needles are shared, and direct immunosupression as the drugs interact with body systems. Respiratory distress is extremely likely, as well, if anyone with pneumocystis carinii pneumonia (PCP) uses narcotic substances.

Stimulant Drugs: These drugs range from amphetamines, to cocaine in its various forms, to psychedelic drugs such as LSD. Cocaine is the most addictive stimulant drug and its use leads to extreme anxiety states which often result in the use of other drugs such as alcohol, opioids, and marijuana concurrently, all with severe immunodepressing results.[16]

Amyl Nitrite: The use of the recreational drug Amyl Nitrite increases the risk in immune-compromised people of developing Kaposi's sarcoma, and severely damages immune function, as well.[17] Surveys regarding the use of nitrites have shown patterns in which about 60 percent of homosexual males used them in 1984, reducing to a figure of 27 percent in 1991, as against less than 1 percent of heterosexual populations of the same age groups during that period.[18] These drugs should be avoided at all costs, and anyone at risk, anyone with signs of immune dysfunction (frequent infections, swollen lymph glands, fatigue, etc.), and anyone who is HIV positive at whatever stage should completely avoid the use of "social/recreational" drugs.

Pharmaceutical Drugs Used to Treat Co-factor Illnesses

Steroid Drugs: Steroid medications (cortisone, hydrocortisone, prednisone, etc.) are commonly used in the treatment of the various co-factor illnesses associated with AIDS and HIV. For example, steroid creams are commonly used on venereal skin infections such as herpes simplex, and are readily absorbed via vaginal, penile, and rectal tissues.[19] Steroids may also be used in the treatment of systemic problems, such as respiratory problems, including asthma, or joint problems (which are frequent in hemophiliacs).[20]

Steroids are extremely fast-acting drugs that can give marked symptom relief, but they are also immune depressants. They can produce a rapid decline in T and B cell numbers and reduce cell-mediated immunity, making the user more susceptible to infection, as well as having other negative influences on the body.

As long as anyone is receiving steroid medication, recovery from immune-depressed situations or from opportunistic infections is almost impossible. Unfortunately, because steroid medication so effectively masks many distressing symptoms, a massive decline in health status may take place before it is apparent. At most, short-term use (meaning days, not weeks) might be sanctioned, although avoiding steroid use altogether would be in the best interests of the patient in almost all instances unless the situation is life-threatening.[21]

Non-steroidal Anti-inflammatory Drugs: Non-steroidal anti-inflammatory drugs such as aspirin have been shown to depress immune function.[22]

Antibiotics: There are times when antibiotics are lifesaving and this should be kept in mind as we consider their negative effects. Without exception, antibiotics damage internal ecosystems, most notably the intestinal flora that are major protectors against invasive pathogenic bacteria and yeasts, as well as having many other beneficial influences on the body in terms of detoxification and nutrient supply.

If antibiotics are being used (and as stated above, there are times when this is appropriate), supplementation with high potency colonizing strains of Bifidobacteria (for the large intestine) and *Lactobacillus acidophilus* (for the small bowel) is highly desirable. This supplementation should continue during, and for some weeks after, antibiotic medication.

AZT: Conventional Treatment for AIDS

AZT (Zidovudine), until recently the most commonly used drug against AIDS, is a reverse transcriptase inhibitor. Reverse transcriptase is an enzyme required to convert RNA to DNA, and in its absence the RNA of the HIV virus is prevented from entering the genetic material of a healthy T cell.[23] By inhibiting the expression of reverse transcriptase, AZT appears to interfere with this process, although many investigators now suggest that the side effects of AZT are more likely than AIDS to kill the patient.

The reasoning behind this controversial assertion is as follows:

- AZT interferes with the process by which HIV-RNA is converted into DNA by inhibiting reverse transcriptase, but this does not happen in all the infected cells, leaving a reservoir of infection.
- If HIV is not the major player in the progression of AIDS then this interference might in itself be of limited value, even if all infected cells were influenced. And this does

not take into account the strong negative trade-off (in terms of side-effects) in return for this possible benefit.[24]

- The HIV virus rapidly develops resistance to AZT, mutating into strains that are not affected by it.

- Most experts believe that even when infection is active, as few as one T-cell in five hundred is infected with the virus. This means that 499 healthy T cells would be killed by AZT for every infected cell that is deactivated.

- Since one of the main medical theories as to how HIV does its main damage suggests that this happens through the destruction of T cells, it is obvious from the scenario outlined above that AZT is nearly 500 times as likely to be killing a major part of the immune system (healthy T cells) of the person infected as it is of killing HIV.

- Setting aside this thought, we should consider the admitted toxicity of AZT, which suppresses the important tasks of bone marrow (without which immune function collapses anyway), causing anemia, neutropenia, and leukopenia in between 20 percent to 50 percent of people given the drug, with up to half of these requiring transfusions within weeks of commencing its use.

- Other common symptoms resulting from AZT side-effects are muscle wasting, extreme nausea, acute hepatitis, headaches, insomnia, dementia seizures, and the appearance of cancerous lymphomas.

Sexual Considerations

There are practices in both homosexual and heterosexual settings which foster immune deficiency, strongly encouraging sexually transmitted diseases in general, and acquisition of HIV in particular. Anal intercourse is highly conducive to infection because rectal tissues are often torn and the mucous membrane of the rectum is too delicate to cope as a defensive barrier, especially when repeatedly exposed to seminal fluids.

Sperm ejaculated into a body cavity represents a foreign protein that would normally be attacked by the body's immune system. Since its sole purpose is procreation and survival of the species, it is protected from this attack by two strongly immunosuppressive factors in the seminal fluid that block rejection of the spermatozoa long enough for one of them to reach the ovum and initiate conception. Obviously, when seminal fluids are ejaculated into the rectum, the same immunosuppressive phenomenon will block the body's defense system and permit invasion of microorganisms, including HIV.[25]

Exactly the same process would take place in the mouth and throat in the case of oral sex. Seminal fluid often contains bacteria, viruses, or yeasts (and the ejaculate from people in high risk groups is commonly found to contain Hepatitis-B, Herpes, Epstein-Barr, Cytomegalovirus, and the organisms which cause chlamydia, syphilis, and candidiasis). These pathogens would certainly find their task of gaining access to the body far easier if the surface tissues were lacerated and if the immune response was suppressed at the same time.

Microorganisms, including HIV, would find it easier to infect through such a portal of entry. And, were lacerations or abrasions present in such tissues, the sperm itself would inevitably enter the bloodstream, provoking a defensive immune response against it. It has been observed that the antibodies which the body produces in response to the presence of sperm in the bloodstream are also specific against T4 helper cells.[26]

This might account for low T4-cell levels observed in many male homosexuals even though there is no evidence of HIV; immune function is therefore already depressed in such people. Safe sex has to mean avoidance of the risks outlined above. Whether condoms can provide total protection is extremely doubtful, since microscopic holes are not uncommon, and these may be big enough to allow some penetration of organisms. And we should not forget that abrasion of anal and rectal tissues will occur with or without a condom, and that this will expose the individual to infection from microorganisms in waste material passing through the bowel, which are usually kept out of the bloodstream by an intact mucous surface.[27]

Lubricants used to prevent abrasions during sex may also lead to problems. These are often petrochemical products such as petroleum jelly. Journalist and activist Gary Null reports that tests on animals have shown that rectal implants of both natural and petrochemical lubricants resulted in the animals dying of AIDS-like symptoms or cancer.[28]

Conclusion

The evidence of this chapter illustrates that our lifestyle choices and traits are critically connected to how well or how poorly our immune systems will function when assaulted by disease-causing organisms and stressors. Our choices and behavior in the past, along with the experiences we were exposed to, have set the scene for what is happening in our lives now.

By engaging in positive actions which initiate the process of healing and repair, and by modifying (or actually stopping) negative practices and habits, we can demonstrate that we have courageously accepted responsibility for, and are not passive bystanders in, what is probably the most critical confrontation of our lives. The experience of those people who have recovered from AIDS and other life-threatening illnesses partly by their own efforts demonstrates that life without dangerous drugs and without potentially-dangerous forms of sex need not be boring or empty, and that the satisfaction of rebuilding health and vitality can infuse a new meaning to life.

4 Prognosis for the Future

It is clear that our understanding of AIDS and its causes has changed substantially from the prevailing viewpoints which existed when the syndrome was first discovered. Many suppositions about the disease which once were regarded as gospel are now being seen as myths that are beginning to unravel. As they do so, a new picture of the illness is beginning to emerge, as the statements below reveal. As we consider them, it is inevitable that we must seriously ask ourselves whether it is time to reconsider what we have been taught about AIDS up to now, letting go of entrenched beliefs and prejudices so that we might move forward in a manner which best serves those who struggle with the illness.

- According to a report published in the *New England Journal of Medicine*, HIV is an extremely difficult virus to transmit and to acquire, with the virus being up to a thousand times less infectious than hepatits viruses.[1]
- People who become HIV positive will not necessarily develop AIDS, according to another report, published in *The Lancet*, and as shown by the many adults and infants exposed to HIV, who have tested HIV positive yet have failed to become ill even fourteen years after infection.[2]
- The HIV virus alone may not be enough to cause AIDS. This is the view of a growing number of researchers, including the discoverer of HIV, Dr. Luc Montagnier of the Pasteur Institute in Paris. Montagnier has stated that HIV is "not a sufficient cause of AIDS on its own."[3] He and other leading scientists now believe that additional "co-factors," such as malnutrition, other infections, and/or drug abuse, are also required in order for AIDS to manifest.[4]
- Many people who have initially tested HIV positive have later tested HIV negative and have remained healthy, as was reported as early as 1988, in the journal *Science*. Such people have controlled and/or eliminated the virus on their own.[5]

- A significant number of people with AIDS have no sign of HIV at all; their condition looks in *every* respect like "HIV-associated AIDS" but without the AIDS virus.[6]
- AIDS does not have to be a fatal disease; an increasing number of people with AIDS *do* recover.[7] As Professor Robert Root-Bernstein, of Michigan State University, states, "Some AIDS patients are alive a dozen years after diagnosis (of full-blown AIDS)."[8]
- AIDS may not even be a new disease, and quite possibly may have been documented for at least the past 130 years.[9]
- There is an increasing degree of doubt as to the accuracy of the testing methods used in assessing HIV status. (See below.)
- A wide and growing range of effective and safe treatment options exist which encourage positive outcomes to immune deficiency conditions, as will be shown in the chapters which follow.

In view of the above, it is important to understand that an HIV positive test result, or even a diagnosis of AIDS, does not necessarily translate into a fatal outcome. The fact is that there can still be a good prognosis if appropriate action is taken in time. In short, as later evidence will make clear, people with AIDS and its attendant illnesses do not have to die from their condition.

An Important Message

Two clear and powerful messages emerge from the evidence gathered in this book, and they must be understood if hope and a positive outcome are to be delivered to those who are suffering from AIDS:

- Diseases which involve immune deficiency are almost always the result of multiple interacting causes, not of a single event or organism.
- The normalization of such a disease state requires the treatment of the multiple causes, as well as support for the immune system. These multiple causes include nutritional deficiency; drug and acquired toxicity; multiple previous and current viral, fungal, bacterial, and parasitic

infections; bowel dysbiosis (toxicity of intestinal tract with consequent malabsorption and toxic problems); emotional stress; damaged organ function (such as in the liver); and inherited genetic traits and weaknesses.

If the complex of interacting causes are successfully treated in ways which create no new problems, and if the immune system is appropriately supported and modulated, the prognosis for anyone who is HIV positive or who has AIDS improves immeasurably. What seems to many to point to an inevitable decline towards disease and death *can* be turned around.

The Courage to Get Well

One message central to this book is that putting right what is wrong requires that each of us accept responsibility for ourselves. We must apply dedicated and persistent efforts to reform what is wrong with our lives, our societies, and our planet. This is undoubtedly a huge task, but the alternative to tackling it is unthinkable since we have seen in AIDS what the future holds for us if we don't turn things around.

Many experts now consider that the emergence of "new" diseases such as Chronic Fatigue Syndrome (CFS) and AIDS can be shown to have multiple causes. This is also true of a condition which is becoming apparent in most industrialized countries in which many people seem to have become "universal reactors" in that they are apparently allergic to multiple factors and substances and suffer from profound chemical intolerances.

People who suffer from "Universal Reactor Syndrome" or CFS or AIDS can all be said to have immune dysregulation of one sort or another, and since it can be shown that such problems usually involve multifactorial causes, the rational management of these conditions should be multifactorial as well.[10]

Living Proof

In Part Two: "Alternative Treatments for AIDS," evidence will be presented which confirms that there are many people who, despite becoming infected with HIV, are able to rid themselves of the virus altogether and test HIV negative again, after appropriate treatment. There are other people who have been

HIV positive for many years and yet remain in almost perfect health, although some of these individuals may simply have been misdiagnosed through faulty HIV antibody tests.

Even more remarkable are the reports in Part Three: "Long-Term Survivors," of actual case histories of people who are alive, well, working, and living life to the fullest, despite their initial prognosis, which, in some cases, was that they only had a few more months to live.

Using various combinations of herbal medicine, nutritional supplements, mind/body medicine, and oxygen therapies, there are a growing number of practitioners in the United States, Canada, and Europe who have successfully reversed many cases of AIDS.

Key Questions about AIDS

The examples given within the answers to the following key questions can help us to better understand the issues which surround AIDS and its acquisition.

Does Exposure to HIV Automatically Lead to AIDS?

In short—no. As Dr. C. Ludlum of the Royal Infirmary, Edinburgh, Scotland explains, "Not everyone exposed to HIV becomes infected and those that do so progress to AIDS at varying rates."[11] The last part of his statement seems increasingly inaccurate, as many people have remained healthy but HIV positive for upwards of fourteen years. It now seems possible that some people with HIV will *never* develop AIDS.

In fact, one of the more interesting aspects of the AIDS issue has been the way in which the "latency" period considered to be necessary before HIV develops into AIDS has been extended. In the mid-1980s, we were cautioned that exposure to HIV to acquisition of AIDS could result within two years. By 1989, this period was extended to ten years, and since 1992, we have been told it was from ten to fifteen years.[12]

In addition, there are numerous other reports which explore low levels of infectivity, suggesting that HIV is not as highly an infectious virus as was previously believed. As we have already seen from the 1987 report in Britain's *General Practitioner Journal*, which investigated accidental exposure to HIV by medical personnel as little as *one out of 1,500* hospital workers in the England and the U.S. became infected after exposure.[13]

A Nigerian report from the same year states that examined semen samples from 12,000 people from different socio-economic and risk groups indicate that "this virus (HIV) is of low infectivity and that risks to health workers are negligible."[14]

And the following research study gives additional evidence which strongly supports the view that HIV infection need not lead to AIDS, or even to illness. In the study, Australian researchers examined the progress of many people who had received HIV-tainted blood. They state: "There have been reported cases of long-term, symptomless HIV infection, but it is not clear whether the benign course was due to host, viral, or other unknown factors. During follow-up of transfusion-acquired HIV-1 infection in New South Wales, Australia, we identified a group of six subjects infected through a single common donor. We were therefore able to study the contributions of various factors to the course of the infection."[15]

Throughout the follow-up period (over ten years in the earliest cases), five of the recipients (of HIV contaminated blood), as well as the donor, remained free of symptoms and maintained normal CD4-cell counts. The other recipient developed pneumonia and died 4.3 years after infection. However, she had previously also received immunosuppressive treatment for Lupus erythematosus.

The longest symptom-free follow-up on any of the recipients was 10.2 years following transfusion, and the donor, who had been infected some time prior to this, was also symptom-free at this time. The only person to suffer negative effects from the contaminated transfusion was already immune-compromised due to having an autoimmune disease (Lupus) and to receiving immune-suppressive treatment.

Was this, as the researchers ask, a less virulent virus? Or, rather, was the HIV virus being controlled by sound immune systems, apart from the one tragic case where immune function was already impaired? Though such questions have yet to be finally answered, at the very least the study shows that an HIV positive test result need not have any negative effects, even after ten years.

Can A Person Be HIV Positive And Not Get AIDS?
A great deal of evidence now points to the possibility that a person who is HIV positive, but who has a healthy immune system, may be able to keep the virus in check indefinitely.[16] In 1974, from a group of nine French recipients of contaminated blood (donated before 1973 by an HIV-infected Portuguese man), four died within months of complications unrelated to AIDS. In 1984, one women tested HIV positive on two different test methods, but as of 1988 she had not developed any symptoms—suggesting that it is possible to be infected for fourteen years with no sign of AIDS. A second woman tested in the same year was found HIV positive by one test, and negative by the other; as of 1988 she, too, had not developed any AIDS symptoms.[17]

There have also been instances in which clear evidence exists of individuals testing positive repeatedly and then becoming seronegative. One such situation occurred in 1987, at Johns Hopkins University, in which five men who had repeatedly tested positive suddenly lost detectable levels of antibodies to HIV. In 1988, after repeated tests, four of the five were pronounced free of HIV antibodies and antigens, nor could the virus be cultured from the cells of any of these four. They had effectively controlled and eliminated their infections.[18]

Similar reports were sent to the CDC from several other hospitals as part of the Multicenter AIDS Cohort Study. After examining the study, Dr. Root-Bernstein states, "At least four other cases of loss of HIV positivity, accompanied by normal T-cell counts, and continued good health are on record among adults and dozens among infants." He continues, "The longer the AIDS epidemic has lasted, the more people there are who are surviving HIV infections for ever-longer periods of time."[19]

Are HIV Test Results Accurate?
There are two currently accepted tests for the presence of HIV antibodies that may indicate the presence of the virus, ELISA and Western Blot. However, both tests are known to be highly erratic and unreliable.[20]

The ELISA (Enzyme Linked ImmunoSorbent Assay) test is the most commonly-used test to determine HIV status. The

CDC (Centers for Disease Control) considers a single positive ELISA test, without any other confirmation, to be proof of HIV infection. The ELISA test, however, is known to give a high rate of false positive results, with readings indicating the presence of HIV infection when, in actuality, it has not occurred. A 1991 study presented at the VII International Conference on AIDS, noted: "In half of the cases in which the subject had a positive p24 test, the subject later had a negative test without taking any medication that would be expected to affect p24 antigen levels." The researchers concluded that the "test is clinically erratic and should be interpreted cautiously."[21] In some studies reported in *The New England Journal of Medicine* and the *Journal of the American Medical Association*, as many as four out of five tests showing a positive result with ELISA fail to subsequently test positive with the more sophisticated Western Blot testing method.[22] In addition, Australian biophysicist, Eleni Papadopulos-Elepulos, notes that out of 20,000 positive ELISA test results in Russia in 1990, only 112 were confirmed using the Western Blot.[23]

The Western Blot test is used for confirmation of the ELISA test, but, unfortunately, the Western Blot technology is no more accurate than ELISA.[24] According to one highly respected AIDS expert, Dr. Max Essex of Harvard University's School of Public Health, some 85 percent of African patients found to be HIV-negative, tested positive to the Western Blot. It was later determined that proteins of the leprosy germ, which infect millions of Africans, can show up as a false positive on both ELISA and Western Blot.[25] A study of Venezuelan malaria patients determined that the rate of false positives was 25–41 percent. Researchers concluded that "HIV is not causing AIDS, even in the presence of the severe immunoregulatory disturbances characteristic of acute malaria."[26]

Why should the test results be so variable in their accuracy? Researchers now believe that there are a number of possibilities which could explain the inaccuracies. The assumption that the detection of an antibody response to the virus is proof of its actual presence may be erroneous, as both the ELISA and Western Blot tests react to many other proteins caused by other diseases. The entire immune system may become confused when confronted by a host of foreign proteins which resemble each other chemically (many proteins have very similar characteristics to HIV), and as a result, false positive tests for HIV are more likely.

For example, the protein p24, generally accepted as indicating the presence of HIV, is found in all retroviruses that live in the human body and cause no harm.[27] Other conditions capable of producing false positive results in ELISA tests include hepatitis B and C, malaria, papillomavirus warts, glandular fever, tuberculosis, syphilis, and leprosy,[28] as well as cytomegalovirus and mycoplasma.

These infections are capable of producing protein markers which can confuse the test results, and may be introduced in some forms of vaccinations, in semen during anal sex, or during blood transfusions. Since some proteins mimic other proteins, the immune reaction (formation of antibodies to these antigens) prevents testing from being always able to detect the difference between HIV antibodies and antibodies to other proteins. In addition, such protein markers can produce further harm beyond inaccurate test results. They can also initiate a great deal of mayhem as the immune system fails to recognize the body's own proteins with similar markers, thereby attacking both foreign and native cells indiscriminately. This may result in an autoimmune reaction that may, in turn, become a chronic disease or syndrome such as AIDS.[29]

The degree of false testing is impossible to estimate, but there is no doubt that it has led to needless confusion and heartbreak on more than one occasion, since one of the criteria for being labeled as having AIDS is a positive HIV test result.

Is AIDS an Autoimmune Disease?

There are many autoimmune diseases which can affect humans, including rheumatoid arthritis, colitis, and lupus erythematosus, and medical science is beginning to understand that in many of these cases there is a situation of "mistaken identity" in which certain types of healthy cells are mistaken for an invading foreign substance and attacked. Now many leading researchers, including Dr. Root-Bernstein, are postulating that much of the damage seen in AIDS is also the result of autoimmune activity. The cause of this mistaken focus of immune attack seems to involve minute protein markers carried by some invading microorganisms, as well as by sperm and some blood products, which are almost identical to the chemical (protein) markers carried by healthy CD4 (and other) cells belonging to the immune system.[24] When confronted with a flood of these look-alike protein antigens (foreign proteins), the body begins to attack and destroy them along its own healthy cells, which become targets because of their similarity to the foreign invaders. Joseph Sonnabend, M.D., a leading, New York researcher, has shown that up to 80 percent of gay men have antibodies which attack their own defensive lymphocytes.[25]

Dr. Root-Bernstein points out that many of the microorganisms active in AIDS have very similar, look-alike proteins, including herpes zoster and herpes simplex virus, cytomegalovirus, Epstein-Barr virus, hepatitis B virus, and mycoplasma. Semen and blood products used in treating hemophiliacs also have similar protein particles in their makeup. When a variety of organisms and factors (such as semen, blood, and viruses), all carrying such protein markers, have been injected into animals simultaneously (even in small quantities, with or without HIV), a powerful autoimmune response has been seen, according to Dr. Root-Bernstein. When this occurs, an attack is launched against the foreign proteins as well as the normal immune cells which they resemble.

"What we think happens is the following," says Dr. Root-Bernstein. "An unfortunate person becomes infected with some appropriate combination of infectious agents, one of which is a CD4 mimic and the other a MHC class II mimic [MHC is the marker protein which tells the immune system whether the antigen—the protein it is examining—is 'self' or 'non-self']. Many possible combinations exist [between different microorganisms and proteins] [and] each infectious agent induces an appropriate antibody response. These antibodies not only recognize their respective antigens as targets, but each other, and CD4 and MHC class II proteins as well. The result is immunological mayhem."[26]

A suitable vaccine may be part of the answer in treating AIDS, according to the findings of this research and other studies. It seems that when a large amount of one of the microorganisms with "confusing" protein is injected into an animal, the autoimmune problem clears up as the immune system turns its attention towards the specific threat rather than the multiple minor ones. Until such a vaccine is found, Dr. Root-Bernstein cautions against drug use and urges safe sex practices and sound nutrition to ensure against contracting AIDS or HIV. And he is working on a vaccine approach to the problem he has defined as being due to a self-destructing immune system.

How Can Co-factors Be Kept in Check?

Prevention of a decline towards AIDS itself after infection seems to be dramatically helped by using methods which either retard other infections, or which enhance the natural protective, detoxifying, and repairing roles of the body, in order to try to maintain balance, health, and homoeostasis. Retarding secondary infections can take the form of prevention of contact, or of direct assault on the infection using nutrition, herbal approaches, oxygen treatment, hyperthermia or drugs; whereas immune enhancement would involve boosting or modulating immune function through the use of a variety of techniques, ranging from nutrition, acupuncture, stress reduction, and herbal approaches.[27]

Whether the virus can be held in check seems to depend on where the individual who is HIV infected starts out. The degree of infectivity of any organism is dependent on two factors—its own nature and the ground on which it operates. Relative low infectivity seems to be a feature of HIV, but it can still present a problem to an immune system which has already been compromised by co-factors such as poor nutrition and toxicity, which act as symbiotic agents capable of greatly increasing the virus's potency. Questions which must be asked when dealing with the virus include:

- How much previous disease or infection is present or has existed in the past?
- What other medical problems are there/have there been?
- How much toxicity from drugs, pollution, and other factors is the patient dealing with?
- What is the patient's level of nutritional status (excellent or poor)?

- What is the patient's emotional state and how good are his or her stress-coping abilities?
- Are lifestyle factors (including sexual) helping or harming the body's defensive efforts?
- Is immune function at a reasonable level?

The answers to these questions provide a good idea of the sort of territory the HIV virus has entered, and of how easy or difficult it will be for it to cause destruction in the immune system. HIV entering a super-efficient immune system may well be overwhelmed and eliminated. On the other hand, when an immune system has already been compromised by poor nutrition, other illnesses, or drugs, the virus can more easily penetrate the body's defenses and proliferate. We only have to look at the six cases from Australia to see a clear example of this: the immune-compromised person succumbed, whereas the five with sound immune systems have almost no sign of HIV and no sign at all of ill-health after up to ten years.

Can a Person with AIDS Get Well Again?
There are numerous case histories of people who have developed advanced signs of AIDS (Kaposi's sarcoma, etc.), or who are HIV positive, who have managed to turn their condition around to regain relative good health.[28] We will be examining some of these cases later on in Part Two and Part Three. Although such stories can be dismissed as anecdotal, the sheer volume of the anecdotes themselves overwhelms the weight of the dismissive arguments of the skeptics.

Continuing long term studies at Basytr University in Seattle, Washington have examined the possibility of keeping people who show early signs of AIDS from degenerating further. The studies indicate that not only does the possibility exist, but often the patients' conditions can be turned around, as well, so that they once again become active, productive, and self-sufficient.[29]

Positive Action for Persons with AIDS
It seems very likely that HIV is not the sole cause of AIDS. Once this is well understood, the co-factors to the virus, many of which are more easily controlled or removed than HIV

itself, can be treated to good effect. And if it is proven that AIDS can occur without HIV, the implications will be enormous, shifting the research focus to a host of issues which we can already do something about now. These include:

- Improving immune function through improved nutritional status.
- Detoxification to improve immune function.
- Using the mind to help boost immune function.
- Introducing effective stress-reduction methods such as biofeedback, meditation, and guided imagery.
- Dealing with other infections safely and effectively.
- Investigating the use of safe herbal and homeopathic medications.
- Investigating the use of acupuncture, massage, oxygen therapy, and other treatments.

Action for Those Who Are HIV Positive
The possibility of being HIV positive and not developing AIDS may well depend on much the same health-enhancing strategies as would be required to treat AIDS (with or without HIV). Presenting HIV and co-factors with a more difficult environment to operate in must be one of the most important objectives of all. Millions of lives could be saved, or at the very least extended in reasonable health, if this were possible—and the evidence is strong that it is.

Summary
The prognosis for anyone with AIDS is certainly less negative than we might think after reading the popular press or watching TV. But effectively dealing with AIDS first requires a changed attitude, an acceptance of responsibility for our own health status and the choices we make, based upon a clear understanding of the issues which surround the disease. Once we achieve this mindset, we then have available to us a menu of alternative approaches which, in many instances, have reversed the course of AIDS, as we shall see in the following sections.

Part Two: Alternative Treatments for AIDS

"The highest ideal of cure is the speedy, gentle, and enduring restoration of health by the most trustworthy and least harmful way."

— Samuel Hahnemann (1755-1844), Founder of Homeopathy

W hile the mainstream view of AIDS treatment focuses almost entirely on the elimination of HIV, the alternative view places the emphasis on restoring overall health by first eliminating the co-factors. Prevention of a decline towards AIDS itself, after HIV infection, seems to be dramatically helped by using methods which either retard other infections or which enhance the natural protective, detoxification, and self-healing roles of the body. This includes boosting the body's immune system, which, together with the other defensive systems, tries to maintain a proper internal balance for health.[1]

Whether the virus can be held in check seems to depend on a number of factors, namely where the individual who is HIV infected starts out—at what level is immune function, how much previous disease or infection has there been, what other medical problems are there, and how much toxicity is there from drugs, pollution, and other harmful environmental elements. Other important factors include the person's nutritional status, emotional state, and stress-coping abilities, as well as "lifestyle" choices, including sexual, that may be helping or harming the defense effort. HIV entering a super-efficient immune system may well be overwhelmed and get nowhere. On the other hand, HIV or any other organism entering a system already compromised by poor nutrition, other illnesses, and drugs will find its task that much easier.

If we see disease in general—and AIDS in particular—as being represented by a dynamic balance, or rather lack of it, between homeostatic forces (including immune function and all other repair and balance mechanisms) on one hand, and the onslaught of varied and multiple stress insults ranging from nutrient deficit to toxic accumulation, drug abuse, multiple infections, emotional anarchy, allergies, bowel dysbiosis, and much more on the other, we can see that normalization (relatively speaking) of the situation demands that either or both ends of the spectrum be addressed. We can try to reduce the multiple stress load or we can try to improve the self-regulating (including immune system) functions—or we can try to do both.

The degree of vulnerability and current vitality, multiplied by the level of the current stress load (inherited and acquired deficiency/toxic/emotional/infective/other—often including HIV) equals the likelihood of survival and decides the speed of decline. The more the two ends of the equation (vulnerability and stress load) can be modified towards the better, the greater the chance of health restoration.

One only has to look at the six cases from Australia previously cited in Chapter Four to see a clear example of this. The immune-compromised individual succumbed, whereas the five with sound immune systems have almost no sign of HIV and no sign at all of ill-health after up to ten years.

Some of the alternative methods being used today to improve the health and immune function of individuals with AIDS and HIV infection include improved nutritional status, detoxification, acupuncture, mind/body medicine, stress reduction therapies, herbal medicine, homeopathy, hyperthermia, as well as ozone and other oxygen-based treatments.

Just as AIDS is a multifaceted, complex syndrome, so is the recovery process. There are no simple "magic bullet" answers, on either the mainstream or the alternative side. But, as we have tried to demonstrate, a diligent, consistent, multifaceted approach to recovery, aimed at detoxifying and reconstructing the diseased body, is far more effective than any pharmaceutical agent taken alone. The proof of this is evidenced by the long-term survival rate of patients who have followed the former course as compared to the limited success achieved by those who have followed the latter. It may be confusing that no single treatment or approach seems to work for everyone, but this is consistent with the philosophy of natural health. Each person is unique, each disease manifestation is unique, and therefore, each recovery is unique.

5 Diet and Nutritional Supplements

There is perhaps no more empowering option for the immune-compromised person than to take charge of his or her health through a better diet. The best ways to do this are by avoiding foods that do more harm than good to the body, emphasizing those that are the most beneficial, and paying attention to how food is prepared in order to take advantage of their maximum nutritional value.

Healthy eating alone may not be enough for someone engaged in a fight to fend off infection, however. A program of nutritional supplementation may usually be needed, as well, to further support the digestive system. Additionally, some of the conditions that a person with HIV or AIDS is prone to are known to respond to particular nutrients. The needs of one person may be similar to those of another, but individual requirements must be assessed and addressed for the best results.

If the digestive system is healthy and ideal forms of food are consumed, a person should be able to acquire all their needs for health from food alone. But when the digestive system is compromised, and when particular nutrient requirements are excessive due to metabolic demands which are greater than normal—such as illness, stress, pollution, or a devitalized diet—supplementation becomes essential for recovery and healing to take place.

Benefits of a Healthy Diet

Although people in the United States consume plenty of food, they do not always eat healthily. Statistically, studies have shown that about two-thirds of the average American's diet is made up of fats and refined sugar having low to no nutrient density. Consequently, the remaining one-third of the typical diet is counted on for the essential nutrients needed to maintain health, which may or may not be from "high-nutrient-density" food.

"Nutrition is the foundation of natural therapy for AIDS," states Laurence Badgley, M.D., of Foster City, California. "Broad segments of the American population have been proven to be deficient in specific vitamins and minerals, which are critical to immune system function. For example, persons with AIDS are often deficient in folic acid, selenium, zinc, and iron."

Because of each person's biochemical individuality (genetic and environmental differences), each patient will have specific nutrient requirements. A qualified health care professional should always be consulted in order to receive specific, individual guidelines.

To illustrate the importance of diet as a healing factor, Dr. Badgley reports of a patient who has been HIV positive for eight years and who was diagnosed with AIDS three years ago. This patient appears to have eliminated his symptoms through diet and detoxification. The patient began a diet of raw organic fruits and vegetables, emphasizing freshness, moderation, and a variety of foods. He also utilizes enemas to rid his system of toxins and to cleanse the colon. He avoids foods that are mucous-forming, like dairy products, eating only cheeses made from sunflower and pumpkin seeds. The patient reports that his T-cell counts have risen to normal levels, and a liver disease with which he had been diagnosed is now in remission.

Understanding Individuality

There is no universal dietary prescription which applies to everyone since we are all starting from different places, with varying histories, both in terms of health and diet, and our own biochemical uniqueness.[1] Some people will have eaten optimally in the past (and present), while others may be grossly nutritionally deficient; some will be able to readily absorb nutrients from their food, while others will have badly impaired digestive and absorption capabilities; some people will be overloaded with toxic debris from past use of drugs, junk food, and exposure to pollutants, while others will have no such burden; and, because of biochemical individuality, some will have specific nutrient requirements vastly different to others due to genetic factors over which they have no control. As a result, only general nutritional guidelines are given in this chapter and they are not meant as a prescription to be followed without expert guidance.

 Advice from a suitably qualified and licensed health care professional is recommended to provide responsible specific nutritional guidelines.

Dietary Guidelines for Better Health

Malnutrition, of whatever severity, is perhaps the most significant AIDS co-factor, influencing the rate of progression of the disease processes and the degree of well-being, stability, and resistance to decline.[2] Without sound nutrition, all other therapeutic efforts are bound to be less likely to succeed.

The key to eating for better health is to follow a balanced whole foods diet. "Balanced" means a diet that offers the full range of vitamins, minerals, amino acids, fats, and carbohydrates that the body needs to maintain health and well-being. "Whole" foods simply mean fresh, unprocessed food, as fresh from the source as possible.

The reason for a disturbed nutritional status can be due to poor choices of what is eaten, poor digestion/absorption of food (even if it is balanced), or problems in the way digestion and absorption occur because of disturbed transportation and assimilation systems within the body.

Dietary awareness requires care, *not obsession*, since economics, lifestyle, and the region a person lives in do not always allow the very best of foods to be available all the time. If indiscretions or lapses occur, guilt should not be imposed upon oneself, as this and similar emotions can have adverse effects upon immune function and are probably more harmful than the odd cup of coffee.

Foods to Avoid

With the focus on whole foods, we can easily come up with a list of "foods" to be avoided (completely, if possible) in our diet. The items listed below have been shown to reduce immune function, interfere with nutrient uptake, and even to create problems of their own.

- **Refined carbohydrates** (sugar of any color, white flour products) have been shown to depress immune function and should be avoided in anything but small amounts.[3]
- **Saturated fats, and a high fat diet** in general, retard digestion. By increasing levels of cholesterol and certain fats, they also lead to a reduction in the efficiency of specific aspects of immune function, such as antibody production and response to infectious agents.[4] Animal fats in general (meat and dairy) should be avoided or reduced, as well as hydrogenated oils (found in margarine and many processed foods), although oils from cold-water fish and many plants are helpful in promoting immune function.
- **Alcohol and caffeine** are known to negatively affect immune efficiency and should be excluded from the diet.[5]
- **Deep-fried and barbecued foods** can be high in dangerous carcinogens, and rancid oils and artificial coloring and flavoring agents should also be avoided.

Cooked Foods Versus Raw Foods

A commonly associated problem for people with HIV or AIDS is malnutrition. This is often due to disruptions in the digestive processes caused by the weakening of the immune system. If the digestive system is not easily able to handle raw foods such as vegetables, then an abundance of these nutrient-rich foods should be consumed lightly cooked (steamed, stir-fried, or in soups, stews, etc.), or juiced in order to better facilitate digestion.

Protein Intake

Protein intake needs to be kept at a high level in order to supply adequate energy needs. Non-fat live yogurt, fish (especially cold-water varieties), free-range poultry, and lean meat are all suggested sources of protein. (For lean meat, game is preferred because it has lower fat levels than domesticated animal sources, and fewer residues of antibiotics and steroid drugs that are commonly fed to farmed animals.)

The ratio of proteins to carbohydrates and fats which are eaten is of notable importance and this has been emphasized by a wide range of health experts.[6] The optimal balance of food intake will ensure 65 percent complex carbohydrates (vegetables, fruits, legumes, and grains), 15 percent protein (fish, yogurt, fertilized eggs, and organic, free-range meat), and 20 percent fat. Variations will exist in terms of requirements for any single nutrient, and a qualified nutritional expert should take the factors of biochemical and metabolic individuality, as well as other individual special needs, into consideration when determining the proper nutritional protocol. These refinements, however, should not effect the overall balancing of the ratios of proteins, carbohydrates, and fats in a person's total food intake.

Many nutritional advisers go a step further and recommend a completely vegetarian diet. If a vegetarian mode has been decided on then protein sources need to ensure a daily combination of legumes (bean family) and grains (unless there is an allergy/sensitivity to these), since they combine to provide a complete protein. A daily supplement of free-form amino acids (powder or capsule) can ensure a good, virtually predigested, source of protein (see supplement suggestions below) for individuals who have difficulty digesting proteins. Vegetarians should be particularly careful to thoroughly clean fruits and vegetables before eating.

Dietary recommendations vary, and ultimately a person has to educate him- or herself and choose the nutritional plan which is best for them. Many health practitioners stress that a key factor in recovery for a person with AIDS is to exercise their own intelligence, will, and decision-making power in every lifestyle choice possible.

 Sensitivity reactions sometimes occur to protein foods and proteins in other foods (carbohydrates, for example) when the digestive system is impaired (by parasites, yeasts, or bacterial agents). These types of problems need to be addressed by an expert who might advise the use of digestive enzymes or other substances to help bowel health, as well as specific means of controlling the underlying problems.

Healing AIDS Research Project (HARP)
Dietary Guidelines

While there is no universal dietary or nutritional prescription for the treatment of AIDS and HIV, there are a few general guidelines that a person can follow. The Healing AIDS Research Project (HARP) at the Natural Health Clinic of Bastyr University in Seattle, Washington (see Chapter Nine) issued the following general ten-point nutritional guideline to participants:[7]

- Eat whole foods with as many essential nutrients and as few additives as possible.
- Fresh, organic vegetables, fruits, and proteins (fish and meat) are suggested whenever possible.
- Avoid processed foods.
- Reduce or eliminate refined carbohydrates (sugars, white flour, etc.) and replace with complex carbohydrates such as vegetables, whole grains, and beans, which are rich in nutrients.
- Reduce polyunsaturated and saturated fats and oils.
- Use monounsaturated oils (olive oil) with special emphasis on omega-3 oils (fish and certain plant oils).
- Eat smaller portions more frequently throughout the day to optimize absorption of nutrients from food.
- Try to keep a balance of food intake which ensures that 65 percent is complex carbohydrates (vegetables, fruits, legumes, and grains), 15 percent protein (fish, yogurt, eggs, and meat), and 20 percent fat.
- Make sure fruits and vegetables are thoroughly clean and free of parasites and bacteria by steaming lightly before eating.
- Eat a wide variety of foods to help avoid becoming sensitized to specific food families through repeated exposure.
- Eliminate chocolate, caffeine, and alcohol.[8]

Most people with AIDS, and most of those at greatest risk of contracting it, are likely to have, or to have had, digestive problems. Sound immune function demands optimum nutrition which is impossible to achieve on a poor or imbalanced diet. Achieving the best from our food calls for making good choices in the diet, preparing our food with care, and making

A Suggested Day's Diet for Anyone HIV Positive or Ill with an AIDS-like Condition

In almost all alternative strategies aimed at healing AIDS, diet is a key factor, because the best treatment in the world cannot help a malnourished immune system to return back to health. What a person eats and absorbs from food provides the raw materials from which the body can rebuild its defensive potentials. The choices made every day in the meal plans are therefore vital. Fortunately, there is a great deal to choose from, enabling our meals to be both nutritious and delicious, as the following outline illustrates.

Note: *This outline is based on Western eating patterns. Many people have found macrobiotic principles a useful guide to their dietary strategy. Anyone interested in such an approach should read one of the books on macrobiotic diets listed in the Recommended Reading section at the end of this chapter.*

Breakfast
Choose two or three selections from the following list. With imagination, they may be combined into an endless variety of great tasting meals:

- Mixed seeds (sunflower, pumpkin, sesame, linseed) and whole grains (wheat, oat, millet, or rice flakes). The seeds can be eaten whole or milled. They can be lightly oven-roasted or soaked overnight in a little water to soften them. Add the seeds to live low-fat yogurt and fresh fruit, or eat them on their own.
- Oatmeal (or millet) porridge plus fresh almonds or walnuts
- Vegetable or fish soup (with brown rice or whole-grain noodles)
- Live low-fat yogurt or kefir together with a teaspoon of cold pressed flaxseed oil
- Sourdough rye or wheat bread or toast (depending on sensitivities/ allergies) with olive oil or low-fat cottage cheese
- Enzyme-rich fruit such as papaya and pineapple
- Tofu (bean curd) stir fried with vegetables
- Two or three eggs weekly (lightly boiled or poached, or scrambled in a little olive oil). If digestion is strong, up to

    eight eggs a week may be tolerated.
- Drink herbal teas, spring water, or fresh juices such as carrot.

Mid-morning and mid-afternoon snacks
Rice cakes or any of the items listed under "breakfast."

Lunch and evening meal
Eating a number (four to six) of smaller meals daily, instead of three large set meals, has been shown to best suit both the digestive system and the body's maintenance of adequate blood-sugar. If work and social demands allow for this sort of eating pattern, then the traditional mealtimes become snack times, with another meal thrown in between breakfast and lunch and another between lunch and the evening meal. A last meal would occur a little before bedtime.

The same overall amount of food would be eaten over the day, but with less of a demand on the digestive system at any one time, and with a better end result in terms of maintenance of energy levels.

Such an eating pattern might look something like this:

8:00 A.M.	Low-fat cottage cheese and flaxseed, plus seeds or grains (as above), and papaya
10:30 A.M.	Rice cakes and herbal tea, or an egg on spinach
12:30 P.M.	Stir fried vegetables and fish or chicken, or mixed salad and jacket potato with tofu
3:00 P.M.	Fruit, seeds, and nuts, or low-fat yogurt and fruit
6:00 P.M.	Stir-fried vegetables or salad. Eat with poultry, game, fish, or rice and lentils (or other member of the bean family). If animal protein was eaten at midday then a vegetarian option should be eaten at this time.
9:00 P.M.	Vegetable, lentil, or fish soup

Obviously, any of the suggestions could be eaten at any of the times—this is just an outline of a typical day's menu. If you intend to stick with the "three set meals" format, then, after eating a breakfast (similar to those suggested above for the 8 A.M. or 10:30 A.M. meal), consider the following:

- One of these meals, at least, should contain an animal protein source such as fish, poultry, or game.

(Vegetarians may get the equivalent amino-acid intake by balancing high-protein sources such as those in the next meal option.) Again, fish should preferably be a cold-water type, such as herring, salmon, sardine, haddock, sole, or cod. Choose free-range poultry or game in order to avoid the antibiotics and steroids given to most farm-reared animals (poultry should have the skin removed).

Cook these meats by boiling, steaming, grilling, stir-frying, poaching, or using them in a casserole or soup. Avoid frying or roasting, as those methods detrimentally alter the nature of the fat. Ideally, protein should be eaten with green vegetables (or seaweed from an Asian-food or health-food store) which are lightly cooked in one of the ways mentioned above. Season with herbs, garlic, and spices, using as little salt as possible (or Asian seasonings such as miso). If any oil is employed in cooking, it should be extra virgin olive oil, which can also be used as a dressing.

- Another protein-balanced option is a meal consisting of a combination of legumes (chickpeas, mung beans, lentils, kidney beans, or any other sort of beans) and grains (millet, brown rice, quinoa, amaranth, buckwheat, or pasta noodles). A soup, stew, roast, or other combination of ingredients from these two categories provides a first-class protein source. Low-fat cheese or tofu may be included in the dish or be eaten at the same time. A variety of starchy vegetables (lightly cooked), such as carrot, beet, squash, or potato, as well as green vegetables, are also highly desirable. There is abundant evidence of the health-enhancing value of the *Brassica* family (cabbage, kale, broccoli). If digestion is sound, include a raw salad as well.

Desserts: Desserts should be low-fat yogurt (live) or enzyme-rich fruit (papaya, apple, or pear).

Note: *This brief "menu" is not definitive, but outlines possibilities and gives a framework in which four or five snack meals daily are consumed, providing ample basic nutrition. In almost all cases of immune depression, additional nutrient support (supplements) is helpful and desirable if financially possible.*

sure that it is well chewed and eaten slowly. At the same time, attention should be paid to any problems affecting the digestive tract, such as enzyme deficiency, which might be retarding the digestion and absorption of nutrients from food. The manner in which the area of nutrition (diet and supplementation) is addressed can determine the rate of recovery or decline in any given case.

Nutritional Support for Immune Function

In almost all cases of immune depression, supplementation of the diet with specific nutrients can be beneficial. Malnutrition is common in people who are HIV positive and is almost universal in people with AIDS.[9] Supplementation by mouth or injection (intramuscular or intravenous as appropriate) are the only ways of ensuring that adequate nutrients get into the body, although the oral route does not always guarantee that what is swallowed will arrive where it is needed until impaired digestive and absorption capabilities can be brought back to normal.

A number of herbal medicines have been shown to have profound beneficial effects on digestion, absorption, and on aspects of immune function. These will be outlined in Chapter Six. Nutritional efforts to improve immune function can usually be safely combined with herbal methods (along with methods which bring into play the immune-modulating power of the mind).

People who are HIV positive and/or who have been diagnosed as having AIDS are most commonly deficient in the following essential nutrients:

- vitamin B_6[10]
- folate[11]
- vitamin B_{12}[12]
- selenium[13]
- zinc[14]

Nutritional supplementation has been shown in clinical studies to offer great benefits to people already seriously ill with AIDS, and it is seen by many as the cornerstone requirement for recovery. In one six-month study, vitamins, minerals, amino acids, and essential fatty acids were all supplemented. Among the observed clinical benefits was a general improvement in well-being and a significant decrease in the p24 antigen, which rises in the presence of increased HIV activity.[15]

Other nutrients commonly supplemented in HIV positive and AIDS cases are vitamins A (beta-carotene), B-complex, and E. The B vitamins thiamine (B_1), riboflavin (B_2), pantothenic acid (B_5), pyridoxine (B_6), and B_{12} are especially essential for improving a weakened immune system. Vitamin C has also proven to be a powerful antioxidant and inhibitor of viruses and bacteria, as well as having specific and potent immune-enhancing effects.[16]

According to Robert Cathcart III, M.D., a pioneer in the use of vitamin C therapy, "Preliminary clinical evidence is that massive doses of ascorbate (a salt of vitamin C) can suppress the symptoms of disease and can markedly reduce the tendency for secondary infections." Working with a group of 102 patients with AIDS/HIV, most of whom were taking vitamin C on their own, Dr. Cathcart reports "considerable improvement" in most of the patients' conditions. Some of the improvements include a reduction of diseased lymph glands and the disappearance of Kaposi's sarcoma lesions.[17]

Supplementation of folic acid, biotin, potassium, magnesium, and manganese is also recommended, as well as amino acids and essential fatty acids, particularly omega-3 and omega-6. A good multivitamin and mineral supplement can take the place of the individual supplements listed above, but the best advice is to always consult with a qualified health practitioner in order to optimize any supplementation regimen.

Joan Priestley, M.D., of Anchorage, Alaska, reports good results from placing an HIV positive patient on a regimen of intravenous nutrition with supplements taken three times a week in an IV-nutrient drip. Dr. Priestley also prescribed high doses of oral vitamin C daily and B-complex shots once a week, as well as garlic capsules, Siberian ginseng, beta-carotene, zinc, and aloe vera. The patient also began exercising, meditating, and receiving acupuncture.

Since beginning treatment, the patient has gained forty pounds and now has much fewer symptoms, despite having a low T-cell count, according to Dr. Priestley, who has contin-

Diet and Nutrition in Treating HIV: A Case History

Jim[18] is a person who has benefited from nutritional therapy. He has regularly taken, on top of the usual daily multivitamin and mineral supplement, such compounds as evening primrose oil, potassium iodide, and B-complex injections.

"In June of 1988," Jim says, "I was diagnosed as HIV positive. My only symptom was swollen glands. But I got on the holistic boat right away. My diet changed . . . no red meat. Dairy intake was very limited. My diet is also very low in fat. For protein, I eat beans, nuts, poultry, and fish. And, of course, I eat vegetables and fruit. I feel more energy now. I'm able to do daily work and have energy afterwards. There's also a psychological boost in knowing a snowball effect is taking place in my health. At the beginning, my T-cell count was 304. Now it's 658. And as a diabetic, I'm only taking half the insulin I used to! So it's helped me there, too."

ued the patient on a course of nutrients and preventative medicines to guard against infection.

Essential Dietary Supplements

The following list provides the commonly advised dosage range of specific nutrients when prescribed as dietary supplements. *This information is not intended to serve as a recommendation for self-treatment, however. Anyone considering beginning such a regimen is advised to consult with a health care professional first, as individual requirements can vary substantially, and for certain individuals supplementation of some of the nutrients may be contraindicated.* Certain of the nutrients listed below are more important than others. These are highlighted with an asterisk*. In addition, a multivitamin and mineral supplement comprising all of the essential vitamin and mineral requirements can often be used, rather than taking the nutrients listed below separately.

Beta-Carotene (Pro-vitamin A)*: A dosage of between 100,000 and 300,000 IUs is used in treating active AIDS conditions. Beta-carotene is a safe substitute for vitamin A as it is basically non-toxic (unlike vitamin A itself, which should only be taken under expert guidance in any but small dosages, due to its potential toxicity). Beta-carotene is metabolized by the body into vitamin A. It is also a powerful antioxidant and is important in minimizing viral damage. Beta-carotene has been shown to boost the immune system of individuals diagnosed with AIDS, increasing CD-4 T-helpers cells by almost 20 percent.[19] Beta-carotene is also capable of actually killing certain other disease-causing viruses.[20]

Vitamin C (Ascorbic acid)*: Vitamin C is a powerful antioxidant and has been shown to be an inhibitor of viruses and bacteria, as well as having specific and potent immune-enhancing effects.[21] Dosage is usually suggested to "bowel tolerance" if any active infection is current. This means stepping up intake day by day until diarrhea or loose stools develop, after which the dosage is reduced to that taken the previous day, and then maintained at this level. Because of biochemical individuality, some people reach bowel tolerance when taking as little as 3 to 4 grams a day, whereas others can take 50 or more grams daily without bowel looseness.[22]

Calcium, sodium, and magnesium ascorbates (forms of vitamin C) are all easily available, with magnesium ascorbate considered by many physicians to be the superior form, due to its greater bioavailability.[23]

A major report on vitamin C's effects on AIDS has shown that it reduced levels of the p24 antigen (which rises in the presence of increased HIV activity) by 90 percent, and levels of reverse transcriptase (the enzyme which allows HIV to combine its genetic material with that of the cell it is infecting) by 99 percent.[24]

Vitamin E*: This is another powerful antioxidant which protects cell wall integrity.[25] A dosage range of 400-800 IUs daily is usually suggested. Supplementation with vitamin E results in an increase in the production of antibodies, especially when taken with the mineral selenium. Deficiency of either of these nutrients can lead to a decline in T and B cells.[26]

Vitamin B-Complex*: One or two slow-release B-complex capsules taken daily are commonly suggested. For best results, these should be formulated to a high potency (50-100 milligrams) of each of the major B vitamins, many of which may also be required individually, as well, depending on the individual's needs.

Some of the individual B vitamins that influence immune functioning are listed below.

- **Thiamine (B1)*:** A deficiency of B1 produces a decline in immune function.
- **Riboflavin (B2)*:** Required for antibody production. A deficiency leads to a decline in T and B cells. It is partially manufactured by healthy bowel flora.
- **Pyridoxine (B6)*:** Also needed for antibody production. A deficiency can lead to T-cell decline and a reduction in the size of the thymus gland. Pyridoxine is involved in many aspects of immune function and is commonly found to be deficient in most diets. Along with folic acid, it is vitally involved in protein synthesis and therefore is of major importance in any attempt to maintain and build body bulk when weight loss is a factor. A number of the medical treatments involved in the treatment of the AIDS complex of conditions can produce a deficiency of pyridoxine, most notably when Mycobacterium Avium Complex (MAC) infections are present and treated with Isoniacin, Cycloserine, L-Dopa, or Penicillamine.[27]
- **Pantothenic acid (B5)*:** When deficient, B5 is involved in altered T and B cell ratios. Viral infection is also more common when this vitamin is in short supply.
- **Vitamin B12*:** A key ingredient for ensuring T and B cell efficiency. Supplementation of this nutrient is essential if digestive function is impaired. People with AIDS are advised to use a sublingual supplement (one that is taken under the tongue) of 1 or 2 milligrams daily.
- **Folic acid (folate)*:** Very important in any attempt to improve weakened immune status. Resistance to infection is poor when folic acid is deficient, which can be the result of certain medical treatments, specifically the use of trimethoprim-sulfamethoxazole, which is sometimes used to treat Pneumocystis carinii. Folic acid is also depressed when toxoplasma gondii infection is treated with Pyrimethamine (Daraprim).[28]

- **Biotin*:** Usually produced by healthy bowel flora. It becomes deficient as a result of damage to the "friendly bacteria" of the intestines (often resulting from excessive use of antibiotics) or due to contact with sperm (as in male "receiver" homosexual behavior).[29] When biotin is deficient, an increase in virulent yeast overgrowth (a common co-factor infection in people who are immune-compromised) can occur.[30] People with AIDS are advised to supplement with a daily dosage of 500 micrograms.[31]

 Requirements for these B vitamins can usually be met by taking a B-complex, as recommended above. Exceptional circumstances may demand that they be taken separately, however. This is something which should be decided by a responsible health care advisor. Yeast-free sources of B vitamins are recommended by many experts in order to avoid possible aggravation of sensitivities resulting from yeast infections such as Candida albicans.[32]

Selenium*: This mineral is symbiotic with vitamin E, and is a vital constituent of important enzymes, such as glutathione peroxidase, which defends cell wall integrity. Many people with AIDS are deficient in selenium, and 100-200 micrograms daily should be supplemented if this is the case.[33]

Zinc*: It has been suggested that practically all people with AIDS are zinc deficient.[34] Nearly one hundred important enzymes, many of them involved in immune function, depend upon an adequate presence of zinc. Tests can determine zinc deficits, which are often evaluated by the range of known associated symptoms. These include skin lesions (ulceration, thickening, dryness), hair loss, loss of appetite, reduced sense of smell, lethargy, and increased susceptibility to infection. Supplementation with 30-50 milligrams daily is usual.

Potassium: This mineral is commonly deficient in people with immune depression. It is adequately replenished by a diet rich in vegetables. Excessive sodium intake (from, in particular, table salt—sodium chloride) can diminish potassium levels by causing its excessive loss via the urine. Coffee, alcohol, and excessive sugar intake can produce similar results, as well.[35]

Magnesium*: Commonly deficient in modern western diets, and especially so in people with immune depression. Supplementation of 500 milligrams daily is usual. Magnesium is vital for normal metabolic processes. It activates important enzymes; promotes the absorption of other minerals, such as calcium and potassium; helps in the utilization of vitamins B, C, and E; and regulates energy production from sugars.

Iron: A mineral concentrate present in every cell of the body, iron's main function is as an oxygen carrier in the blood. Any deficiency leads to lowered resistance to stress and infection. Iron is commonly deficient when there is immune depression, but it should be supplemented only under expert guidance.

Manganese: A trace element which activates many vital enzymes, manganese is a catalyst in the synthesis of cholesterol and fatty acids, taking part in many body processes, including hormonal, nerve, and brain functions. Deficiency is common. A typical recommendation is 5-10 milligrams a day.

N-acetyl-Cysteine (NAC)*: Evidence suggests that HIV infection is closely associated with the depletion of the amino acid glutathione from leukocytes, which play a vital role in immune system defenses.[36] This deficiency is thought to promote replication of the HIV virus. Supplementation of NAC enhances stores of glutathione. Because NAC is a modified amino acid, or protein fraction, which encourages synthesis of glutathione, it is now widely used in the treatment of people who are HIV positive to help restore immune function. Recommended dosages are from 500-1,500 milligrams daily.

Glutamine, another amino acid, also plays an important role in helping to preserve glutathione levels. It can be supplemented along with NAC at a dosage of 1 gram daily, taken outside of meals.[37] A good level of protein in the diet also helps to achieve this aim.

Full Spectrum Amino Acids: In the report on the one year HARP study,[38] it was stated: "Malnutrition is a significant contributory factor in the progression and pathology of AIDS. The immune deficiencies, such as profound depression of cellular immunity, the multiple infections, are similar to those seen in protein calorie restriction." This finding underscores the necessity of maintaining protein intake at adequate levels.

An effective means of doing so is through the use of free form amino acids taken supplementally. These provide the body with a predigested source of protein, bypassing the need for the digestive processes to become involved. Since many cases of AIDS/HIV are accompanied by impaired digestion due to infection or side effects from medication, the value of receiving protein from this form of supplementation is readily apparent. Depending upon the degree of protein deficiency, 5–20 grams daily are suggested (taken outside of meals).

Essential Fatty Acids*: Supplementation with essential fatty acids was a major component of a recent study in which clinical benefits were observed in twenty nine people with AIDS/ARC or HIV.[39]

The omega-3 and omega-6 essential fatty acids must be provided in the diet as humans cannot manufacture them. Omega-3 is found in fish and flaxseed oil, while omega-6 is found in seeds from warm climates, such as sunflower seeds. Their importance as aids to malabsorption problems and immune dysfunction is well-established, as is their ability to modify inflammatory processes.

Alpha and gamma linolenic acid (GLA) and linoleic acid are other essential fatty acids. Good sources of these can be found in evening primrose oil, black currant seeds, borage, and flaxseed, as well as in certain fish oils (which also provide eicosapentenoic acid (EPA) and docosahexanoic acid (DHA), which vegetarians can convert from the oils found in flaxseed). Anyone who is suffering from compromised digestion or immune dysfunction should consider supplementation with essential fatty acids. Between one and three grams daily are commonly recommended. However, advice should be sought from a qualified nutritional expert in order to determine one's particular needs and most appropriate sources.[40]

Probiotics ("Friendly Bacteria"): Nearly everyone suffering from immune dysfunction has a compromised internal ecology affecting their bowel flora. When the flora are healthy, they help detoxify the bowel, manufacture B vitamins, and keep yeasts and undesirable bacteria in check. But these flora can be easily damaged by antibiotics, steroids, an unbalanced diet, and stress.

Restoration of healthy flora in the intestines requires two organisms in particular, both of which should be regularly supplemented. These are *Lactobacillus acidophilus* (for the small intestine) and Bifidobacteria (for the colon). Supplementation with these friendly bacteria is especially urgent if yeasts (such as *Candida albicans*) are present and active. Dosage depends on the type of formulation used, and expert advice is suggested.[41]

Multivitamin and Mineral Supplements: As an added "insurance" against nutrient deficiency, and in place of a number of the individual nutrients cited above, a soundly constructed multivitamin and mineral supplement was used in the HARP study,[42] and such a choice provides a useful option to insure an adequate, underlying source for one's nutritional requirements.

The Future of Dietary Supplements

Since nutritional supplements cannot be patented, there is little financial incentive for pharmaceutical companies to invest the millions of dollars needed to meet the government's stringent requirements in order to receive FDA (Food and Drug Administration) approval for treatment of specific conditions.

The FDA is currently producing new regulations for vitamins, minerals, and herbs which will ultimately restrict public access to these safe, natural products. Because supplements are a vital element of restoration and good health, write your representative to let him or her know that you use supplements and support nutritional supplement freedom. Demand that funds be allocated for research in nutritional and other alternative approaches to treating AIDS.

Where to Find Help

Alternative Medicine Yellow Pages. **The Burton Goldberg Group. Puyallup, WA: Future Medicine Publishing, Inc., 1994.**

Lists over 16,000 practitioners of alternative medicine in the United States and Canada. Practitioners are listed by therapy, city, and state. See sections on "Diet," "Environmental Medicine," "Enzyme Therapy," "Nutritional Supplements," and "Orthomolecular Medicine."

Locating a Physician Trained in Nutritional Medicine

**American Association of Naturopathic Physicians
2366 Eastlake Avenue, Suite 322
Seattle, Washington 98102
(206) 323-7610**

Contact them for the location of a licensed naturopathic physician in your area.

**American College of Advancement in Medicine
P.O. Box 3427
Laguna Hills, CA 92654
(714) 583-7666**

ACAM provides a directory listing physicians worldwide who have been trained in nutritional and preventative medicine. The directory also provides an extensive list of books and articles on nutritional supplementation.

**American College of Nutrition
722 Robert E. Lee Drive
Wilmington, North Carolina 28480
(919) 452-1222**

A membership organization which produces a journal and newsletter. Annual meetings open to the general public. Provides lectures on nutrition research.

Food and Allergy Testing and Information

Meridian Valley Clinical Laboratory
24030 132nd Avenue S.E.
Kent, Washington 98042
(800) 234-6825
Offers a wide variety of specialized testing, including: micro-parasitology, allergies, food, essential fatty acid, and mineral and amino acid analysis.

MetaMatrix Medical Laboratory
5000 Peachtree Industrial Boulevard, Suite 110
Norcross, Georgia 30071
(800) 221-4640 (For doctors only)
(404) 446-5483
A full-service laboratory specializing in nutritional status, toxicology, and allergy testing.

Doctor's Data, Inc.
P.O. Box 111
West Chicago, Illinois 60185
(800) 323-2784
Offers mineral and allergy testing.

Immuno Laboratories, Inc.
1620 West Oakland Park Boulevard
Fort Lauderdale, Florida 33311
(800) 231-9197
This laboratory specializes in allergy and immunological testing.

Learning More About Organics

The Organic Foods Production
Association of North America
P.O. Box 1078
Greenfield, Massachusetts 01302
(413) 774-7511
(413) 774-6432 (Fax)
Publications and memberships are available.

Becoming Vegetarian and Cooking Vegetarian

Vegetarian Journal
Vegetarian Resource Group
P.O. Box 1463
Baltimore, Maryland 21203
(410) 366-8343
A nonprofit vegetarian resource group, whose main goal is to educate the public on health, nutrition, and the environment.

Vegetarian Times
1140 Lake Street, Suite 500
Oak Park, Illinois 60301
(708) 848-8100
A glossy, color magazine that offers recipes as well as informative articles and the latest news in vegetarian lifestyles.

Water Testing

National Testing Laboratories
6555 Wilson Mills Road
Cleveland, Ohio 44143
(800) 458-3330
(216) 449-2525
A certified water testing facility, serving consumers, the beverage industry, and municipal customers. Call for laboratories in Michigan, Florida, and New Hampshire.

Watertest Corporation of America
28 Daniel Plummer Road
Gottstown, New Hampshire 03045
(800) 458-3330
(603) 623-1780

Sources of Organically Grown, Hormone-Free, Nitrite-Free Meat and Poultry

Center for Science in the Public Interest
Americans for Safe Food Project
1875 Connecticut Avenue N.W., Suite 300
Washington, D.C. 20009-5728
(202) 332-9110 Ext. 384
You can obtain a list of suppliers—both mail order companies and supermarket chains—from this organization.

Eden Acres
Organic Network
12100 Lima Center Road
Clinton, Michigan 49236-9618
(517) 456-4288

Organic Network, a division of Eden Acres, offers a 150-page international directory and local statewide directories of suppliers of organic meats, poultry, fruits, and vegetables.

 # Recommended Reading

Alternative Medicine: The Definitive Guide. The Burton Goldberg Group. Puyallup, WA: Future Medicine Publishing, Inc., 1993.

The most comprehensive reference on alternative medicine ever compiled. Provides in-depth, easily understandable coverage of 43 alternative therapies and over 200 health conditions, with advice from nearly 400 alternative physicians worldwide. See chapters on "Diet," "Nutritional Supplements," and "Orthomolecular Medicine."

Diet

AIDS, Macrobiotics, and Natural Immunity. Kushi, Michio. Briarcliff, MA: Japan Publications, 1989.

An excellent introduction to building the immune system of AIDS patients with Kushi's macrobiotic diet.

Cooking With Rachel. Albert, Rachel. Oroville, CA: George Ohsawa Macrobiotic Foundation, 1989.

Rachel Albert studied macrobiotics at the Kushi Institute of Great Britain, taught cooking classes, and owns a cafe. This book appeals to a wide range of tastes and food preferences.

Coping with Your Allergies. Golos, Natalie; and Golbita, Francis. New York, NY: Simon and Schuster, 1986.

An excellent resource on food allergies.

Diet for a New America. Robbins, John. Walpole, NH: Stillpoint Publishing, 1987.
John Robbins provides a well-documented, factual account of the unhealthy and inhumane conditions animals are subjected to when they are raised for food. He discusses the physical, emotional, and economic ramifications of these conditions.

The McDougall Plan. McDougall, John., M.D.; and McDougall, Mary. Piscataway, NJ: New Century Publishing, Inc., 1983.
This book encourages an adaptation of a specific vegetarian diet and lifestyle. This diet is centered on starchy plant foods such as rice, potatoes, pasta, and all fresh fruits and vegetables.

Perfect Health. Chopra, Deepak, M.D. New York: Harmony Books, 1990.
By determining your body type, Chopra seeks to restore inner balance to the body. He uses Ayurvedic techniques, diet, stress reduction, and exercise to strengthen the mind/body connection.

Staying Healthy with Nutrition. Haas, Elson M., M.D. Berkeley, CA: Celestial Arts Publishing, 1992.
A comprehensive guide to diet and nutritional medicine. Includes an analysis of the building blocks of nutrition and their uses in medicine, an evaluation of diets around the world, the environmental aspects of nutrition, nutritional therapies, and help in creating individualized diets.

Still Life with Menu. Katzen, Mollie. Berkeley, CA: Ten Speed Press, 1988.
Fifty original still lives accompanied by menus and recipes of meatless delicacies.

Transition to Vegetarianism. Ballantine, Rudolph. Honesdale, PA: Himalayan Publishers, 1987.
This book provides solid information on how to design an optimal vegetarian diet with advice on how to approach it gradually and wisely.

Nutritional Supplementation

Dr. Wright's Guide to Healing with Nutrition. Wright, Jonathan V., M.D. New Canaan, CT: Keats Publishing, Inc., 1990.
A very readable and informative book, it contains many case histories describing how Dr. Wright approaches patients' problems.

He describes the patients' exams, tests, and treatments that solved long-standing disorders.

The Healing Nutrients Within. Braverman, Eric R., M.D.; and Pfeiffer, Carl C., M.D., Ph.D. New Canaan, CT: Keats Publishing, Inc., 1987.

This book focuses on protein and amino acids and their function in treatment of depression and insomnia, addiction, detoxification, and nutritional support for surgery. The author has found amino acid therapy effective in cases of cancer, arthritis, allergy, physical and emotional health problems, and other disorders. This book is useful to health care professionals and understandable to lay readers.

The Nutrition Desk Reference. Garrison, Robert H., Jr., M.A.R., Ph.D.; and Somer, Elizabeth, M.A., R.D. New Canaan, CT: Keats Publishing, Inc., 1990.

Reference for personal health and professional research. Basic nutritional information. Research findings on vitamins and minerals and their role in disease treatment and prevention.

Nutritional Influences on Illness. 2nd Edition. Werbach, Melvyn A., M.D. Tarzana, CA: Third Line Press, 1992.

This is a sourcebook that abstracts and organizes many studies dealing with the way nutrition affects illness.

Prescription for Nutritional Healing: A Practical A-Z Reference to Drug-Free Remedies Using Vitamins, Minerals, Herbs, and Food Supplements. Balch, James, M.D.; and Balch, Phyllis, R.N. Garden City Park, NY: Avery Publishing, 1990.

A complete guide to dealing with health disorders through nutritional, herbal, and supplemental therapies written by a medical doctor and a nutritionist. It provides all the information needed for the average person to design his or her own nutrition program.

6 Herbal Medicine

Herbs have provided humankind with medicine from the earliest beginnings of civilization. Throughout history, various cultures have handed down their accumulated knowledge of the medicinal use of herbs to successive generations, and this vast body of information serves as the basis for much of traditional medicine today.

Many herbal medicines work in much the same way as do conventional pharmaceutical drugs, i.e., via their chemical makeup. Herbs contain a large number of naturally-occurring chemicals that have biological activity. In the past one hundred and fifty years, chemists and pharmacists have been isolating and purifying the "active" compounds from plants in an attempt to produce reliable pharmaceutical drugs. Examples include such drugs like digoxin (from foxglove [*Digitalis purpurea*]), colchicine (from autumn crocus [*Colchicum autumnale*]), and morphine (from the opium poppy [*Papaver somniafera*]).

Yet, for the most part, modern medicine has veered from the use of pure herbs in its treatment of disease and other health disorders. One of the reasons for this is economic. Since herbs, by their very nature, cannot be patented and drug companies cannot hold the exclusive right to sell a particular herb, they are not motivated to invest any money in that herb's testing or promotion. In addition, the collection and preparation of herbal medicine cannot be as easily controlled as the manufacture of synthetic drugs, making its profits less dependable. Most importantly, the demand for herbal medicine has decreased in the United States because Americans have been conditioned to rely on synthetic, commercial drugs to provide quick relief, regardless of the side effects which many of these drugs are known to cause.

Today, there is extensive scientific documentation worldwide regarding the therapeutic use of herbs for a wide range of health conditions, including premenstrual syndrome, indigestion, insomnia, heart disease, cancer, and AIDS and

HIV infection. Herbal medicine forms the basis of the treatment programs in many forms of alternative medicine, including naturopathic medicine and the ancient and time-tested systems of Traditional Chinese Medicine and Ayurvedic medicine.

Chinese Herbal Medicine and AIDS/HIV

AIDS can be managed by the use of Chinese herbal remedies, often in conjunction with Western drugs, according to Subhuti Dharmananda, Ph.D., Director of the Institute for Traditional Medicine in Portland, Oregon. Although his studies do not reflect the long-term manageability of this relatively new disease, Dr. Dharmananda has theorized that for some individuals, HIV infection can become a chronic disease rather than an acutely fatal one. "A large proportion of the long-term survivors of this infection have used Chinese medicine and attribute their survival to a combination of their positive attitudes towards life and the use of this type of medical intervention," he says.

Acupuncture (See Chapter Eight), best known for its influence on pain, is commonly used in conjunction with herbal medicine for the treatment of HIV and AIDS.

Combination Herbal Formulas

Much of our knowledge of using herbs in treating immune depression is derived from Traditional Chinese Medicine. A major contributor in sharing this knowledge is Dr. Dharmananda, a leading herbal expert, who maintains that skilled blending of various herbs is more effective than herbs used individually.[1] As he explains, "Combining herbs provides a substantial benefit over using herbs individually [because] herbs from different categories of therapy can address a syndrome more effectively than approaching treatment from just one direction."[2] Dr. Dharmananda employs a variety of herbal formulations in his work with patients with AIDS or who are HIV positive. These include:

Composition-A

Dr. Dharmananda's primary recommendation for treating people with HIV is Composition-A, an herbal formulation used to bolster the immune system, protect the organs from damage, promote blood circulation, and inhibit infections. Dr. Dharmananda prescribes Composition-A along with daily nutritional supplements and food therapy items, to ensure that his patients' needs are met with a complete protocol. Additional adjunctive treatments are sometimes also employed to address specific patterns of dysfunction unique to each patient.

Composition-A is a blend of twenty-eight herbs, with the following herbs serving as its major ingredients, according to Dr. Dharmananda: astragalus, licorice, ganoderma, salvia, isatis, curcuma, deer antler, and hu-chang.

Dr. Dharmanada reports that during 1991 an average of one thousand HIV-infected people in the United States were taking Composition-A daily. Of these, many were also taking a second combination suitable for their particular condition.

Studying these cases reveals the efficacy of this approach. Their "symptoms" are listed below, together with the number of patients involved in each category, and the percentage of cases with full resolution or partial improvement.[3] Most of the patients in the study also received acupuncture. The length of treatment time needed to achieve these results was three months, according to Dr. Dharmananda.

Symptom	Number of People	% Resolved	% Improved
Diarrhea	56	62%	12%
Sinus infection	66	41%	29%
Fatigue	60	40%	35%
Anxiety	60	47%	18%
Depression	47	45%	25%
Insomnia	46	56%	11%
Headache	38	68%	8%
Skin rashes	36	42%	14%
Herpes	19	68%	26%
Night sweats	25	68%	16%
Pharyngitis	26	62%	15%
Cough	21	81%	0%

Minor Bupleurum Combination

Minor Bupleurum Combination is used to treat hepatitis and other conditions associated with immune depression. According to Dr. Dharmananda, this formula is extremely popular in Japan for treatment of hepatitis and many other chronic infections. "It has been studied in laboratory evaluations of HIV-infected cells in Paris and shown to have anti-retroviral activity," Dr. Dharmananda reports. "It is not, however, often prescribed for HIV patients, but some are self-administering it, mainly in San Francisco, based on the French studies."

Minor Bupleurum Combination contains bupleurum, scutellaria (an anti-inflammatory containing antioxidant flavonoids), ginseng (an adaptogen), jujube, licorice, pinellia (an anti-inflammatory and mucolytic), as well as citrus and ginger (for their essential oils, which promote digestion and reduce nausea). Overall, the combination improves digestion, regardless of the factors which may have previously impaired it.

Astra Isatis

Astra Isatis, another formulation developed by Dr. Dharmananda, contains the following herbs: astragalus, conodopsis, licorice, atractylodes, dioscorea, broussonetia, isatis, laminaria, bupleurum, lycium, and cynamorium. Of these, researchers believe that astragalus and isatis are the most important (see below for their individual characteristics.)[4]

Astra Isatis was employed by the Healing AIDS Research Project (HARP) at Bastyr University in Seattle, Washington, as part of their protocol for a study conducted on the effectiveness of a naturopathic approach to AIDS. Due to the positive outcome of this study (see Chapter Nine), Astra Isatis can be regarded as having significant value in the fight against the disease and its related conditions.

Individual Herbs Used to Treat AIDS and Associated Illnesses

Herbs cannot be said to offer a "cure" for AIDS. Even so, a surprising number of traditional Western and Chinese herbs are considered beneficial in modifying and balancing body processes, in addition to controlling a range of invading

Different Systems of Herbology

There is a great diversity and richness in the various herbal traditions of the world, most of which still thrive today. Native American cultures contain a cornucopia of healing wisdom, as do European traditions, from the Welsh to the Sicilian. There are a number of other highly developed medical systems around the world that utilize medicinal plants in their healing work, as well. These include ancient systems such as Ayurvedic medicine from India and Traditional Chinese Medicine. The essential differences between these various systems of medicine are their cultural contexts rather than the goals or effects which they strive to achieve.

Traditional Chinese Medicine (TCM): The restoration of harmony is integral to Chinese herbal medicine. Harmonious balance is expressed in terms of the two complementary forces known as *yin* and *yang*; and in the five elements of fire, earth, metal, water, and wood. The five elements are of particular importance to the Chinese herbalist, as they give rise to the five tastes by which all medicinal plants are evaluated. Fire gives rise to bitterness, earth to sweetness, metal to acridity, water to saltiness, and wood to sourness. Each taste is said to have a particular medicinal action. Bitter-tasting herbs clear heat and remove toxins; acrid herbs disperse; salty-tasting herbs soften masses; sour-tasting herbs are astringent; and sweet-tasting herbs tonify and nourish.

Herbs that have none of these tastes are described as bland, a quality that indicates that the plant may have a diuretic effect. The taste of a plant can also indicate the organ to which it has a natural affinity. Besides defining particular herbal tastes, the Chinese ascribe different "natures" to herbs, i.e., hot, warm, neutral, cool, and cold.

Ayurvedic Medicine: Ayurvedic medicine has ancient roots in the Indian subcontinent. It also recognizes five elements: ether, fire, water, air, and earth. These five elements manifest themselves in the body to form the *tridosha* or three basic humors: *vata* (the principle of air or movement); *pitta* (the principle of fire); and *kapha* (the principle of water). Ayurvedic medicine sees all universal energies as having their counterparts within the human being. The healing process seeks to achieve a balance in individuals between the elements of air or wind *(vata)*, fire or bile *(pitta)*, and water or phlegm *(kapha)*.

Ayurvedic medicine holds that the taste of an herb is indicative of its properties. The Sanskrit word for taste, *rasa*, means "essence." There are six essences: sweet, sour, salty, pungent, bitter, and astringent. For example, herbs which are pungent, sour, and salty-tasting cause heat, thereby increasing *pitta* (fire). Sweet, bitter, and astringent herbs, on the other hand, have precisely the opposite effect, cooling and decreasing *pitta*. As in Traditional Chinese Medicine, Ayurvedic texts categorize all plants according to this system, so that herbalists can prescribe herbs more easily.

Western Medicine: The use of medicinal plants is also fundamental to Western society's pharmacologically-based approach to medicine. The majority of our medicinal drug groups were discovered or developed from the plant kingdom, even if they are now manufactured synthetically. However, most conventional health professionals view medicines as biochemical "magic bullets," which are expected to provide instant results. This approach has been very successful in certain areas, such as in the treatment of acute illness, but it has been shown to have major limitations when it comes to treating chronic or degenerative disease.

organisms, making these herbs worthy of further research into the roles they might play in the fight against AIDS. As it is, the use of individual herbal medicines in the treatment of AIDS is already widespread, with additional studies now underway to assess their possible additional applications and effectiveness.

Some of the herbal remedies most often employed as treatments for AIDS and its related illnesses include astragalus,[5] carnivora (venus fly trap),[6] echinacea,[7] licorice,[8] and goldenseal.[9] Garlic[10] and isatis root[11] are also commonly used because of their broad antibacterial and antiviral qualities, as is ginseng, due to its tonic effects on the thymus gland and its ability to help those who take it to resist all forms of stress.[12] St. John's Wort is used, as well, because of its specific retrovirus-blocking actions.[13] Chinese bitter melon, monolaurin, and lentinan (an extract of *shiitake* mushrooms) have also shown dramatic anti-HIV effects.[14]

Some of the leading herbs currently being used in treatment of immune deficiency and associated illnesses include the following:

Aloe Vera *(Aloe vera)*

This plant has been used medicinally for nearly five thousand years. As with a number of herbs, researchers have begun to explore its properties in the laboratory and to isolate the key ingredients which operate as healing agents. The most important therapeutic ingredient in aloe is called acemannan, a polysaccharide found in the leaf, which is reported to have antiviral capabilities, through its immune-enhancing action.[15] However, Dr. Dharmananda reports that it is almost impossible to get enough acemannan from aloe vera or aloe juice alone in order to achieve the desired effects of health restoration.

Acemannan is currently licensed in the United States as a veterinary drug in oral and injectable forms. It is effective against feline leukemia, which suggests it may be useful for treating HIV infection. Belgian and Canadian studies have shown that patients who use acemannan gain an average of nine to ten months longevity, whether or not they simultaneously use AZT. Intravenous administration is recommended.[16]

In a summary of several human studies, presented at the Sixth International Conference on AIDS, it was reported that patients who took oral acemannan for four years showed increased T4 counts, gained weight if they had previously lost it, experienced "an elimination or reduction in frequency of bacterial, viral, or fungal infection, [and had] rapid responses to appropriate antimicrobial therapy when infection occurred."[17]

Indications: Bacterial, fungal, and viral infections. Immune enhancement.

Astragalus *(Astragalus membranaceus)*

Astragalus membranaceus is an immune system enhancer. It induces:[18]

- increased phagocytosis ("swallowing" of bacterial invaders by white blood cells)

- enhanced T-cell transformation (activation of T cells to target specific antigens, thus initiating the immune response to the invading pathogens)
- increased numbers of macrophages (a type of immune system cell which scavenges foreign particles and cells and, after digesting them, presents the antigens to the T cells to commence the immune response)
- increased levels of the immunoglobulins, IgA and IgG (antibodies produced by certain immune responses that are important in the defense against infection)
- formation of interferon (a substance produced in the body which increases the resistance of cells to penetration by viruses)
- enhanced lymphocyte blastogenesis (increased formation of defensive white blood cells) in cancer patients

Indications: Swellings, night sweats, skin ulcers, detoxification, cancer, and the need for immune enhancement.[19]

Carnivora (*Dionaea muscipula*)
Carnivora, also known as Venus Fly Trap, is an immune stimulator and modulator known to increase the number and activity of T cells, and to increase phagocytosis of the macrophages. It has been shown to reduce the viability of the HIV virus, and to improve clinical response in patients with HIV infection at all stages of the illness. Carnivora can be used intravenously, intramuscularly, orally, or by inhalation.[20]

Indications: To enhance immune function, and for treatment of HIV and other infections.

Chinese Bitter Melon (*Momordica charantia*)
There is increasing scientific evidence indicating Chinese bitter melon's broad range of anti-HIV effects. It is considered capable of destroying HIV-infected cells, and blocking cell-to-cell infection, while protecting other T cells and white cells from invasion by the virus.[21]

Bitter melon has been tried orally, but very few patients with HIV infections report positive benefits when taking the herb in this manner. A further deterrent to this approach is the fact that it is also very bitter and unpleasant to drink, and may cause nausea, as well. The recommended method of using the herb is via a rectal retention enema. This method ensures that the herb maintains its potency, which does not always occur when it is ingested orally, due to reactions which can result from contact with stomach acids. Since the rectal retention enema therapy bypasses the stomach acids and is absorbed through the colon and large intestines in order to pass directly into the blood stream, this form of treatment is considered most effective.

Indications: HIV infection.

Echinacea *(Echinacea angustifolia)*
This herb has long been valued by traditional cultures, including those of Native Americans, for its immune-enhancement properties. Research has shown that echinacea results in macrophage activation, and that it is a potent inhibitor of viral infection.[22]

Indications: Viral and fungal infection, and the need for immune enhancement.

Garlic *(Allium sativum)*
Garlic is one of the most widely employed herbs in the world. Research has shown that it has strong antibacterial, antifungal, and antiviral properties, and that it is effective against worms and protozoa, including organisms resistant to standard antibiotics.[23]

Indications: Any of the indicated infections (see Chapter Eight for more information).

Goldenseal (Hydrastis canadensis)
Goldenseal is another potent immune enhancer that is recognized by many cultures. It is used to stimulate macrophage and natural killer cell activity; enhance gastrointestinal function (especially as an antidote for diarrhea); and also works as an antibacterial, antifungal, antiprotozoal agent, including being effective against *Giardia lamblia*, *Cryptococcus neoformans*, and *Candida albicans*.[24]

Indications: Need for immune enhancement, or to combat intestinal infection.

Isatis *(Isatis tinctoria)*

Isatis is a broad spectrum antibacterial and antiviral agent which calms inflammation and lowers body temperature.
   Indications: Inflammation, fever, detoxification.[25]

Licorice *(Glycyrrhiza glabra)*

Licorice is another well-known immune system enhancer.[26] It improves both macrophage activity and the production of interferon, and acts as an inhibitor of DNA and RNA viruses.[27] It has also been shown to be a reverse transcriptase inhibitor and to result in significant anti-HIV activity (in vitro).[28] In addition, licorice extract has broad spectrum antimicrobial effects.[29]
   It is also useful as an antioxidant, protecting tissues from free radical damage, especially the liver.[30] Glycyrrhizin, a component of licorice, is also an anti-inflammatory agent, and protects against allergy and its effects, most notably those related to skin conditions.[31]
   Finally, licorice helps protect the thymus gland from shrinking when steroids such as cortisone are used, and actually enhances the anti-inflammatory effects of this steroid.[32]
   Indications: Need for immune enhancement, inflammation, allergy, cortisone medication, liver dysfunction.

Siberian Ginseng *(Eleutherococcus sentiocosus)*

Siberian ginseng is particularly well-known in Asia. It is a powerful adaptogen, and has been shown to enhance resistance to all forms of stress, as well as producing tonic effects on the thymus gland.[33]
   Indications: Illness and stress.

St. John's Wort *(Hypericum perforatum)*

Hypericin, a component of St. John's Wort, is known to act against retroviruses. Its action against HIV in a test-tube is described as "dramatic," as it has been shown to prevent infected cells from releasing the virus and to stop free-floating HIV from infecting healthy cells, without toxicity. In addition, it is a known antibacterial and antiviral agent, with specific antiretroviral effects.[34]
   Indications: Bacterial and viral infections; HIV infection.

All herbal compounds, and many individual herbs, are toxic if used in excessive amounts. Many produce mild digestive side effects, as well.[35] Advice from an expert in the use of herbal medicine is always prudent if consideration is being given to the use of herbal products for health-related issues.

 # Where to Find Help

***Alternative Medicine Yellow Pages.* The Burton Goldberg Group. Puyallup, WA: Future Medicine Publishing, Inc., 1994.**

Lists over 16,000 practitioners of alternative medicine in the United States and Canada. Practitioners are listed by therapy, city, and state. See sections on "Aromatherapy," "Ayurvedic Medicine," "Flower Remedies," "Herbal Medicine," "Naturopathic Medicine," and "Traditional Chinese Medicine."

**American Association of Acupuncture and Oriental Medicine
4101 Lake Boone Trail, Suite 201
Raleigh, North Carolina 27607
(919) 787-5181**

The AAAOM is a national professional trade organization of acupuncturists who meet acceptable standards of competency. They also can provide you with the names and locations of local members.

**American Association of Naturopathic Physicians
2366 Eastlake Avenue, Suite 322
Seattle, Washington 98102
(206) 323-7610**

Provides referrals to a nationwide network of accredited or licensed practitioners. Publishes a quarterly newsletter for both professionals and the general public. Also offers a series of brochures and pamphlets on a variety of subjects.

Herb Research Foundation
1007 Pearl Street, Suite 200
Boulder, Colorado 80302
(303) 449-2265
Co-publishes HerbalGram *with the American Botanical Council. Provides research materials for consumers, pharmacists, physicians, scientists, and industry.*

 # Recommended Reading

Alternative Medicine: The Definitive Guide. The Burton Goldberg Group. Puyallup, WA: Future Medicine Publishing, Inc., 1993.

The most comprehensive reference on alternative medicine ever compiled. Provides in-depth, easily understandable coverage of 43 alternative therapies and over 200 health conditions, with advice from nearly 400 alternative physicians worldwide. See Chapters on "Herbal Medicine," "Aromatherapy," "Ayurvedic Medicine," "Flower Remedies," and "AIDS."

Chinese Herbal Therapies for Immune Disorders. Dharmananda, Subhuti, Ph.D. Portland, OR: Institute for Traditional Medicine, 1993.

Presents a technical description of the selection of herbs and herbal formulas for the treatment of various disorders involving immune dysfunctions, and provides some information about the active constituents of herbs and their pharmacology. The book has four sections: a description of basic therapeutic approaches, an examination of the main groups of active constituents, a quick review of several disease categories with sample herbs and formulas, and an appendix of detailed articles on specific immune problems.

The Healing Herbs. Castleman, Michael. Emmaus, PA: Rodale Press, 1991.

An A to Z guide on herbs and their medicinal qualities, along with a history and description of each herb. Castleman includes a paragraph or two on the safety factor and dosage, as well as on how to grow the herbs.

HerbalGram
American Botanical Council
P.O. Box 201660,
Austin, Texas 78720
(512) 331-8868
(800) 272-7105 (Phone orders)
The quarterly magazine of the American Botanical Council and the Herb Research Foundation. Loaded with information on the medical and scientific updates on herbs; feature articles; reviews on medicinal plants; reviews of media coverage; updates on legal and regulatory matters, conferences, book reviews, networking, and more.

The Herbs of Life. Tierra, Lesley. Freedom, CA: Crossing Press, 1992.
A concise, well-organized book of both Western and Chinese herbs and their uses.

The New Holistic Herbal. Hoffmann, David. Rockport, MA: Element Books, 1992.
A revised and updated version of the best-selling comprehensive guide to the use of herbs in healing. The New Holistic Herbal *is an indispensable reference work for all those who want to find out more about the healing properties of plants.*

"Let thy food be thy medicine and thy medicine be thy food."

—*Hippocrates (460–377 B.C.)*

7 Nutritional and Herbal Treatments for Illnesses Associated with AIDS

As we have seen, according to the Centers for Disease Control (CDC), there are at least twenty-eight conditions which are now associated with AIDS, many of them bewildering and seemingly unconnected to each other. The best known of these conditions which can now fall under the umbrella of AIDS include Kaposi's sarcoma (KS) and Pneumocystis carinii pneumonia (PCP), but alongside of these are a number of more general conditions which often befall people with AIDS, as well. Among them are diarrhea, weight loss, night sweats, fevers, rashes, and swollen lymph glands.

All of these more generalized conditions and their related symptoms are known to be linked to a host of opportunistic microorganisms which a healthy immune system can usually keep in check, but which can pose grave risks to one which has already been compromised. Of themselves, many of these conditions are relatively minor, or at least not life threatening. Occurring together and cumulatively, however, they can initiate a very sharp decline in one's health.

The problem which these conditions can present was summarized in a report published in the journal *Nutrition Research* in 1985, which stated: "The evidence worldwide suggests that the immunodeficient state which results from malnutrition and/or the interplay between (multiple) bowel infections and malabsorption is probably the precursor of the next stage of AIDS—initiated by HIV infection."[1]

While certain researchers now suggest that the HIV virus alone may not be enough to precipitate the condition into the "next stage," the statement remains important if for no other reason than the fact that it pinpoints the area in which the problems listed above usually start, namely, the digestive tract.

For instance, long before AIDS was recognized and defined, it was clear that something was seriously wrong with the health of many gay men. As far back as 1977, a New York research study reported on two hundred and fifty gay men and their bowel problems, using the term "Gay Bowel Syndrome" for the first time.[2] A wide selection of protozoa, parasites (such as worms), bacteria, fungi, and viruses were involved in this syndrome, setting the scene for lowered immunity, malabsorption of nutrients, and an increased likelihood of further ill-health and infection.

A combination of sexually acquired diseases, drug use (see Chapter Three), and sexual practices such as anal intercourse and various forms of aberrant rectal play were also implicated as causes of this particular constellation of bowel problems and infections. The earliest general symptoms, apart from gastrointestinal distress, were fatigue, weight loss, fevers, and diarrhea. Today, these symptoms remain at the center of conditions associated with AIDS, along with other infections involving a host of other organisms.

The earlier these "minor" symptoms can be identified, treated, and checked the better, as early treatment can often ensure that immune function does not become severely compromised. Symptoms such as fatigue and night sweats can be the result of many possible underlying conditions and tend to respond when those conditions are addressed. A combination of approaches, ranging from nutrition, herbal medicine, homeopathy, stress reduction, relaxation, and visualization techniques, acupuncture, and bodywork, are all potentially helpful in treating such broadly-based problems.[3]

 If unconventional methods are being employed alongside orthodox approaches to any of these conditions, nutritional supplementation (for example, with beta-carotene, vitamin C, and other immune system enhancing nutrients, details of which can be found in Chapter Five) may be included in a treatment program.

General Immune Enhancement and Anti-HIV Methods

Rather than focusing on each of the symptoms which are associated with AIDS and HIV infection, it first makes sense to try to enhance the normal defense mechanisms of the body so that they can act in their appropriate ways, dealing with infections and any particular detoxification or repair requirements, thus preventing the symptoms from becoming entrenched. Such an approach, if not always able to succeed in eradicating the symptoms, at least ensures that they do not wreck further havoc on the body. This is what makes overall nutritional excellence and lifestyle (behavior) factors the bedrock from which all other therapeutic strategies can be constructed.

Anyone with AIDS or HIV infection, or who is a member of one of the high risk groups linked to these conditions, should take note of the guidance offered in this chapter, as well as in Chapters Five and Six, and apply it as is deemed appropriate after consulting with a health care professional.

The nutritional and herbal methods most likely to be helpful in immune enhancement and/or inhibition of AIDS/HIV are as follows:

Beta-Carotene
See Chapter Five for more information and references. A daily dose of 300,000 units per day will have antiviral effects, protect against tissue damage, and raise levels of CD4 lymphocytes.[4]

Vitamin C to Bowel Tolerance
The use of vitamin C in high dosages has been shown to act against retroviruses in general, and HIV in particular; to protect tissues against inflammatory damage resulting from bacteria and virus activity; to have specific antiviral activity; and to boost immune function, specifically of macrophages and neutrophils (a type of leukocyte or white blood corpuscle).[5]

The dosage of vitamin C when used for this purpose is stepped up by a gram per day, starting at one or two grams per day. When diarrhea or loose bowel motion is noted (a condition known as bowel tolerance), the dosage taken the previous day is reverted to and maintained.[6] Some people find they reach bowel tolerance when taking as little as 5 to 10 grams daily, whereas others seem able to exceed 50 grams without such symptoms. Biochemical individuality (see Chapter Five) plays a part in this difference.

Monolaurin
This fatty acid is active against particular classes of viruses similar to HIV, which are known as "enveloped viruses." Monolaurin is also known to be effective against the Epstein-Barr virus, Herpes 1 and 2, and cytomegalovirus (see Herpes below).[7]

Astragalus *(Astragalus membranaceus)*
Long used to enhance immune function in Chinese medicine, astragalus has been shown by research to improve T-cell levels and function, along with improving phagocytosis.[8]

Astragalus *(Radix astragalus)*
Widely used against infection, this form of astragalus stimulates immune production of interferon which inhibits viral replication.[9]

Carnivora *(Dionaea muscipula)*
This extract of the Venus Fly Trap plant is widely used in cancer treatment in Europe and has been shown to be active against HIV. It is used orally, by inhalation, and as an intravenous or intramuscular injection.[10] (See also Chapter Six.)

Chinese Bitter Melon *(Momordica charantia)*
Extracts of this and related plants have been shown to have anti-HIV effects in laboratory studies. Recent case history reports also show bitter melon extracts to be capable of helping to stabilize CD4 cell levels in infected individuals.[11] (See also Chapter Six.)

Garlic *(Allium sativum)*
Garlic is a powerful antibacterial, antiparasitic, and antifungal agent with recent evidence of anti-HIV potential.[12] (See also Chapter Six and Chapter Eight.)

Isatis *(Isatis tinctoria)*
Isatis acts as a broad spectrum antibacterial and antiviral agent against a number of known pathogens active in immune-compromised individuals, including infectious mononucleosis.[13] (See also Chapter Six.)

Licorice (Glycyrrhiza glabra)

As far as immune function and HIV are concerned, this remarkable herb improves macrophage activity. In test tube settings it has shown anti-HIV potential (influencing reverse transcriptase activity which AZT also targets), and it has a broad spectrum antimicrobial action against numerous undesirable pathogenic bacteria (Staphylococcus aureus for example, and *Candida albicans*).[14] (See also Chapter Six.)

St. John's Wort *(Hypericum perforatum)*

St. John's Wort is known to act against retroviruses, blocking some of the behavior of HIV (but not acting as a reverse transcriptase inhibitor). (See also Chapter Six.)

Shiitake Mushroom Extract *(Lentinan)*

There are case reports of HIV positive individuals reverting to HIV negative status, and recovering fully, following use of this mushroom extract.[15]

Candidiasis

Recurrent candidiasis (an overgrowth of the yeast *Candida albicans* throughout the intestinal tract and/or the vagina) is common in people who are immune-compromised. Candidiasis is a condition which can become almost universal and constant as immune efficiency declines, and is often a major problem for people with AIDS/ARC.[16]

In many women, vaginal candidiasis may be stubbornly present for between six months and three years before a positive diagnosis of HIV infection is made. Eileen Stretch, N.D., a Canadian naturopathic physician, reports that unexplained vaginal candidiasis which is resistant to treatment is often the only clinical indication of severe underlying immunodeficiency.[17]

As the problem of candidiasis progresses, in both men and women, the yeast often spreads to the mouth, larynx, and pharynx, and sometimes to the stomach and esophagus. It may be accompanied by obvious herpes infection, swollen lymph glands, and low resistance to infection, as well as profound exhaustion.

One of the side effects of chronic candidiasis is the damage it causes to the intestinal walls. This allows absorption into the blood stream of multiple antigenic and toxic substances, resulting in allergies which are commonly seen in people who are HIV positive and from high risk groups.

Dr. Eunice Carlson, of Michigan University, has shown that when candidiasis is actively present in the system at the same time as an infectious agent, such as *Staphylococcus aureus*, the toxicity of the latter is greatly enhanced and can result in fatal toxic shock syndrome.[18] Therefore, it is vital for people with immune depression to try to get the candida organism under control.

Conventional Medical Treatment of Candidiasis

Conventional medical treatment of candidiasis usually involves the following drugs:

- **For local treatment:** Chlortrimazole.
- **For bowel overgrowth:** Nystatin.
- **For systemic involvement:** Fluconazole and Itraconazole.

For many people, these drugs can result in side effects. This highlights the chief flaw in the conventional approach to treating candidiasis, namely that little attention is paid to restoration of the natural ecological controls of the yeast while the antifungal drugs are being used. This almost inevitably means that yeast overgrowth will return soon after drug treatment ceases, and that the cycle will eventually repeat itself.

Alternative Treatments for Candidiasis

In order to avoid this repetitive cycle, practitioners of alternative medicine use a multipronged approach. Attempts to kill the yeast are made, using a variety of herbal products such as garlic, caprylic acid (coconut plant extract), aloe vera juice, licorice, goldenseal, and/or echinacea. At the same time, steps are taken to restore the normal bowel flora, using viable colonizing strains of the friendly bacteria *Lactobacillus acidophilus* (for the small intestine) and Bifidobacteria (for the colon). These friendly bacteria, often damaged through the use of antibiotics or steroid drugs, normally keep the growth of candida in check.[19] Cultured dairy products such as kefir and live low-fat yogurt are also good sources of these friendly bacteria.[20] Selective use of *Lactobacillus bulgaricus*, a non-colonizing bacteria with powerful antifungal and antibiotic potentials which are employed as the bacteria passes slowly through the digestive tract (requiring three weeks or so of transit time), can also be beneficial.

Finally, a nutritional strategy which discourages the proliferation of the *Candida albicans* is also adopted. Usually this involves an extremely low intake of simple carbohydrates and sugars, with an emphasis placed on complex carbohydrate intake (from vegetables, grains, legumes),[21] together with cultured (live) dairy products. In addition, an anticandidiasis strategy commonly employs antifungal foods such as garlic and olive oil (oleic acid). Such methods tend to be extremely successful, but may take six months or more before full control of the the yeast overgrowth is achieved.

Diarrhea

Diarrhea of a serious nature occurs in around 50 percent of people with AIDS and leads to weight loss, nutritional deficiency, and weakness.[22] Among the most common infecting agents in diarrhea associated with AIDS and HIV infection are *cryptosporidiosis*, *microsporidiosis* (parasite), cytomegalovirus, *giardia lamblia* (amoeba), *B. hominis* (amoeba), *mycobacterium avium* (MAI), as well as *Candida albicans* (yeast).

Conventional Medical Treatment of Diarrhea

Once the main infecting organism which is causing the diarrhea is identified, a specific drug is employed to deal with it. When such a treatment approach is unsuccessful, the diarrhea may be considered to be due to whatever metabolic and systemic disturbances have resulted from the HIV infection itself.

Bernard Bihari, M.D., of New York City, states that when treating diarrhea of an undetermined cause (meaning that no identification of an infecting agent has been made following laboratory tests), he has been successful in at least half the cases using the drug Humatin, which is usually prescribed for intestinal parasites.[23] He finds this drug useful in two thirds of cases of cryptosporidiosis diarrhea, as well, despite the fact that it is commonly considered to be untreatable. Presumably, the response to Humatin in patients whose stool cultures are negative reflects the presence of parasites that escaped laboratory detection (possibly microsporidiosis).[24]

Alternative Approaches to Diarrhea
Alternative approaches for treating diarrhea employ nutritional, herbal, and homeopathic methods, as well as those from Traditional Chinese Medicine.

Extracts from the herbs goldenseal and garlic are commonly prescribed for their multiple antiamoebal, antiviral, and antifungal potentials,[25] along with probiotic friendly bacteria such as Bifidobacteria and *Lactobacillus acidophilus*, which both control fungi and produce their own antibiotic substances to destroy many bacterial pathogens.[26]

Candida overgrowth is another common factor in bowel problems and conventional and alternative medical approaches to this are outlined. Candida is arguably the easiest (and one of the most important) organisms to control using dietary and simple supplementation strategies.

Homeopathic methods (including the use of Bach Flower Remedies) have been shown clinically to help restore normal bowel activity, as well. A qualified homeopathic practitioner who uses these methods should be consulted for advice on the specific remedies indicated.[27]

In cases of diarrhea where parasites are the cause, the invaders are often successfully treated using extracts of grapefruit seeds (known as microcidin) and the plant Artemesia (wormwood).[28] As for cases of cryptococcosis, Chinese medical experts have used extracts of garlic intravenously with very good results.[29]

Herpes Infections
The family of viruses which belong to the herpes group includes herpes simplex (HSV-1 causes cold sores and HSV-2 genital herpes), herpes zoster (chicken pox and shingles), cytomegalovirus (CMV), Epstein Barr virus (EBV), as well as human herpes virus 6.[30] Most adults harbor three or more of

these viruses, which usually remain inactive unless immune function declines. They are extremely common in people who are HIV positive or who have AIDS.[31]

Raymond Keith Brown, M.D., author of *AIDS, Cancer, and the Medical Establishment*, reports that the Epstein Barr virus which causes mononucleosis is found in 20 percent of healthy adults with no symptoms, and in 100 percent of people who are HIV positive.[32] And in laboratory conditions when any of the herpes viruses are added to HIV, the cell destruction caused is greatly increased.

Conventional Medical Treatment of Herpes

Conventional medical treatment normally involves the use of the drug acylclovir, which is relatively non-toxic for most people, but which can cause severe liver and kidney damage in some people. Acylclovir is now frequently prescribed for people who are HIV positive whether or not herpes is known to be present, since if infection recurs, it can trigger HIV activity.[33]

Alternative Treatment of Herpes

Clinical experience has shown that a diet rich in the amino acid arginine encourages the activity of the herpes virus, whereas a diet rich in another amino acid lysine discourages its activities. Supplementation with one to two grams daily of lysine, taken outside of mealtimes, helps tilt the balance away from arginine, as does a dietary strategy which emphasizes lysine-rich foods, such as fish, chicken, lamb, cheese, beans, brewer's yeast, and bean sprouts, and which discourages arginine rich foods (peanuts, cashew nuts, pecan nuts, almonds, chocolate, carob, wheat germ, coconuts, oats, gelatin, edible seeds, peas, cereals, and garlic). Since many of the arginine rich foods are commonly part of a healthy eating pattern, it is probably desirable to supplement with lysine rather than avoiding nuts, seeds, and grains.[34]

Other alternative approaches to treating herpes include the above dietary modifications in conjunction with the following antiviral herbs: Echinacea, goldenseal, licorice, St. John's Wort. (See Chapter Six.)

Herpes Simplex: Lysine supplementation and a high lysine/low arginine diet. Glycyrrhizin (licorice) can be applied to the skin lesions, as well.[35]

Herpes Zoster: Diet and licorice as above, plus supplementation with vitamin B12.[36]

Cytomegalovirus (CMV): Garlic extract has been shown to inactivate CMV and many other viruses during active infections.[37]

All Herpes Viruses, Including Cytomegalovirus and Epstein Barr: The plant extract monolaurin is used with excellent results.[38]

Kaposi's Sarcoma (KS)

Kaposi's sarcoma involves a tumor on the walls of blood vessels or in the lymphatic system which results in multiple pink to purple lesions on the skin. KS may also occur internally in addition to, or independent of, lesions. The methods outlined above under the heading "General Immune Enhancement and Anti-HIV Methods" gives an indication of the alternative methods used in the treatment of Kaposi's sarcoma. Rather than targeting the lesions directly, treatment is usually focused on enhancing overall well-being.

According to Robert Cathcart III, M.D., of Los Altos, California, high dosage Vitamin C supplied intravenously can reverse KS in many instances.[39] By contrast, the current conventional approach is the use of alpha interferon, a treatment which is highly toxic and appears to damage CD4 cells.[40] Newer non-toxic drugs are claimed to be working their way through the patent and legal processes, however, and should soon be available.[41]

Liver Dysfunction

Liver dysfunction is common in immune-compromised individuals, many of whom may have had previous infections with hepatitis.

Alternative medical methods use herbs such as silymarin (milk thistle), glycyrrhizin, Minor Bupleurum Compound (see Chapter Six), and detailed nutritional counseling.[42]

Pneumocystis carinii pneumonia (PCP)

Originally the organism causing PCP was thought to be a protozoan, but it is now known to be a yeast-like agent. Other yeast-type infections which are commonly associated with AIDS include *toxoplasmosis*, *cryptococcosis*, *histoplasmosis*, and *candidiasis*.

Between 60 and 80 percent of all AIDS patients contract PCP. As protection against developing PCP, the antibiotic trimethoprim-sulfamethoxazole (Bactrim or Septra/TMP-SMX) is given. Previously, pentamidine was prescribed.[43]

This and other drug approaches have undoubtedly saved many lives, since PCP was at one time considered virtually untreatable, whereas many people have survived several bouts using current methods. Side effects from these drugs, however, include rashes, which can be very severe, and massive depletion of the B vitamin folic acid. As an adjunct to conventional treatment of PCP infection, alternative methods stress the use of general immune enhancement using nutrition and herbal approaches, with immune system modulators such as echinacea possibly being prescribed.[44]

Specific use of folic acid supplementation is also indicated during and after medical treatment (with a dosage range of between 800 and 1,200 mg daily), and use of quercetin (a bioflavonoid often associated with vitamin C) is suggested to reduce rashes resulting from histamine release. Nutritional supplementation with beta-carotene, vitamin C, and other immune system enhancing nutrients (see Chapter Five) would be included if alternative methods were being employed alongside of conventional approaches to this infection.

Skin Rashes

Supplemental zinc, essential fatty acid supplementation, and the use of retinoids (Vitamin A) in the form of beta-carotene (see notes above under "General Immune Enhancement and Anti-HIV Methods" in this chapter, as well as Chapter Five) are helpful in restoring skin health, which is often impaired due to malnutrition, toxicity, and the use of various medications.

When yeasts are responsible for the skin problem, an anticandidiasis protocol is also called for. In addition, individ-

ualized homeopathic remedies may be useful, while local
application of extracts of comfrey, echinacea, or calendula, in
the form of creams or gels, can soothe skin lesions and promote healing.[45]

Weight Loss

The dietary approach outlined in Chapter Five, with specific
emphasis on free form amino acid supplementation, will help
to serve as a foundation for other nutritional efforts to maintain weight.[46] Specific attention can also be given to the individual's digestive process through the use of digestive
enzymes and hydrochloric acid supplementation, as required.

If weight loss is related to circulation of the hormone
cachetin, which is released in response to a very low CD4 cell
count, it can often be helped by use of the amino acid N-
acetyl-l-Cysteine (NAC). (See Chapter Five.) Dronabinol, a
cannabis extract, has recently been licensed by the FDA for
treatment of weight loss associated with AIDS, as well.[47]

Conclusion

Many medical experts now believe that it is vital that we confront and more adequately deal with the host of co-factor diseases and influences (deficiency, toxicity, etc.) which are so
much a part of the majority of AIDS cases. By taking these
associated conditions more seriously, by not simply attempting to suppress or mask them, or treating them in a way that
add further burdens to the defense mechanisms of the body,
we can dramatically assist in the restoration of health.

This should not be taken to imply that conventional
approaches are never needed or appropriate, however.
Obviously this is not so, as we have seen with respect to PCP,
where conventional treatments are literally life-saving. Rather,
what should be realized is that many of the non-life threatening conditions which are an increasing part of the AIDS picture should be seriously tackled, as well. It is here that alternative health care has compiled an excellent track record, with
minimal side-effects, when dealing with many aspects of the
co-factor phenomenon. Whether we consider herbal medicine,
Traditional Chinese Medicine (including acupuncture), nutri-

tional therapy, hyperthermia, stress reduction, or oxygen-based therapies, a variety of possibilities exist (as we will see in the following chapters) which offer great promise for people with AIDS and HIV, especially when they are administered under expert guidance.

"Health is the proper relationship between the microcosm, which is man, and the macrocosm, which is the universe. Disease is a disruption of this relationship."

— Dr. Yeshe Donden,
physician to the Dalai Lama

8 Acupuncture and Traditional Chinese Medicine

Traditional Chinese Medicine (TCM) is a complete system of healing, utilizing herbs, acupuncture, food therapy, massage, and therapeutic exercise to achieve and maintain health. The philosophy of Traditional Chinese Medicine is very different from that of modern Western medicine. TCM is more preventative in nature than conventional medicine, and views the practice of waiting to treat a disease until after the symptoms are fully developed as being similar to "digging a well after the drought has begun." In addition, practitioners of TCM search for the underlying causes of imbalances and patterns of disharmony in the body and view each patient as unique. Whereas practitioners of conventional western medicine generally provide treatment for the specific illness in question, those who practice TCM address how the illness manifests in each particular patient and treat the patient as a whole, not just the disease.

Of the many alternatives to conventional medicine, TCM is one of the more frequently used methods of treatment by people with AIDS and HIV. "Although AIDS does not arise as a disease entity in TCM literature, it presents itself as a constellation of symptoms especially amenable to diagnosis and treatment by TCM," says Qingcai Zhang, M.D. (China), Lic. Ac., of New York City. People with AIDS and HIV can benefit from a number of TCM treatment strategies, according to Dr. Zhang. These include the use of antiviral herbs to combat HIV; herbal immune regulators to help restore the immune system; and specially designed herbal formulas to treat AIDS-related opportunistic infections, malignancies, and non-specific constitutional symptoms (such as night sweats, fatigue, and weight loss).

According to Mary Kay Ryan, N.C.C.A., Dipl. Ac., co-founder of AIDS Alternative Health Project and Northside HIV Treatment Center in Chicago, Chinese herbal medicine is most effective for individuals in the early and middle stages of

HIV infection. "Early stages are when there are moderate symptoms, or fatigue, but there has been no infection. I think of middle stage as people with one or more infections who may also be experiencing other early stage symptoms," explains Ryan, who has treated AIDS patients since 1986. "I find herbs to be especially helpful in dealing with the symptoms that are generic to AIDS, such as fatigue, night sweats, anxiety, and sleeplessness."

Acupuncture is also an effective treatment for AIDS and associated illnesses, due to its ability to reduce pain, increase immune response, and influence external and internal co-factors. Acupuncture treatment is based on the long-standing Chinese medical belief that health is determined by a balanced flow of the vital life energy present in all living organisms (referred to as *qi* or *chi*). Although it cannot be said that acupuncture cures AIDS, it remains a beneficial adjunctive therapy for reducing uncomfortable or dangerous symptoms, including night sweats, fatigue, and digestive disturbances, particularly when coupled with Chinese herbs or other alternative therapies.

In Chinese medical theory, *qi* is said to circulate in the body along twelve major energy pathways, called meridians or channels, each linked to specific internal organs and organ systems. According to William Michael Cargile, B.S., D.C., F.I.A.C.A., Chairman of Research for the American Association of Acupuncture and Oriental Medicine, there are over one thousand acupoints within the meridian system that can be stimulated to enhance the flow of *qi*. When special needles are inserted into these acupoints (just under the skin), they help correct and rebalance the flow of energy and consequently relieve pain and/or restore health.

Immune Enhancement

Traditional Chinese Medicine has a wealth of knowledge concerning the issue of immune suppression. Drawing upon this knowledge, Subhuti Dharmananda, Ph.D., Director of the Institute for Traditional Medicine in Portland, Oregon, proposes a multifactorial approach rooted in Traditional Chinese Medicine in treating people with HIV and AIDS. He stresses a protocol of Chinese herb combinations (usually consisting of eight to twelve herbs) and acupuncture, food therapy, massage, and exercise. Of particular value in treating patients with AIDS or with HIV is a combination herbal formulation called Composition-A (see Chapter Six), according to Dr. Dharmananda.

Acupuncture should also be seriously considered by those who are immune-compromised, as clinical studies confirm that multiple immune-related effects occur from skillful application of acupuncture needles. Chinese and Western research shows that a needle placed into a point below the knee (known as Stomach Point 36) will increase white blood cell counts by up to 70 percent three hours later. And after a day, the levels are still about 30 percent higher than before the acupuncture. When non-acupuncture points are needled, no rise in immune defense takes place, showing that the benefit observed is not a reaction to having needles placed merely anywhere on the body surface.[1]

"According to client observation at the Quan Yin Healing Arts Center in San Francisco, acupuncture appears to increase immune function, helps stabilize white and red blood counts, and, in some cases, T-cell counts," states Misha Cohen, O.M.D., L.Ac., the Center's clinical director.[2] Dr. Cohen uses acupuncture as an adjunct to her Traditional Chinese protocol, and adds that it can also stimulate relaxation and meditation, helping people begin the vital "inner" work that is increasingly being shown to be a necessary aspect of the healing process.

Dr. Cargile has worked with AIDS patients for many years, and reports that he has been able to increase T-cell counts with acupuncture treatments. "One of these patients had a T-cell count of 30 to 40," he recounts. "We eventually brought it up to 270, and although this is half the level a person is said to need, the patient has been doing great for the last six months." Dr. Cargile adds that the key to understanding acupuncture's influence on blood values and cell counts lies partly in its ability to minimize stress and strengthen the body's adaptive mechanisms. "I think that if we had more acupuncture and less AZT, we would see a qualitative improvement in patient health," he states.

Antiviral Effects of Chinese Herbs

Dr. Zhang has reported significant success in restoring immune function with the antiviral herb, Chinese bitter melon (*Momordica charantia*). Chinese bitter melon has been found effective in raising CD4 counts in many patients. One of Dr. Zhang's patients has used bitter melon in a retention enema treatment for four and a half years, and his CD4 count has increased from 480 to 1,120. This patient has been stable for two years, as a result. Another of Dr. Zhang's patients increased his CD4 level from 0 to 12 in six months. In addition, many people using the herb report enhanced energy after undertaking the treatment, as well as a reversal of weight loss.

Garlic is another herb widely prescribed in TCM for its immune-enhancing abilities. Garlic has strong antimicroorganism properties and is effective in treating the opportunistic infections that accompany AIDS, according to Dr. Zhang. It can inhibit or kill many types of viruses, bacteria, fungi, and protozoa that prey on the system.[3] Garlic's toxicity level is very low, and its purified active ingredient, allicin, can be used intravenously, as an aerosol spray, or retention enema. Dr. Joan Priestley, M.D., reported at the IX AIDS Conference in Berlin in 1993 of a patient brought out of a deep coma caused by Cryptococcal meningitis through the use of an intravenous solution of allicin as an antifungal agent.

Other Chinese herbs commonly used as antivirals by practitioners of TCM include:

- Isatis root (broad antibacterial and antiviral qualities)[4]
- Licorice (inhibitor of DNA and RNA viruses, a reverse transcriptase inhibitor, significant anti-HIV activity [in vitro])[5]
- Shiitake Mushroom Extract (used for dramatic anti-HIV effects)[6]
- St. John's Wort (specific retrovirus blocking actions)[7]

Relief of Associated Illnesses of AIDS

TCM and acupuncture also alleviate many of the symptoms related to HIV infection and AIDS. According to a published report, "Many patients report a reduction in fatigue, abnormal sweating, diarrhea, and acute skin reactions after only four to

Diagnosis in Traditional Chinese Medicine

Unlike Western medicine, which seeks to destroy a pathogen or a disease process in a specific part or parts of the body, Traditional Chinese Medicine (TCM) seeks to identify an illness by deducing the overall functioning of the body. The TCM practitioner arrives at a diagnosis by analyzing the observed pattern of the patient's symptoms. This symptom pattern is referred to as "patterns of disharmony." But patterns of disharmony should not be confused with disease; rather, they comprise a total picture of the patient's physiological, mental, and emotional states. Integrating the Western medical disease diagnosis with the TCM diagnosis of patterns of disharmony can produce a better treatment protocol and is a standard procedure in the health care system of modern China. The combined use of both systems has yielded better therapeutic results than those achieved by either system alone.[8]

A first-time patient, accustomed to Western medicine, may be surprised that TCM diagnosis does not require procedures such as blood tests, x-rays, or exploratory surgery. Instead, the practitioner performs the five following, non-invasive methods of investigation:

- Inspection of the complexion, general demeanor, body language, and tongue.
- Questioning the patient about symptoms, medical history, diet, lifestyle, history of the present complaint, and any previous or concurrent therapies received.
- Listening to the tone and strength of the voice.
- Smelling any body excretions, the breath, or body odor.
- Palpation (or feeling with the fingers) of the pulse at the radial arteries of both wrists (pulse diagnosis), the abdomen, and the meridians and/or acupuncture points.

Through pulse diagnosis, a skilled practitioner can examine the strength or weakness of the *qi* and "blood" (which in TCM includes lymph and other bodily fluids), and assess how these affect each of the organs, tissues, and layers of the body. The practitioner will also look at the impact of a wide range of personal and environmental factors. Mood influences, activity, sex, food, drugs, weather, and seasons of the year can each affect health and the healing process.

six acupuncture treatments. Many describe an improved sense of well-being; some report weight gain and are able to return to longer hours of work."[9]

Sir Jay Holder, M.D., D.C., Ph.D., founder and Medical Director of the Exodus Treatment Center in Miami, Florida, has also achieved significant results using acupuncture. He describes the case of a man with AIDS, suffering from Kaposi's sarcoma, and given just twenty-two months to live. Within three weeks of treatment with acupuncture and Chinese herbs, his T-cell count returned to normal and his lesions disappeared.

Numerous studies attest to acupuncture's effectiveness in improving immune function and relieving the associated symptoms of AIDS:

- Acupuncture was found to reduce levels of secondary opportunistic infections and to have a general beneficial influence upon two hundred patients in New York with AIDS or ARC.[10]
- At Lincoln Memorial Hospital in New York City, twenty out of twenty-seven people with AIDS who received acupuncture treatments reported a reduction of fatigue and an improvement in night sweats and diarrhea after one to three weeks. Many also gained substantial amounts of weight. Michael Smith, M.D., who oversaw the patients, reports that in some cases T-cell ratios rose dramatically over a two to three month period with acupuncture alone.[11]
- Fifteen patients who received acupuncture treatments regularly at Somerville Centre near Boston all reported improvement in general symptoms and six reported reduced side effects of medical treatment for Kaposi's sarcoma.[12]

These and other studies, along with the continuing results achieved by physicians such as those mentioned above, suggest the need for more research into the value that TCM, acupuncture, and Chinese herbal medicine offer those afflicted with AIDS and its associated disease symptoms.

Where to Find Help

Alternative Medicine Yellow Pages. **The Burton Goldberg Group. Puyallup, WA: Future Medicine Publishing, Inc., 1994.**
Lists over 16,000 practitioners of alternative medicine in the United States and Canada. Practitioners are listed by therapy, city, and state. See sections on "Acupuncture," "Herbal Medicine," "Qigong," and "Traditional Chinese Medicine."

**American Association of Acupuncture
and Oriental Medicine
4101 Lake Boone Trail, Suite 201
Raleigh, North Carolina 27607
(919) 787-5181**
The AAAOM is a national professional trade organization of acupuncturists who meet acceptable standards of minimum competency and can provide you with the names and locations of local members. Referrals by written request only. A fee of five dollars is charged.

**Institute for Traditional Medicine and
Preventive Health Care
2017 S.E. Hawthorne
Portland, Oregon 97214
(503) 233-4907**
The Institute's goals are to determine the nature and practices of traditional medicine and to make this information and the associated practices available to the public, mainly by training practitioners and providing traditional health care services to clients. Publishes technical books and produces video programs and other educational opportunities that train health professionals in the proper utilization of Chinese herbal medicine, which was determined to be the most accessible traditional health care method that could be integrated with our modern medical system.

**Quan Yin Healing Arts Center
1748 Market Street
San Francisco, California 94102
(415) 861-4964**
Offers a program for people with AIDS or who are HIV positive. Services include acupuncture, herbal medicine, yoga, and massage

*therapy. Also provides lecture series and discussion groups to
provide support and nutritional information. Available on a sliding
scale fee basis.*

 # Recommended Reading

AIDS and Its Treatment by Traditional Chinese Medicine.
Translated by Di, Fu; and Flaws, Bob. Boulder, CO: Blue
Poppy Press, 1991.

*A clincial manual on the treatment of AIDS by Traditional Chinese
Medicine. Designed for the professional TCM practitioner, this book
covers the diagnosis and treatment of the HIV latent phase, ARC,
and nineteen opportunistic infections and conditions associated with
AIDS. These include emaciation, fatigue, fever, diarrhea, night
sweats, lymphadenopathy, thrush, Kaposi's sarcoma, and dementia.
Treatment plans include both Chinese herbal formulas and acupuncture protocols. There are also sections on Chinese dietary
therapy and lifestyle modifications.*

Acupuncture: Is It for You? Worsley, J. R. New York:
Harper & Row, 1973.

*An in-depth question and answer session with the founder of the
College of Traditional Chinese Acupuncture (UK) and the
Traditional Acupuncture Institute.*

Alternative Medicine: The Definitive Guide. The Burton
Goldberg Group. Puyallup, WA: Future Medicine Publishing,
Inc., 1993.

*The most comprehensive reference on alternative medicine ever
compiled. Provides in-depth, easily understandable coverage of 43
alternative therapies and over 200 health conditions, with advice
from nearly 400 alternative physicians worldwide. See Chapters on
"Acupuncture," "Traditional Chinese Medicine," and "Qigong."*

Between Heaven and Earth: A Guide to Chinese Medicine.
Beinfield, Harriet, L.Ac.; and Korngold, Efrem, L.Ac.,
O.M.D. New York: Ballantine Books, 1991.

*Combines Eastern tradition with Western sensibilities. The authors
address three vital areas of Traditional Chinese Medicine—theory,
therapy, and types—to present a comprehensive, yet
understandable, guide to this ancient system.*

Chinese Herbal Therapies for Immune Disorders.
Dharmananda, Subhuti, Ph.D. Portland, OR: Institute for
Traditional Medicine, 1993.

*Written in 1988 and extensively revised and updated in 1993, this
book presents a technical description of the selection of herbs and
herb formulas for the treatment of various disorders that involve
immune dysfunctions, and provides some information about active
constituents and their pharmacology. The book has four sections: a
description of basic therapeutic approaches, an examination of the
main groups of active constituents, a quick review of several disease
categories with sample herbs and formulas, and an appendix of
detailed articles on specific immune problems.*

Nine Ounces: A Nine Part Program for Prevention
of AIDS in HIV Positive Persons. Flaws, Bob. Boulder,
Colorado: Blue Poppy Press, 1989.

*Describes a nine-part program designed to boost the immune system
using the age-old wisdom of Traditional Chinese Medicine.
Discusses HIV infection and AIDS from the Chinese point of view
and then, based on these theories, discusses Chinese dietary
therapy, exercise, deep relaxation, abdominal self-massage,
acupuncture, Chinese herbal medicine, sexual pacing, visualization,
and the cultivation of a healthy attitude. Using these mostly self-
applied therapies, individuals can help bring yin and yang, qi and
blood, and the functioning of their viscera and bowels into balance,
thus preventing the arising of disease. This book treats HIV infection
as a controllable, chronic condition which does not have to be fatal.*

Plain Talk About Acupuncture. Mitchell, Ellinor R. New
York: Whalehall, Inc., 1987.

*A book for prospective acupuncture patients who would like to learn
what acupuncture can do for their health.*

Tao of Nutrition. Ni, Maoshing, D.O.M., Ph.D., L.Ac.; and
McNease, Cathy. Santa Monica, CA: Seven Star
Communications, 1993.

*Based on traditional Chinese principles of using food for healing,
this book explains the energies and therapeutic properties of foods
and details how to create a diet that is most appropriate for health
and well-being. Includes sample meal plans, recipes, and dietary
recommendations for over-forty health conditions.*

Treating AIDS with Chinese Medicine. Ryan, Mary Kay; and
Shattuck, Arthur D. Berkeley: Pacific View Press, 1993.

*This comprehensive handbook offers a theoretical framework for
understanding the HIV phenomenon, and presents herbal and*

*acupuncture treatment strategies found in clinical practice to be
most effective. Organized for ease of use, it cross-references
information about symptoms, infections syndromes, and treatment
drugs associated with AIDS to Traditional Chinese Medicine's
diagnostic approach. There is detailed information on herbs,
formulas, and herbal patents developed for HIV. It also addresses
the special problems of women, persons with hemophilia, and IV
drug users. For practitioners of Chinese and alternative medicine,
for persons exploring alternative therapy for HIV, and for medical
doctors.*

***The Web That Has No Weaver: Understanding Chinese
Medicine.*** Kaptchuk, Ted. New York: Congdon and Weed,
1992.

*An excellent introduction to Acupuncture and Traditional Chinese
Medicine for the layperson familiar with Western medicine. It
contains detailed case histories comparing Acupuncture and
Traditional Chinese Medicine with conventional Western medicine.*

9 Naturopathic Medicine

Naturopathic medicine offers a multifactorial approach to treating AIDS. By prescribing a combination of therapies to meet each individual patient's medical needs, naturopathy offers a precise, non-invasive method of treatment for the person with AIDS that allows for greater patient involvement in his or her own care.

The most commonly utilized naturopathic therapies in the treatment of AIDS include nutrition, herbal medicine, homeopathy, Chinese medicine, hydrotherapy, physiotherapy, manipulation, and counseling, according to Steven Bailey, N.D., Assistant Professor of Pharmacognosy and Nutrition at National College of Naturopathic Medicine in Portland, Oregon. "Every patient presents different needs," Dr. Bailey notes. "Although I do have a basic AIDS protocol, I individually assess the lifestyle, diet, mental outlook, and spiritual status of all patients. I do more teaching and counseling than prescribing, although there are many natural products with well-documented benefits to the immune system."

In his private practice, Dr. Bailey has treated over one hundred HIV positive and fifty symptomatic AIDS patients over the past eleven years.[1] He reports a high percentage of success in treating HIV positive patients who have not progressed to a symptomatic level or who are only mildly symptomatic. However, he has not achieved good success with many late stage AIDS patients who have already used AZT, ddI, or ddC, have a history of opportunistic infections, have experienced severe weight loss, or who have been taking multiple medications. Such patients' immune systems are usually already severely impaired and, as a result, "They come [to me] with so little energy," Dr. Bailey says, "that they are often able to be only minimally involved in their treatment."

Dr. Bailey's Basic AIDS Protocol

Dr. Bailey's basic daily protocol for HIV positive and AIDS patients is as follows:

- Start the day with the "power blend" smoothie (see recipe later in this chapter).
- One quart of fresh vegetable juice daily with equal parts carrot, celery, and beet with two cloves of garlic
- Vitamin C: HIV positive (2-6 grams), ARC (6-10 grams), AIDS (15 grams)
- Glandular support: spleen, thymus, and liver glandulars
- Multi-species intestinal flora (*Lactobacillus acidophilus*, etc.)
- Yeast control products as needed
- Herbs: Deglycerated licorice root

Alternate the following formulas. Take herbs plain, with juice, or with water (cold or warm, not boiling):

Formula 1: Combine beforehand a 50/50 mixture of echinacea and ligusticum. $^1/_2$ teaspoon 3 times a day.

Formula 2: Mix the following: 1 oz. lomatium, $^1/_2$ oz. hypericum, $^1/_2$ oz. berberis. $^1/_2$ tsp. 3 times a day.

In addition to his basic protocol, Dr. Bailey develops individualized programs for his patients drawing from the following therapies:

Counseling

Dr. Bailey feels that the most important first step in returning to health is removing the helpless, victim consciousness and maintaining a positive attitude. "Self empowerment and personal responsibility are paramount to health and survival," he says. " Education is essential to self-empowerment. It is important to forgive yourself, remove guilt, learn to love and nurture yourself, and to detach yourself from the failure of other AIDS patients."

Dr. Bailey educates patients on the dangers of recreational and excessive prescription drug use and helps establish safe-sex practices and an exercise program. He also emphasizes the importance of leisure and fun in a patient's daily routine and helps establish goals and a sense of purpose in one's life.

Nutrition
Nutritional support for AIDS patients in Dr. Bailey's protocol involves diet, vitamins, minerals, enzymes, herbs, fresh juices, and glandulars. He recommends minimizing meat, and moderation in sugars, processed foods, and fats, as well as an abundance of crunchy vegetables, fruits, cereals, grains, and legumes.

Herbal Medicine
Many herbs are widely accepted for boosting the immune system, combatting infections, aiding digestion and sleep, as well as managing pain. (See Chapter Six, "Herbal Medicine," and Chapter Seven, "Nutritional and Herbal Treatments for Illnesses Associated with AIDS," for more information.)

Chinese Medicine
Traditional Chinese Medicine (TCM) is increasingly being shown to be of value in dealing with AIDS and HIV infection. Acupuncture, a subset of TCM, is effective for detoxification; support and normalization of spleen, liver, and thymus function; and for support of the emotional aspects surrounding disease. In addition, the production of endorphins which results from acupuncture treatment has a strong positive effect on mood and immune function. Many Chinese herbs are also included in Dr. Bailey's basic herbal protocol. (See Chapter Eight, "Acupuncture and Traditional Chinese Medicine.")

Homeopathy
While homeopathic prescribing involves individual assessment, Dr. Bailey has found the following remedies to be invaluable in the care of AIDS:

- *Medorrhinum:* Sleep problems, attention deficit
- *Natrum mur:* Grief, closed emotions
- *Tabacum:* Nausea, loss of appetite, vomiting
- *Cinchona:* Night sweats
- *Tuberculinum:* Pneumonia, lower respiratory infections
- *Pulsatilla:* Grief, mood swings, craving personal support

Secondary remedies for other symptoms include: Skin rashes *(Sulphur, Cantharis, Rhus. Tox., Urtica, Psorinum)*;

Depression *(Aurum, Nat. mur.)*; Trauma, bruising (Arnica); Bleeding *(Phos., Ferrum phos., Belladona)*; Drug reactions *(Petrolium)*; Reactions to Immunizations *(Ledum, Pulsatilla)*.

Physiotherapy, Hydrotherapy, Manipulation

Spinal manipulation and massage are of great benefit for immune function, digestive function, stress management, and a broad range of musculo-skeletal and physiologic functions, notes Dr. Bailey. The use of heat and hydrotherapy to improve immune function also plays a significant role in his treatment approach. (See Chapter Twelve, "Hyperthermia.")

Dr. Bailey's Power Blend

Dr. Bailey's Power Blend

Steven Bailey, N.D., recommends that his AIDS patients start the day with a basic smoothie that is prepared as follows:

In Blender, add:

- Medium whole fruit, i.e., apple or banana
- 1/2 cup fruit juice (use 100 percent juice)
- 1-2 tablespoon yogurt (if dairy sensitive, use acidophilus product)

For qualities of intestinal balance, consider:

- 1/2 cup raw goats milk (contains secretory A, lactoferon, and IgG's)

To this, add:

- 1 tablespoon cold-pressed flax oil (source of quality essential fatty acids)
- 1 heaping teaspoon of lecithin granules
- 2-4 capsules of Nutrizyme™ * (or equivalent powdered vegetable enzyme products with full-spectrum vitamins and minerals) *Product of Tyler Encapsulations, (800) 869-9705.
- 7 drops liquid beta-carotene (70,000 IUs) *(Available through many professional clinics, or contact Naturopathic Formulations, (800) 547-4891.)*
- 1 tablespoon protein powder *(Dr. Bailey uses Naturade® soy free vegetable protein. Egg albumin provides another quality form of protein.)*

Patient Case Histories

Jim was diagnosed as being HIV positive in 1985 and began working with Dr. Bailey at that time. The initial treatment approach was conservative, involving vitamins, minerals, herbs, and a decrease in the stress of normal life (he moved to the Oregon coast and decreased his work schedule).

As he was experiencing no symptoms of illness or opportunistic infections, he maintained this conservative approach until 1991, at which time his T-cells were significantly reduced and his Helper/Suppressor ratio was .28 (greater than .9 is normal). At that point, he accelerated his treatment program to Dr. Bailey's full protocol. By January 1993, his T-cell counts returned to a high normal level with a complete reversal of the Helper/Suppressor ratio, now at 1.39. He continues to be symptom-free today, and his T-cell counts remain in the normal range.

Ray and Bernie comprise a case of two partners who came in together for an initial consultation in 1988, after having been tested HIV positive earlier in the year. Both were asymptomatic at the time but had not done any T-cell counts or other diagnostic tests. Ray was a lean 130 pounds, while Bernie was a very muscular 150. Bernie began a very conventional treatment program with another physician, while Ray chose to pursue a natural approach.

Ray's T-cell counts were in the 400s, although he had experienced no AIDS-related conditions. He followed a program that consisted of nutrition, herbal and homeopathic medicine, glandular products (oral thymus, spleen, and liver), physiotherapy, and counseling. Throughout the next three years, his T-cell counts remained stable, his energy improved, and he experienced fewer of the common infections that he saw in friends surrounding him.

"In August of 1990, Ray asked if I would be willing to work with Bernie, who had had numerous opportunistic infections," Dr. Bailey recounts. "When Bernie arrived, he was carting an oxygen tank with tubes to his nose. He reported no ability to hold foods, estimating that he could keep only 5 percent of his food down. He was on over a dozen medications and had lost nearly forty pounds.

"Over the next few months, Bernie integrated natural approaches and soon was off the oxygen, holding down over 90 percent of his food, and removing some of the medicines. In November, however, he began to discontinue all supplementation. His health worsened and his medical doctor discontinued all care, as he had lost a good percentage of liver and kidney function. Ray, in the meantime, brought Bernie home and was a twenty to twenty-two hour a day nurse during Bernie's last four months. As he could no longer tolerate most of the prescription pain medicines and drugs, he was treated primarily with herbs, homeopathic medicine, and nutrition."

During this period, until Bernie's death in February of 1991, Ray had been experiencing the death of a friend or an acquaintance in his support group and his community every two weeks. Shortly after Bernie's death, Ray himself began to experience more illness. His T-cell count began to drop and he began to get more frequent infections. Ray was experiencing tremendous grief over the loss of his mate, in addition to having already lost everyone in his primary support group and then having lost half of his friends in his second group.

"He began to have a more defeatist attitude about his own health care and began to lose significant amounts of weight the following year," says Dr. Bailey. "It was very difficult to keep Ray's attitude focused towards believing that he could be healthy, and he had tremendous fear of losing weight, as that was a sign which most of his friends who had died had also experienced. He was equally fearful of CMV (cytomegalovirus) retinitis.

"We began to accelerate the program with Ray, and treated some of the opportunistic infections, particularly in the digestive tract, so it could absorb foods more efficiently. He was given oral medications, but at this point, he was also receiving vitamin injections and some intravenous nutrition. As he reached a low of 96 pounds, he also had recently experienced CMV and had come to grips with the fact that he had gotten the two worst conditions that he had feared most.

"As we had been working for years since his exhausting nursing and stress, we were able to maintain a strong program and, by integrating a few additional products, his weight began to return," continues Dr. Bailey. "Over the past eight months, Ray has now returned to 125 pounds, which is within five pounds of his original weight. He has discontinued going to most of the support groups. He feels that they have been reinforcement for the fallibility of the medical system for most people and realizes that he needs to focus and accentuate a more positive outlook. He has been disabled for three years, but is now finally returning to being able to do more work in his field [at the same time that he] continues to be stable with regards to his retinitis."

Karl, another HIV positive patient, was diagnosed as having pneumonitis. When he came to see Dr. Bailey, he was on many medications, including 65 mg/day of Prednisone, a steroidal medication known to depress immune function. "The patient had felt a great degree of guilt about the circumstances surrounding his infection," says Dr. Bailey, "and was looking for reassurance and an opportunity to do something to allow him to breathe more easily so that he could get off of his medicines.

"We began natural therapeutics, including a number of juice fasts, and concentrated on his respiratory condition and on removing the steroid medications so that his immune system could get back to normal. He had also been having chronic problems with his teeth and ended up having a number of them extracted, which seemed to greatly benefit his health. Within one year's time, his generalized lymphatopathy had gone into almost total remission; he had gotten off all his steroids, and, in fact, had tested HIV negative on two occasions."

He returned to work full time and then took on a second job. The insurance policy with his new job did not cover Dr. Bailey's care and Karl discontinued visiting him and following the protocol. "One year later I received a phone call from him asking if I could do a home visit," Dr. Bailey relates. "I returned to his home only to find him on oxygen, and back on 65 mg/day of Prednisone. He had been rediagnosed as having AIDS after being told by his medical doctors (after testing HIV negative) that he must have had an initial misdiagnosis. He was receiving free food through disability that consisted entirely of processed foods, high sugar, high additives, and he had gotten off his program of nutrition and juices."

Dr. Bailey attempted to re-integrate nutritional therapeutics, including as much liquid and non-tablet forms as possible. However, Karl's condition was too far progressed, and he passed away in three months.

Karl's tale is important for what it illustrates. As soon as he was able to work, Karl choose not only to return to his normal job, but to take on an additional twenty to thirty hours of work per week in order to create his own business. Dr. Bailey has observed this pattern in a few of his patients whose conditions deteriorated. He finds that people sometimes get frantic to complete their life, instead of being patient to do the things that are necessary to reduce the stress, to optimize health, and to progress with their condition before they re-integrate a full workload back into their lives. He has found it very useful to help patients realize that they do not have to do everything all at once. "If they can get stronger," says Dr. Bailey, "they will experience less dependency and less need for other people to help them than if they bull-headedly use their remaining energy to work for a couple of months and drive themselves into severe illness."

Healing AIDS Research Project (HARP)

Bastyr University in Seattle, Washington conducted a one-year study, the Healing AIDS Research Project (HARP), on the effectiveness of a naturopathic approach to HIV Disease. In successfully treating sixteen male patients diagnosed with ARC (AIDS-related complex), the actual treatments consisted of a combination naturopathic protocol: constitutionally prescribed homeopathic medicines for five patients and the use of herbal medicines and glandulars for eleven patients, the use of therapeutic nutrition for each patient, periodic application of hyperthermic hydrotherapy, and regular access to psychological counseling. Individual symptoms or patient side effects were treated with the appropriate non-drug treatment, often herbal remedies.

Dietary Guidelines

Malnutrition is a significant factor contributing to the progression of AIDS. The HARP study issued general ten-point nutritional guidelines to participants.[2] Although the guidelines were specifically tailored for participants of this study, it is an excellent program to improve and maintain health in general.

A slightly modified version of the HARP guidelines is as follows:

- Eat whole foods (foods in their original, unprocessed form) which are more nutritionally dense and contain fewer additives.
- Emphasize organic and fresh vegetables, fruits, and proteins (fish/meat) wherever available.
- Reduce or eliminate simple sugars and replace them with complex carbohydrates (vegetables, whole grains, legumes) which are rich in essential nutrients such as zinc.
- Reduce polyunsaturated and saturated fats and oils.
- Use monounsaturated fats and oils such as olive oil, with special emphasis on omega-3 oils (fish and certain plant oils).
- Eat many small meals throughout the day to optimize the absorption of nutrients from food.
- Try to keep a balance of food intake which ensures 65 percent is complex carbohydrates (vegetables, fruits, legumes, grains), 15 percent protein (fish, yogurt, eggs, meat), and 20 percent fat.
- Make sure fruits and vegetables are thoroughly clean and free of parasites and bacteria by steaming lightly, at least, before eating.
- Eat a wide variety of foods to help reduce the chances of developing sensitivities to foods and to increase nutrient absorption.
- Eliminate chocolate, caffeine, and alcohol.[3]

Natural Products: Herbs, Nutritional Supplements, and Glandulars

Each participant in the HARP study was prescribed a basic supplement program which included vitamin C (ascorbic acid powder or tablets) to bowel tolerance, beta-carotene, egg lethicin, and a multiple vitamin and mineral supplement.

Eleven of the sixteen participants were assigned to the "botanical/natural product group" and received the herbs lomatium, St. John's Wort (*Hypericum perforatum*), licorice (*Glycyrrhiza glabra*), and the combination herbal product "Astra Isatis," an American-made Chinese herbal combination in tablet form. It contains the following herbs: Astragalus, conodopsis, glycyrrhiza, atractylodes, dioscorea, broussonetia, isatis, laminaria, bupleurum, lycium, and cynamorium. This group also received monolaurin and calf thymus extract.

The remaining five participants received homeopathic prescriptions instead of the herbs and glandulars. Symptomatic improvement in the homeopathic group was similar to those who received the herbal medicines and glandulars.

Hyperthermia

Hyperthermia is commonly used in the treatment of HIV and other chronic and acute viral infections at the National Health Clinic at Bastyr University. Hyperthermia treatment was also included as part of the treatment protocol developed for the HARP study because of its immune stimulating, detoxifying, and disinfecting properties.

HARP participants were given a series of hyperthermia baths (104 degrees Fahrenheit) for thirty to forty minutes. The baths were designed to raise the body temperature to between 102 and 104 degrees Fahrenheit, at which point bacteria and viruses begin to die. The results from this type of rise in body temperature are similar to the effects which occur when the body generates a fever. The baths were administered twice weekly for three week periods extended over the course of a year.

According to Leanna Standish, Ph.D. N.D. (who oversaw the HARP study), when participants in the study were asked what aspect of the treatment had the greatest impact, the overwhelming response was hyperthermia. There was a reported decrease in night sweats and in the frequency of secondary infections, as well, and many of the participants claimed to have a greater sense of well-being after receiving hyperthermia treatments.

Psychological Counseling

There was also a major emphasis on psychological counseling in the HARP study. "Patients were requested to begin some form of individual or group psychotherapeutic process. A HARP support group met weekly and focused on open discussion of emotional, physical, and spiritual issues, as well as meditation and positive affirmation strategies modeled after the work of Louise Hay.

Results of the HARP Study

Within the twelve-month period of the HARP trial, significant results were reported.[4] Most patients expressed a general improvement in their sense of overall well-being, and found a reduction in the degree of fatigue and diminished night sweats. The most impressive outcome, however, was the fact that after the one year trial, none of the sixteen had moved from an ARC diagnosis to AIDS, and none had died. On the other hand, in standard AZT studies involving similar patient groups, the progression (decline) rate was between 3 and 7 percent.

The HARP researchers concluded that: "The fact that mortality and morbidity rates were so low suggests the possibility that progression to more serious immune dysfunction and AIDS-defining illness was slowed and perhaps even halted." These results will be closely monitored as a ten-year follow-up is currently underway to monitor the long-term outcome.

Where to Find Help

***Alternative Medicine Yellow Pages*. The Burton Goldberg Group. Puyallup, WA: Future Medicine Publishing, Inc., 1994.**
Lists over 16,000 practitioners of alternative medicine in the United States and Canada. Practitioners are listed by therapy, city, and state. See sections on "Naturopathic Medicine," "Herbal Medicine," "Homeopathy," "Hydrotherapy," "Hyperthermia," "Acupuncture," and "Detoxification Therapy."

American Association of Naturopathic Physicians
2366 Eastlake Avenue, Suite 322
Seattle, Washington 98102
(206) 323-7610
Provides a directory of naturopathic physicians and offers referrals to a nationwide network of accredited or licensed practitioners. Publishes a quarterly newsletter for both professionals and the general public. Also offers a series of brochures and pamphlets on a variety of subjects.

Bastyr University
Natural Health Clinic
1307 North 45th Street, Suite 200
Seattle, Washington 98103
(206) 632-0354
Bastyr University is an accredited educational institution that offers degree programs in the natural health sciences. These include programs in naturopathic medicine, homeopathy, midwifery, acupuncture, nutrition, Chinese herbal medicine, marriage and family counseling, and applied behavioral sciences. Bastyr also offers a limited number of Distance Learning courses in these areas for students unable to attend classes at its Seattle, Washington facility. The physical medicine department of the Natural Health Clinic of Bastyr University uses hyperthermia treatment for detox and in conditions ranging from upper respiratory infection to chronic fatigue syndrome and HIV infection.

The Institute for Naturopathic Medicine
66 1/2 North State Street
Concord, NH 03301-4330
(603) 225-8844
A non-profit, charitable organization dedicated to increasing public awareness of the options and solutions provided by natural medicine in solving the underlying causes of our health care crisis. The Institute's mission is to change the emphasis of the health care system from strictly disease management to health promotion and disease prevention. It serves the needs of consumers, the media, policy makers, medical educators, and others for accurate and reliable information about health care alternatives. In addition, the Institute promotes research into the clinical outcomes and cost effectiveness of natural therapeutics.

National College of Naturopathic Medicine
11231 SE Market Street
Portland, Oregon 97216
(503) 255-4860
Offers postgraduate training in naturopathic medicine and supports teaching clinics. The teaching clinic uses hyperthermia for a wide variety of conditions.

Northwest Naturopathic Clinic
2606 Vaughn Street
Portland, Oregon 97210
(503) 224-7366
Dr. Steven Bailey offers private care for HIV, ARC, AIDS, and other immune disorders. His clinic also specializes in fasting programs. Dr. Bailey will provide initial consultation over the phone at no charge, and has materials on HIV, AIDS, and immune disorders that he will send to interested parties.

 # Recommended Reading

Alternative Medicine: The Definitive Guide. The Burton Goldberg Group. Puyallup, WA: Future Medicine Publishing, Inc., 1993.
The most comprehensive reference on alternative medicine ever compiled. Provides in-depth, easily understandable coverage of 43 alternative therapies and over 200 health conditions, with advice from nearly 400 alternative physicians worldwide. See chapters on "Naturopathic Medicine," "Hydrotherapy," and "Hyperthermia."

Divided Legacy, A History of the Schism in Medical Thought, Vol. 3. Coulter, Harris L. Washington, D.C.: Wehawken Book Company, 1973.
Coulter thoroughly explains the history of natural medicine and the battle between its supporters and the American Medical Association and pharmaceutical companies.

Encyclopedia of Natural Medicine. Murray, Michael, N.D.; and Pizzorno, Joseph, N.D. Rocklin, CA: Prima Publishing, 1991.
A definitive guide for the layperson on naturopathic medicine.

Lectures in Naturopathic Hydrotherapy. Boyle, Wade, N.D.; and Saine, Andre, N.D. East Palestine, OH: Buckeye Naturopathic Press, 1988.
A useful book on general hydrotherapy topics.

Textbook of Natural Medicine, Vols. 1-2. Murray, Michael, N.D.; and Pizzorno, Joseph, N.D. Seattle: John Bastyr College Publications, 1989.
A comprehensive two-volume textbook for the health professional interested in natural medicine. Chapters on the therapeutic modalities used in naturopathic medicine, and descriptions and treatments of certain diseases.

10 Mind/Body Medicine

Mind/body medicine recognizes the profound interconnection of mind and body, the body's innate healing capabilities, and the role of self-responsibility in the healing process, utilizing a wide range of therapies, such as meditation, biofeedback, guided imagery, hypnotherapy, and yoga.

Mind/body medicine is a crucial part of the treatment process when dealing with HIV/AIDS, as it is essential to address the mental and emotional state of the patient for full healing to occur. Anyone with AIDS needs emotional support, as well as stress-coping strategies, counseling, relaxation, and, above all, hope. Because the media insistently portrays the HIV positive person as doomed, and AIDS as invariably fatal, these assumptions can predestine an individual to the type of negative thinking that makes the person feel victimized.

The anxiety that these notions create can lead to a kind of self-fulfilling prophesy: If a person is told often enough that he or she will get sick, eventually, he or she will. But if an individual is told that he or she may survive, that there are steps which can be taken to improve health, the very possibility that such a suggestion conveys can provide the inspiration and strength to recover. This has been observed time and time again. Thus, it is not surprising that several studies have shown what a profound impact the emotional state can have on the immune system.[1]

Long-term AIDS survivor, Michael Callen, traveled the country interviewing other long-term survivors of AIDS for his book, *Surviving AIDS*. He found that although their treatment strategies differed, the one thing they all shared was the belief that AIDS was survivable.[2] Callen's findings are supported by the work of George Solomon, M.D., of the University of San Francisco School of Medicine. Dr. Solomon's interviews with long-term survivors of AIDS indicate that "survivors accepted the reality of their diagnosis, but refused to see the condition as a death sentence. . . . They thought of their physicians as collaborators and tended to take responsibility for their health. They were inclined to think they could influence their health outcome."[3]

Psychoneuroimmunology

In the 1970s, great advances in the study of the immune system helped to clarify the relationship between body and mind, which gave rise to the rapidly expanding field of psychoneuroimmunology (PNI). Researchers found that naturally-occurring substances, known as peptides or neuropeptides (messenger molecules made up of amino acids) could cause alterations of mood, pain, and pleasure.[4] Among the first of these substances identified were endorphins, which is shorthand for endogenous morphines, meaning "the brain's own morphine." When endorphins are released they produce pleasurable responses, similar to those associated with opiates.

"We have come to theorize that these neuropeptides and their receptors are the biochemical correlates of emotions," says Candace Pert, Ph.D., visiting Professor at the Center for Molecular and Behavioral Neuroscience, Rutgers University, and former Chief of the Section on Brain Biochemistry of the Clinical Neuroscience Branch at the National Institute of Mental Health. "It took us fifteen years of research before we dared make that connection," adds Dr. Pert, "but we know that these neuropeptides are released during different emotional states.

"But the astounding revelation is that these endorphins and other chemicals like them are found not just in the brain, but in the immune system, the endocrine system, and throughout the body. When people discovered that there were endorphins in the brain that caused euphoria and pain relief, everyone could handle that. However, when they discovered they were in the immune system, as well, it just didn't fit, so these findings were denied for years. The original scientists had to repeat their studies many, many times to be believed."

Emotions, previously thought to be purely psychological, could now be linked to specific chemical processes taking place throughout the body, not just in the brain. Likewise, these peptides were seen to affect the functioning of all the systems of the body, including the immune system. "Viruses use the same receptors [as a neuropeptide] to enter into a cell," explains Dr. Pert, "and depending on how much of the natural peptide for that receptor is around, the virus will have an easier or harder time getting into the cell. So our emotional state will affect whether we'll get sick from the same loading dose of a virus. You know the data about how people have more heart attacks on Monday mornings, and how death peaks in Christians the day after Christmas and in Chinese people the day after the Chinese New Year. I never get a cold when I'm going skiing.

"The AIDS virus uses a receptor that is normally used by a neuropeptide," continues Dr. Pert. "So whether an AIDS virus will be able to enter a cell or not depends on how much of this natural peptide is around, which, according to this theory, would be a function of what state of emotional expression the organism is in. Emotional fluctuations and emotional status directly influence the probability that the organism will get sick or be well."

AIDS and the Mind/Body Connection

In cases of AIDS and HIV infection, the vital relationship between a person's emotional state and their immune system has a profound impact on whether the individual maintains or recovers health, or whether he or she slips further down into the disease state.[5]

A tremendous negative mental and emotional burden is placed on patients diagnosed as HIV positive or with AIDS, often because of the fears and prejudices which accompany these diagnoses. Emotions such as guilt, hopelessness, suppressed anger, and fear—common among many persons with AIDS—further burden the immune system.

At the University of California at San Francisco, School of Medicine, Biopsychology AIDS Project, specific findings have emerged about people who are HIV positive:

- Most people exhibited a common tendency towards denial or unexpressed emotions (such as feelings of anger).
- Most people had a number of extremely stressful events in the previous year.

- Many felt guilt over past sexual experiences.
- Many gay individuals had not acknowledged their homo-
  sexuality to family, workmates, friends; and of those that
  had, many had not resolved the issues of "coming out."

Emotional stress can be translated into very precise scientifically measurable effects. One study recorded in *The Lancet*
showed that when stressed by exams, some students show
specific decline in immune system defenses (mitogen and
NKCA decline) which invites infection. These negative
immune system changes imply that it is the individual's
response to stress that determines the effect on immunity,
rather than the stress itself.[6] Yet, most negative emotions can
be resolved with some effort and attention. Any stress-coping
strategy which reduces these negative influences on the nervous system—be this relaxation, meditation, visualization, or
some form of psychotherapeutic counseling, treatment, or
group work—will help immune function.

Gerald Epstein, M.D., of New York City, reports that the
imagery processes he has done with patients with HIV have
been quite useful, reducing anxiety and leading to an increase
in their white blood cell count. "I think imagery and visualization have a very prominent place to play in the AIDS healing
process," notes Dr. Epstein. "It is the most promising healing
tool that's known to humankind. However, you need to practice it faithfully and in a consistent manner over a period of
time to see the effects."

Garry F. Gordon, M.D., past President of the American
College of Advancement in Medicine, concurs. "Studies are
finding that patients who practice mind/body techniques such
as guided imagery and relaxation live longer and require far
less conventional medicine for pain control," he points out.

Individual Responsibility and Psychological Support
Steven Bailey, N.D., Assistant Professor of Pharmacognosy at
National College of Naturopathic Medicine in Portland,
Oregon, finds that the most important first step in returning
HIV positive or AIDS patients to health is to remove the help-
less, victim consciousness and to maintain a positive attitude.
He emphasizes that self-empowerment and personal responsi-

bility are vital to one's health and that they also play a significant role in the recovery process. Herb Joiner-Bey, N.D., of Bastyr University in Seattle, agrees, noting that, "Without spiritual and mental involvement, people find it difficult to generate the commitment to getting themselves well."[7]

Jon Kaiser, M.D., is a primary care physician who makes mind/body medicine an essential part of his practice in San Francisco. Nearly 70 percent of his patients are HIV positive. One patient came to him after continually having his anxiety about being diagnosed HIV positive dismissed by other doctors. Dr. Kaiser addressed the man's stress-related symptoms in conjunction with a protocol of diet, nutritional supplements, and herbs. As a result, the man regained control over his emotions and his health has improved to the point where he has been asymptomatic for the last four years. Among the points Dr. Kaiser emphasizes to his patients are the following:

- AIDS is not a death sentence.
- Begin a sound, alternative program early on to increase the possibility of living out a normal life span.
- Maintain a positive attitude.
- Don't panic or give into the negative programming that the media and the medical establishment promote.
- Follow a balanced, focused treatment program.

Alice Hiatt, R.N., of Berkeley, California, reports that the patient's understanding of his or her situation is a determining factor in treatment. "How they perceive their disease, their support system, their alternatives to Western medicine, their financial situation, and how they got AIDS—for example, being angry about someone exposing them to it without their knowledge—is crucial," she says.

De-stressing and Restoring Immune Function

The restoration of a positive, hopeful, and realistic outlook which encourages self-reliance is a common feature of most alternative medical approaches to AIDS. According to Erik Peper, Ph.D., Associate Director, Institute for Holistic Healing Studies, San Francisco State University,[8] this can be done as simply as by changing the way a person thinks. "Let's say you're a slightly older person and it's fall and the health professional says, 'I'm looking forward to what kinds of plans you have for this spring.' That implies that you may live through spring," Dr. Peper explains.

Another basic tenet of mind/body medicine is that the negative emotions that are burdening the immune system need to be addressed and resolved with counseling. The way a person handles stress also needs to be identified, taking into account the characteristics of his or her personality. Once a pattern of behavior has been identified, the task remains to balance these responses so that the person can learn to deal with stress in a more positive and constructive manner.

Developing Mindfulness

Many strategies can be used to develop mindfulness, meaning a control of mind and attention, according to Dr. Peper. "Let's say it's late at night and all of a sudden you feel an ache or an itch. Your brain can say, 'I wonder if this is this, this, or that,' and it pulls in all these negative pictures. Relaxation techniques can teach you to control your attention so that instead of going down negative alleys, you choose a path that helps you take better care of yourself," he says.

Dr. Peper's example illustrates how much what individuals "think" about the things that happen can be as significant as, and even greater than, the actual events themselves. Therefore, just as certain emotions and attitudes can negatively influence the immune system, learning to consciously develop other, more positive emotions can achieve the opposite, helping to enhance immune function in a manner that the individual can both control and incorporate as part of his or her own daily health care regimen.

To fully achieve this, Dr. Peper believes that mind/body practices must be undertaken with a sense of joy and enthusiasm. "I believe that the error many people make is to perform them like a chore, saying 'I have to do it.' That is the language of powerlessness and helplessness," he says. By making a positive choice to take charge of his or her health, a person experiences a greater sense of empowerment. Yet it is not merely a matter of choosing between good and bad responses, but between constructive and destructive ones. Whatever the de-stressing method may be, the most important thing is that it feels right to the person involved and that the method does no harm.[9] And, Dr. Peper adds, "Hope is also critical. It means looking forward to living today, and to have a potential plan for tomorrow and three months from now."

Many Possiblilities

There are a variety of methods within the mind/body field, including relaxation therapies, meditation, visualization and guided imagery, neurolinguistic programming (NLP), hypnotherapy, biofeedback training, qigong, and yoga. A person must choose a treatment that he or she is physically and psychologically comfortable with and, ideally, one that can be practiced at home. According to Alice Hiatt, having a positive support system during this period is a most beneficial addition to treatment.

Patricia Norris, Ph.D., and the Life Sciences Institute of Mind-Body Health

"Attitude is a very important factor in survival time for AIDS/HIV patients," according to Patricia Norris, Ph.D., Director of Clinical Psychoimmunology at the Life Sciences Institute of Mind-Body Health in Topeka, Kansas, and a pioneer in mind/body approaches to enhancing immune system competence.[10] "Emotions are biochemical activities. Every emotion is simultaneously subjective and neurochemical, involving neuropeptides, neurotransmitters, and neurohormone events. All known neurochemicals, neurotransmitters, neuropeptides, and neurohormones have receptors on lymphocytes. Our emotions are constantly modulating the behavior of all of the cells in our body, as well as those of the immune system. In fact, our thoughts and emotions are constantly modulating everything that goes on in the body, including heart rate, blood flow, and visceral responses."

Dr. Norris continues, "Mind/body medicine can play a crucial role in the general treatment plan of an AIDS patient. From one perspective, you could say that its role is paramount, in the sense that attitude determines a person's choices of lifestyle and treatment. In our practice we employ mind/

body medicine to improve immune functioning in AIDS, cancer, and autoimmune disorders. Our patients utilize mind/body therapies that include biofeedback, relaxation, meditation, imagery, and visualization in helping to learn self-regulation skills for symptoms such as anxiety and pain, and to increase health and manage stress. The appropriate therapy or combination of therapies that is best for an individual is discovered in the therapeutic process. We recommend these practices for everyone seeking high-level wellness."

A total treatment plan should address every aspect of health, notes Dr. Norris. "A total treatment plan would include behavioral and lifestyle changes, a nutritional program, detoxification (including ending all toxic substances like smoking and drinking and drug use), appropriate alternative therapies, and repairing emotional fences through love, self-acceptance, forgiveness, and letting go of bitterness and hatred. It is important to release the energy that can get bound up in the 'poor me, why me?' victim consciousness. Fear and despair are probably the most devastating factors on the immune system, more devastating than the pollutants that we face.

"I would recommend that a newly diagnosed, HIV positive patient immediately do everything possible to boost their health," adds Dr. Norris. "If a person is in general good health, then they can have low T4 counts and still do very well for a long time. In fact, one patient I have been working with has had very low T4 counts for a number of years and has been quite healthy. He is not undergoing any particular treatment protocol. He has a happy lifestyle. His life is full of love and music, he is eating well, he is very interested in the things that he is doing in his life.

"AIDS is frightening because so many people think that this is an automatic death sentence, which is untrue," continues Dr. Norris. "Most people diagnosed with HIV have a longer prognosis than for many kinds of cancers. I think that when people who are in good health find out that they have HIV, and then die in one or two years, it seems to be a kind of voodoo death. They believe they are going to die and just continue to move in that direction. The most important thing is for the individual to believe that AIDS/HIV is not an automatic death sentence and to feel, 'I can live, I can live long, I can live healthy, and I can have a good quality of life.'

"For example, one patient came to us at the very beginning of his diagnosis with a tremendous amount of fear and his immune system was down," says Dr. Norris. "He was getting colds and feeling terrible. He embraced all the parts of our program and has been healthy now for four years. We see him occasionally. He looks wonderful and reports he has not had any illnesses at all.

"Another of my patients who chose to discontinue AZT about two years ago has been gaining in health and strength and is now able to heal rapidly. Recently he had a bout with a bacterial infection that resulted in boils inside and outside his body, but he recovered and is back working. I have been working with him continuously, and his program includes vitamins, exercise, and excellent nutrition in addition to stress management and emotional work. He has changed his whole attitude toward life, death, relationships, work, and his family. His judgmental and perfectionist attitude has transformed into one of acceptance and compassion, and he is much more peaceful within himself."

NLP and AIDS: University of Miami School of Medicine

Janet Konefal, Ph.D., M.P.H., C.A., Associate Professor at the University of Miami School of Medicine,[11] has developed a series of counseling interventions to help deal with the emotional turmoil of HIV infection. Her counseling protocols utilize Neuro-Linguistic Programming (NLP), a mind/body therapy that allows people to detect and reprogram unconscious patterns of thought and behavior. This reprogramming alters or shifts the psychological and physiological responses, thus enhancing the healing process. Dr. Konefal's work is directed toward expanding sets of limiting beliefs and altering behaviors among individuals who are HIV positive.

Dr. Konefal's protocols include shifting internal visual images, altering internal dialogue, and actually changing the language patterns used. Typically, a person who is HIV positive makes visual images that are morbid in nature and main-

A Simple Meditation Exercise

Meditation is an easily learned and very important component of mind/body medicine. The first step to practicing meditation is learning to breathe in a manner that facilitates a state of calmness and awareness. The following exercise is recommended by Jon Kabat-Zinn, Ph.D., founder and Director of the Stress Reduction Clinic at the University of Massachusetts Medical Center, as an effective method for achieving this state. Find a quiet place where you will not be disturbed and practice the following for several minutes each day:

- Assume a comfortable posture lying on your back or sitting. If you are sitting, keep the spine straight and let your shoulders droop. Close your eyes if it feels comfortable.
- Bring your attention to your belly, feeling it rise or expand gently on the in-breath and fall or recede on the out-breath.
- Keep the focus on your breathing, "being with" each in-breath. Every time you notice that your mind has wandered off the breath, notice what it was that took you away and then gently bring your attention back to your belly and the feeling of the breath coming in and out.
- If your mind wanders away from the breath, then your "job" is simply to bring it back to the breath every time, no matter what it has become preoccupied with.
- Practice this exercise for fifteen minutes at a convenient time every day, whether you feel like it or not, for one week and see how it feels to incorporate a disciplined meditation practice into your life. Be aware of how it feels to spend time each day just being with your breath without having to do anything.

tains an internal dialogue which supports these thoughts of death and dying. This inclination is in turn reinforced by others, even those with good intentions. Research indicates this resulting hopelessness is a suppressor of the immune system.[12]

Finding out that one is HIV positive has also been found in various studies to be an immunosuppressor.[13]

Based on the knowledge, then, that thoughts and feelings affect the immune system, Dr. Konefal's protocol enhances an individual's abilities to create a way of thinking about HIV infection that fosters the will to live, thus enabling one to be emotionally stronger and more optimistic.

For over ten years, Dr. Konefal has worked with patients in all phases of HIV infection, from recent diagnosis to AIDS. One client has had full-blown AIDS for over ten years; several others have been symptomatically HIV positive for five to nine years. Dr. Konefal explains, "The focus of NLP is to determine the client's goals and then to work with the client to achieve these goals. Several of my clients have made a career of getting healthy; after that goal is reached, they go on with their lives. One who recently returned to work said, 'I've done the impossible—what's next?'"

"Sometimes when clients have lived longer than expected, a sense of doom sets in. They begin to talk about living on borrowed time. When I hear this, it is a sign that additional work is necessary. Others have been successful in getting cancer into remission, so there is no reason that this can't be done with AIDS. To help retain a positive attitude about survival, I warn clients about telling everyone they know about their intent to live. Some people will argue about whether survival is possible; this kind of debate is detrimental to the client's health because it wastes valuable energy and creates stress. Instead, I suggest that they form a small circle of friends and health care providers who will genuinely support their convictions."

In her private practice at the University Outpatient Program, Dr. Konefal has had success by combining NLP with other complementary therapies: acupuncture and a clinical nutritional system called contact reflex analysis. She explains, "I don't like to depend on only one treatment modality, especially with serious conditions like AIDS. As a complementary medicine specialist, I must work with a combination of treatment modalities. If I don't, I become a stress factor in the healing process of my clients."

Where to Find Help

Alternative Medicine Yellow Pages. **The Burton Goldberg Group. Puyallup, WA: Future Medicine Publishing, Inc., 1994.**

Lists over 16,000 practitioners of alternative medicine in the United States and Canada. Practitioners are listed by therapy, city, and state. See sections on "Mind/Body Medicine," "Meditation," "Guided Imagery," "Biofeedback," "Hypnotherapy," "Qigong," and "Yoga."

The Center for Applied Psychophysiology
Menninger Clinic
P.O. Box 829
Topeka, Kansas 66601-0829
(913) 273-7500 Ext. 5375

The Center for Applied Psychophysiology has research and treatment in all phases of mind/body medicine. They work with disorders of the cardiovascular, gastrointestinal, immune, and respiratory systems. They also work with programs on peak performance for athletes, as well as drug and alcohol abuse.

The Center for the Improvement of Human Functioning
3100 North Hillside Avenue
Wichita, Kansas 67219-3904
(316) 682-3100

A medical research educational organization, the center offers clinical services, diagnostic testing, educational classes, conferences, and seminars. The center publishes books, has a large library, and performs clinical and basic research.

Mind-Body Clinic
New Deaconess Hospital
Harvard Medical School
185 Pilgrim Road
Cambridge, Massachusetts 02215
(617) 632-9530

Treatment program at a medical center where the relaxation response can be learned. The Mind-Body Clinic uses yoga, meditation, and stress reduction as part of its program.

Stress Reduction and Relaxation Program
University of Massachusetts Medical Center
55 Lake Avenue North
Worcester, Massachusetts 01655
(508) 856-2656
The oldest and largest hospital-based stress reduction clinic in the country, this pioneering center uses mindfulness training to help patients to work with their own stress, pain, and illnesses more effectively. The Stress Reduction and Relaxation Program is an outpatient behavioral medicine clinic in the form of an eight-week long course taken to complement whatever treatments one may be receiving. People are referred to the clinic by their doctors for conditions such as heart disease, cancer, AIDS, HIV infection, chronic pain, gastrointestinal distress, anxiety, fatigue, sleep disturbance, and skin disorders. The mind/body program is based on intensive training in mindfulness meditation and yoga, and is directed by Jon Kabat-Zinn, Ph.D., and was featured on Bill Moyer's "Healing and the Mind" series on PBS.

Biofeedback

Biofeedback Certification Institute of America
10200 West 44th Avenue, Suite 304
Wheat Ridge, Colorado 80033
Runs the major certification program for biofeedback practitioners and provides information about certified local practitioners.

Hypnotherapy

The American Society of Clinical Hypnosis
2200 East Devon Avenue
Suite 291
Des Plaines, Illinois 60018
(708) 297-3317
Membership is comprised of M.D.'s and dentists trained in the use of hypnosis for treating health conditions. Send a stamped, self-addressed envelope for referrals to practitioners in your area.

International Medical and Dental
Hypnotherapy Association
4110 Edgeland, Suite 800
Royal Oak, Michigan 48073
(313) 549-5594
(800) 257-5467 Outside Michigan
Trains and certifies M.D.'s, dentists, and hypnotherapists in the
therapeutic use of hypnotherapy for treating health challenges. Has
members throughout the United States, Canada, Europe, Japan,
Mexico, and the Virgin Islands. Provides a referral list of certified
practitioners throughout the United States and Canada, available by
sending a stamped, self-addressed envelope.

The American Institute of Hypnotherapy
1805 East Garry Avenue, Suite 100
Santa Ana, California 92705
(714) 261-6400
Trains and certifies hypnotherapists in a wide range of
hypnotherapy applications. Also the only institution of its kind to
be authorized to grant a doctorate degree in hypnosis. Provides a
comprehensive range of books and tapes on all aspects of
hypnotherapy.

Neuro-Linguistic Programming

Dynamic Learning Center
P.O. Box 1112
Ben Lomond, California 95005
(408) 336-3457
(408) 336-5854 (Fax)
The Center provides NLP certification training, as well as NLP
classes open to the general public. Dynamic learning publications
provides books, audio tapes, and educational materials.

Western States Training Associates
346 South 500 East, Suite 200
Salt Lake City, Utah 84102
(801) 534-1022
(801) 532-2113 (Fax)
WSTA provides NLP training to individuals, businesses, and
government organizations. Founders Tim Hallbom and Suzi Smith
can be contacted for further information about their training
seminars and NLP certification programs. References are provided
for people with health-related issues.

Recommended Reading

Alternative Medicine: The Definitive Guide. The Burton Goldberg Group. Puyallup, WA: Future Medicine Publishing, Inc., 1993.

The most comprehensive reference on alternative medicine ever compiled. Provides in-depth, easily understandable coverage of 43 alternative therapies and over 200 health conditions, with advice from nearly 400 alternative physicians worldwide. See chapters on "Mind/Body Medicine," "Meditation," "Guided Imagery," "Biofeedback," "Hypnotherapy," "Qigong," and "Yoga."

Guided Imagery

Healing Yourself: A Step-by-Step Program for Better Health through Imagery. Rossman, Martin L. New York: Pocket Books, 1989.

A simple how-to book on unleashing the body's natural healing powers.

Imagery in Healing Shamanism and Modern Medicine. Achterberg, Jeanne. Boston: Shambala Publications, Inc. 1985.

The author explains how the systematic use of imagery can help patients through painful events ranging from childbirth to burn treatment, as well as act as a positive influence on disease states such as cancer.

Hypnotherapy

Hypnosis, Acupuncture, and Pain. Tinterow, Maurice M., M.D. Wichita, KA: Bio-Communication Press, 1989.

Dr. Tinterow's techniques combine hypnosis and acupuncture to relieve pain and physical suffering.

Meditation

Full Catastrophe Living: Using the Wisdom of Your Body and Mind to Face Stress, Pain, and Illness. Kabat-Zinn, Jon. New York: Delta, 1990.

An excellent description of the stress reduction and relaxation program at the University of Massachusetts Medical Center, a pioneering center using mindfulness training for addressing stress and pain. Offers a comprehensive look at how meditation can be applied to modern life, and provides a variety of self-help exercises, along with actual case histories which illustrate how the mind can be used to create wellness in daily life.

The Meditative Mind. Goleman, Daniel. Los Angeles: Jeremy P. Tarcher, Inc., 1988.

A very helpful book surveying the way in which meditation has been used in different religious traditions, both East and West.

The Relaxation Response. Benson, Herbert. New York: Outlet Books, Inc., 1993.

Still a classic in the field, this book explains the relaxation response, a meditative technique derived from Transcendental Meditation, and its ability to relieve stress, anxiety, and stress-related illness.

Transcendental Meditation. Roth, Robert. New York: Donald I. Fine, Inc., 1988.

A simple, readable introduction to Transcendental Meditation.

Neuro-Linguistic Programming (NLP)

Beliefs: Pathways to Health and Well-Being. Dilts, Robert; Hallbom, Tim; and Smith, Suzi. Portland, OR: Metamorphous Press, 1990.

The first book of its kind to demonstrate how the advanced technology of neuro-linguistic programming can be used to identify limiting or destructive beliefs, and how to rapidly and effectively alter these ideas and promote positive change.

Heart of the Mind. Andreas, Connie Rae; and Andreas, Steve. Moab UT: Real People Press, 1989.

An accessible introductory book that provides examples of common NLP patterns, including easy-to-apply techniques, to deal with weight loss, stage fright, phobias, abuse, grief, as well as tools for becoming more independent, creating motivation, and promoting self-healing.

Stress Reduction and Mind/Body Medicine

***Creating Wholeness: A Self-Healing Workbook Using
Dynamic Relaxation, Images, and Thoughts.*** Peper, Erik;
and Holt, Catherine. New York: Plenum, 1993.
*A simple and accessible self-help program that teaches physical,
cognitive, and imagery-based techniques to reduce stress and
promote health.*

Head First: The Biology of Hope. Cousins, Norman. New
York: Thorndike Press, 1991.
*Based on hundreds of interviews with doctors, patients, medical
students, and research scientists, this book chronicles how an
optimistic outlook, faith, hope, laughter, the will to live, and a
strong relationship with the doctor can make illness less painful and
increase a person's chances of survival.*

The Healer Within. Locke, Steven; and Colligan, Douglas.
New York: Mentor, 1986.
*An accessible, authoritative, and complete study of how emotions
and attitudes can affect health and the treatment of diseases from
the common cold to cancer.*

Healing and the Mind. Moyers, Bill. New York: Doubleday,
1993.
*The transcripts of fifteen interviews with different doctors who are
investigating the power of the mind. An investigation by Moyers of a
new approach to illness.*

***Love, Medicine & Miracles: Lessons Learned about Self-
Healing from a Surgeon's Experience with Exceptional
Patients.*** Siegel, Bernard. HarperPerennial, 1986.
*In this powerful and inspiring book, Dr. Siegel confronts time-
honored perceptions, eloquently explores the link between mind and
body, and shows how you can become an exceptional patient—a
survivor. He finds that survivors share common characteristics:
taking control of their lives, having the courage to work with their
doctors to participate and influence the course of their illnesses,
examining the role illness plays in their lives, and learning the
power of love.*

***Mind/Body Medicine: How to Use Your Mind for Better
Health.*** Goleman, D.; and Gurin, Joel. New York: Consumer
Reports Books, 1993.
*A comprehensive informative book on the power of the mind. A well-
researched collection of essays and case histories by more than
twenty-four different researchers and doctors.*

Minding the Body, Mending the Mind. Borysenko, Joan.
New York: Bantam Books, 1988.

*Based on ground-breaking work at the Mind/Body Clinic at New
England Deaconess Hospital, this book tells of dramatic success
with conditions ranging from allergies to cancer. A unique blend of
physical and mental exercises are explained, which show how to
elicit the mind's relaxation response, boost the immune system,
overcome chronic pain, and alleviate stress-related illnesses.*

**Peace, Love & Healing: Bodymind Communication and the
Path to Self-Healing.** Siegel, Bernard. HarperPerennial, 1989.

*Dr. Siegel challenges us, whether we are ill or well, to recognize
how our mind influences our body and how to use this knowledge
to our advantage. Through accounts of many exceptional patients
he shows us that we, ourselves, play a critical role in communicat-
ing to our mind, body, and self-healing systems, and he teaches us
how to give ourselves healing messages through the techniques of
meditation, visualization, relaxation, and peace of mind.*

Quantum Healing. Chopra, Deepak. New York, Bantam
Books, 1989.

*Draws from Western medicine, neuroscience, physics, Ayurvedic
medicine, ancient wisdom, and case histories, including recoveries
from severe illnesses, to explain mind/body medicine in a thought-
provoking and personal way.*

**Why Me? Harnessing the Healing Power of the Human
Spirit.** Porter, Garrett; and Norris, Patricia, Ph.D. Walpole,
NH: Stillpoint Publishing, International 1985. (Available from
Dr. Patricia Norris, Life Sciences Institute of Mind-Body
Health, 2955 S.W. Wanamaker Drive, Topeka, Kansas 66614,
(913) 271-8686).

*In this book, Garrett Porter tells the story of his battle with an
inoperable brain tumor and the process of overcoming his
condition. Throughout the book, Dr. Norris has woven the
philosophy of mind/body/spirit healing and the dynamics of
biofeedback, visualization, and imagery in healing. Many useful
strategies and techniques for attaining high-level wellness in the
midst of illness are contained in the last three chapters of the book.*

11 Oxygen Therapy

Oxygen therapy refers to a wide range of therapies which utilize various forms of oxygen to promote healing and destroy pathogens (disease-producing microorganisms and toxins) in the body. Ozone therapy, hyperbaric oxygen therapy, and intravenous hydrogen peroxide therapy are the most widely recognized forms of oxygen therapy. These therapies have been found to be effective in treating a wide range of conditions, including infections (viral, fungal, parasitic, bacterial), chronic fatigue syndrome, allergies, arthritis, circulatory problems, and cancer.

In 1988, a group of prominent doctors came out in support of using oxygen therapy as a primary treatment for AIDS and HIV infection. Kenneth Wagner, M.D., former head of the Naval Hospital's AIDS unit in Bethesda, Maryland, Steven Kleinman, M.D., Medical Director of the American Red Cross Blood Services for Los Angeles, along with Michael Carpendale, M.D., of the Veterans Administration Medical Center in San Francisco, California, and Mark Rarick, M.D., an AIDS researcher at the University of Southern California had a direct and simple message: oxygen therapy is the safest and most effective method of treating AIDS and its associated infections.[1]

Oxygen therapies are grouped according to the type of chemical process involved: the addition of oxygen to the blood or tissues is called "oxygenation," and the reaction of splitting off electrons (electrically-charged particles) from any chemical molecule is called "oxidation." Oxidation may or may not involve oxygen (oxidation refers to the chemical reaction and not to oxygen itself). Hyperbaric oxygen therapy, which introduces oxygen to the body in a pressurized chamber, utilizes the process of oxygenation. Hydrogen peroxide therapy, on the other hand, uses the process of oxidation. Ozone therapy utilizes both chemical processes.

Although oxygen therapies have been used in Europe for many years for a wide range of conditions, most remain controversial in the United States and are currently unapproved by the FDA (Food and Drug Administration). Legality of oxygen therapies varies from state to state.

How Oxygenation Therapy Works
All human cells, tissues, and organs need oxygen to function. Oxygenation saturates the body with oxygen through the use of gas, sometimes at high-pressure (hyperbaric), increasing the total amount of available oxygen in the body. Insufficient oxygenation may promote the growth of pathogens, whereas excessive oxygenation may damage normal tissues. However, oxygenation employed under strictly controlled conditions can have very positive therapeutic effects.

Otto Warburg, Director of the Max Planck Institute for Cell Physiology in Germany and a two-time Nobel laureate, proposed that a lack of oxygen at the cellular level may be the prime cause of cancer, and that oxygen therapy could be an effective cancer treatment.[2] He showed that normal cells in tissue culture, when deprived of oxygen, become cancer cells, and that oxygen can kill cancer cells in tissue cultures.

Oxygen therapy may be professionally administered in many ways: orally, rectally, vaginally, intravenously (into a vein), intra-arterially (into an artery), through inhalation, or by absorption through the skin. High concentrations of oxygen gas can also be given orally through masks or tubes, via oxygen tents, or within pressurized hyperbaric chambers. Oxygen may also be injected subcutaneously (beneath the skin). Ionized oxygen, both positively and negatively charged, is administered by inhalation or dissolved in drinking or bath water.

How Oxidation Therapy Works
Oxidation is a process by which the body overcomes invading pathogenic microbial organisms. Controlled oxidation in the proper amounts alters the chemical structural integrity of pathogens while leaving normal cells intact. The word "oxidation" refers to a chemical reaction whereby electrons are transferred from one molecule to another. Oxygen molecules

are frequently, but not always, involved in these reactions. The molecules that "donate" electrons are said to be oxidized, whereas the molecules that accept electrons are called oxidants.

A healthy state of oxidative balance is necessary for optimal function of the body, but when the body is exposed to repeated environmental stresses, its oxidative function is weakened. When oxidation is partially blocked by toxicity in the body or pathological (disease-causing) organisms, oxidation therapy, using intravenous hydrogen peroxide, may help by "jump-starting" the body's oxidative processes and returning them to normal, according to Charles H. Farr, M.D., Ph.D., of Oklahoma City, Oklahoma, Medical Director of the International Bio-Oxidative Medicine Association.[3]

When properly administered, oxidation therapy selectively destroys pathogenic (disease-producing) bacteria, viruses, and other invading microbial organisms, and deactivates toxic substances without injury to healthy tissues or cells.[4] For example, if diluted hydrogen peroxide is placed on a wound, the normal cells thrive while the pathogens die. Oxidation therapy must be administered under clinical supervision, since uncontrolled oxidation may be destructive to the body.

While oxygen free radicals are deadly to viruses and bacteria, they can also do damage to healthy tissue if left unchecked. When the body manufactures these oxygen-based defense substances, it follows this immediately by sending protective antioxidant enzymes to quench the process before harm to healthy tissue can take place. Nutritional support is also generally recommended with any oxygen therapy, particularly vitamin C supplementation, which acts as a stabilizing antioxidant agent.

Ozone Therapy

Ozone therapy relies on the process of oxidation as well as oxygenation. Approximately one-fifth of the air humans breathe is comprised of two atoms of oxygen (O_2). Ozone (O_3) contains three oxygen atoms and is a less stable form of molecular oxygen. Because of this added molecule, ozone is more reactive than oxygen and readily enters into reactions to oxidize other chemicals. During oxidation in the body, the extra oxygen molecule in ozone breaks away, leaving a normal O_2 molecule, and increasing the oxygen content of the blood or tissues. For this reason, ozone therapy is a combination of both oxygenation therapy and oxidation therapy.

Ozone is a common substance in nature, but can also be a source of air pollution when produced by man-made combustion. Medical grade ozone is made from pure oxygen. Used medically, ozone increases local oxygen supply to lesions, improves and accelerates wound healing, deactivates viruses and bacteria, and increases local tissue temperature, thus enhancing local metabolic processes, according to Gerard Sunnen, M.D., of New York City.

Ozone can be administered intravenously, intra-arterially, intramuscularly (within the muscle), intra-articularly (into the joint), and subcutaneously. In the case of an intravenous or intramuscular injection, up to a quart of blood is removed from a vein and mixed with ozone gas, then re-injected into the body. Ozone may also be applied topically as a gas or dissolved in water or olive oil. As a gas it may be insufflated (blown in) vaginally or rectally. It may also be taken orally, rectally, or vaginally in the form of ozonated water.

Claims are made for ozone to be effective in:[5]

- Disinfecting open wounds
- Raising oxygen levels in the blood
- Killing 100 percent of viruses it comes into contact with in the blood
- Removing the fatty (lipid) coat of viruses (including herpes, influenza, Epstein Barr, cytomegalovirus, and others) making them vulnerable to body defenses
- Treating hepatitis, cholera, and dysentery
- Treating donor blood (Ozone is claimed to make this clear of infectious agents which cause hepatitis and syphilis.)
- Treating water supplies (Ozone inactivates polio virus and *giardia lamblia* and cleans water without chlorine. It is used by utility companies in many cities including Los Angeles for this purpose.)
- Disinfecting the mouth during dentistry (a method used since the 1920s)

Ozone Therapy for AIDS and Associated Illnesses

The claims made for the benefits of ozone therapy in the treatment of AIDS are extraordinary. Unfortunately, since the FDA has not approved the practice of ozone therapy in the United States, it is difficult to get data on its use, and few clinical studies are as yet available in the English language to support the claims. However, the scientific literature is growing and numerous patient anecdotal cases are available.

Laboratory studies have shown that ozone is capable of inactivating HIV in solution.[6] It has also been shown to inhibit the growth of human lung, breast, and uterine cancer cells in tissue culture.[7]

A recent study found that when HIV-infected blood was removed from the body and treated with ozone, the virus was completely deactivated.[8] One current AIDS treatment method mimics this approach, removing blood from the body, infusing it with ozone, and then replacing it. Usually this is done at least twice weekly for simple infections and conditions during treatment periods. For more serious illnesses, such as AIDS, it is also applied in other ways. Another treatment approach has been to simply inject a diluted form of ozone into the bloodstream. This treatment can be done daily for several weeks at a time.

French researchers Bertrand Vallancien and Jean-Marie Winkler studied ozone therapy with a group of patients with HIV, herpes, and hepatitis. After nine weeks of transfused ozone, T4 and T8 cells moved toward normal levels in all cases, and the ozone treatments caused no other problems.[9] The late German physician, Alexander Preuss, M.D., used ozone in a regimen including vitamins, minerals, and other treatments of the immune system and achieved remission in a number of patients with AIDS-associated infections.[10]

Ozone Therapy and AIDS in the U.S.

Like many oxygen therapies, ozone therapy is widely used and practiced in Europe, but is still not readily available in the United States. According to Dr. Sunnen, prospective patients and doctors in America must await two further animal studies before the FDA sanctions a phase-one clinical trial with humans, and ultimately approves the therapeutic use of ozone.

For this reason, many physicians have been forced to use ozone therapy without calling attention to themselves, for fear of FDA reprisals.

One doctor, who preferred to remain anonymous, reports of good results with HIV positive patients. He gave these patients three ozone treatments a week for seven weeks. For each treatment, 250 to 300 cc's of blood were removed, treated with ozone, and injected back into the patient. This helped reduce opportunistic infections. Other treatments were also employed to help strengthen the immune system.[11] Patients who have difficulty tolerating AZT treatments may also benefit from ozone therapy.

John Pittman, M.D., of Salisbury, North Carolina, initiated a study with nine HIV positive patients whom he treated with a regimen of ozone one day, hydrogen peroxide the next, and chelation therapy on the third day for twenty-three days (the study was then stopped for legal reasons). In patients whose T-cell count was greater than 100 initially, a 20 to 30 percent rise was seen. There was no effect on those with initial T-cell counts below 100. He believes ozone is helpful in AIDS because it is known to damage viruses which have a lot of fat in their membranes (HIV membranes have a high fat content). Healthy cells have antioxidant enzymes to break down ozone and prevent damage; viruses do not. He believes ozone may also stimulate the immune system.

Jonathan Wright, M.D., Director of the Tahoma Clinic, in Kent, Washington,[12] finds ozone therapy very effective against chronic infections, particularly viruses and candidiasis. He also treats hepatitis B with ozonation of the blood along with the herbal remedy, Phyllanthus, and high doses of intravenous ascorbate (a salt of ascorbic acid—vitamin C). "You can't just use ozone alone," says Dr. Wright. "You need to combine it with a proper diet, [nutritional] supplements, herbs, botanicals, acupuncture, and chiropractic." He adds that antioxidants (chemicals or substances that can donate, or give up, electrons) such as vitamin C should be given along with any oxidative therapy since they prevent uncontrolled oxidation which is detrimental to the body.

Dr. Wright uses ozone therapy with AIDS patients by ozonating the blood and returning it to the patient, or by rectal insufflation. In 1985, he treated an HIV positive patient who was feverish and had swollen glands. The patient was given ozone twice a week for six months, along with vitamin and mineral supplements and botanicals. The patient's symptoms were greatly relieved, and he continues doing well, returning for ozone treatment whenever he has a fever or other symptoms.

Patient Success Stories

Len developed acute sinusitis in 1985. "The next year," he says, "I had swollen glands. That lasted five years. In 1991, I was very sick with AIDS. I was in bed for a month with a high fever, had several bad flus, and was withering away. My T cells went as low as 200. The T4/T8 ratio was .4. I didn't want to take AZT. I had seen so many people on it who died. So I went to see a doctor I thought was intelligent, and went on a protocol involving ozone. I've now gained twenty-five pounds and I've maintained it for a year. I take a few antioxidants and vitamins. My T cells have gone up to 900, and the T4/T8 ratio is .8, which is much better. I've had another series of treatments since the first one . . . I'm thinking of going back for a third series now. If I feel a little worn, I get more treatments."

Kevin became HIV positive seven years ago. "I had night sweats, muscle ache, and my T cells, which had been about 700, went down to 150 pretty quickly. I started on AZT. I was on it for two weeks. My system couldn't tolerate it. I had trouble walking. They took me off it. Then I did ten to twenty treatments with ozone. The T cells jumped up to 400 or 500. For the next two years, I did a number of ozone treatments, where they take a pint of blood out, ozonate it and put it back in. About seventy treatments. My T cells slowly climbed to 928. Of course, I was also doing IV vitamin C, and I was on a healthy diet. I did a lot of things. The symptoms, the night sweats and muscle ache, all had gone after the first week of ozone treatments . . . Now I work with other people, helping them with their ozone treatments. I don't think ozone is best for people with full-blown AIDS. It's best with people who just became HIV positive and their T cells aren't too bad. If people have very low T cells, you should give them less ozone. The regular quantity could be not good for them. If a person has very heavy AIDS symptoms, the ozone could help, but I wouldn't say it would cure them . . . "

CAUTION *Adverse effects associated with intravenous ozone have been reported to include phlebitis (inflammation of a vein), circulatory depression, chest pain, shortness of breath, fainting, coughing, flushing, cardiac arrhythmias, and gas embolus (bubbles). Rectal administration of ozone can lead to inflammation of the lower intestinal tract. Although it is easily tolerated in other tissues, the inappropriate use of ozone in high concentrations causes inflammation of the lung tissues.*

Hydrogen Peroxide Therapy

Hydrogen peroxide is a liquid with a molecular structure which is made up of two atoms of hydrogen and two atoms of oxygen (H_2O_2). Because it is less stable than water (H_2O), hydrogen peroxide readily enters into oxidative reactions, ultimately becoming oxygen in water.

Dr. Farr first characterized the oxidative effects of hydrogen peroxide in humans in 1984, and described his discovery in a 1987 monograph entitled, *The Therapeutic Use of Intravenous Hydrogen Peroxide.*[13] Today, its use has spread to over thirty-eight countries.

Hydrogen peroxide, like ozone, can be administered intravenously, and can also be taken rectally by enema, vaginally, or transcutaneously (absorbed through the skin while bathing), according to Dr. Farr. However, he advocates the intravenous method of delivery, and his current treatment protocol involves eight or ten treatments, once a week—the protocol varying depending on the patient and illness.

Oxidation administered through hydrogen peroxide therapy regulates tissue repair, cellular respiration, growth, immune functions, the energy system, most hormone systems, and the production of cytokines (chemical messengers that are involved in the regulation of almost every system in the body). Oxidation therapy can also work as a defense system, directly destroying invading bacteria, viruses, yeast, and parasites, according to Dr. Farr.

Hydrogen Peroxide Therapy for
AIDS and Associated Illnesses

With regards to AIDS patients, he believes treatment with hydrogen peroxide best benefits those with a very low T-cell count *before* they have full-blown AIDS. "We'll hold them in check for a while," he says, adding, "I don't believe in oral peroxide, because the enzymes of the stomach don't process it properly. Some doctors are using combinations of ozone and peroxide and reporting good results, because of a sympathetic response in cells."

According to Dr. Farr, some other conditions that may benefit from hydrogen peroxide therapy include allergies, lung infections, herpes simplex, herpes zoster (shingles), fungal, bacterial, viral and parasitic infections, acne, and wounds.[14] Hydrogen peroxide injections have been used for inflamed, damaged, and injured tissues, inflamed nerves such as in herpes, or trigger points causing pain and muscle spasms.[15]

Dr. Farr has demonstrated rapid recovery from Type A/Shanghai influenza with intravenous hydrogen peroxide treatments. Two-thirds of his patients recovered after only a single injection. One-third returned for a second injection and only 10 percent required a third. Recovery time was half that of a control group treated with conventional methods: antibiotics, decongestants, and analgesics.[16]

There are few side effects with hydrogen peroxide therapy. In rare cases, a problem involving inflammation of veins at the site of injection will occur. Hydrogen peroxide should not be taken orally as it causes nausea and vomiting, and rectal administration can lead to inflammation of the lower intestinal tract. Other side effects observed include temporary faintness, fatigue, headaches, and chest pain.

Most problems stem from the use of either an inappropriate administration route, administration above patient tolerance, the mixing of oxidative chemicals with other substances, or using oxidative chemicals in too great a concentration, reports Dr. Farr.

Hyperbaric Oxygen Therapy

Hyperbaric oxygen therapy (HBOT) dates back to the beginning of this century, although its modern use in the United

States dates only to the formation of the Undersea Medical Society in the United States in 1967. HBOT may be administered in individual oxygen chambers or in multiplace chambers.

The individual chambers consist of acrylic tubes about seven feet long and twenty-five inches in diameter. The patient lies on a stretcher which slides into the tube. The entry is sealed and the tube pressurized at up to two and a half Atmospheres Absolute (two and a half times the pressure of the atmosphere at sea level) with pure oxygen for thirty to 120 minutes. The increased pressure makes it possible to breathe oxygen at a concentration higher than that allowed by any other means. After treatment, the chamber is depressurized slowly with the patient resting inside. Most of the hyperbaric facilities in the United States are either part of, or affiliated with, hospitals or the military.

Multiplace chambers accommodate many patients at once, the oxygen being delivered by mask, and are now used at the University of Maryland, Duke University, the University of Texas, Scripps Institute, and the Hyperbaric Oxygen Institute in San Bernardino, California. These chambers allow nurses and technical personnel to attend to patients during the treatment. An added advantage of multiplace chambers is that a patient can be removed immediately if problems arise, whereas in individual chambers, the patient cannot be removed until the entire chamber is depressurized.

Today in the United States, HBOT is primarily used for traumas such as crash injuries, stroke, burns, wounds, gangrene (death of tissue, usually due to deficient or absent blood supply), carbon monoxide poisoning, decubitus ulcers (bed sores), stasis (the stagnation of the normal flow of fluids), radiation necrosis (death of an area of tissue or bone surrounded by healthy parts), and recalcitrant skin grafting (skin grafting that doesn't take). Some microsurgical procedures for the repair and restoration of severed limbs are made possible only by the use of HBOT during the surgery.

Hyperbaric Oxygen Therapy for AIDS and Associated Illnesses

According to David Hughes, D.Sc., of the Hyperbaric Oxygen Institute, in San Bernadino, California, HBOT has also demonstrated its value as an adjunct to antibiotics in the treatment of anaerobic (able to live without oxygen) infections. HBOT has begun to be used experimentally to treat the symptoms of HIV infection and its accompanying fatigue. "HBOT is a valuable adjunct in treating opportunistic infections which threaten the immunosuppressed patient," says Dr. Hughes.

Hyperbaric oxygen therapy may cause problems for those with a history of middle ear infection, emphysema, or spontaneous pneumonthorax due to the pressure it requires, according to Dr. Hughes. The use of HBOT for illnesses including AIDS, heart disease, and detoxification from recreational drug addiction and alcoholism is in debate. Yet HBOT is gaining acceptance and is used by both alternative and conventional physicians. Its broad spectrum of applications gives it enormous potential to be used as an adjunct therapy in the future.

Where to Find Help

Alternative Medicine Yellow Pages. **The Burton Goldberg Group. Puyallup, WA: Future Medicine Publishing, Inc., 1994.**
Lists over 16,000 practitioners of alternative medicine in the United States and Canada. Practitioners are listed by therapy, city, and state. See section on "Oxygen Therapy."

The American College of Hyperbaric Medicine
Ocean Medical Center
4001 Ocean Drive, Suite 105
Lauderdale-by-the-sea, Florida 33308
(305) 771-4000
A group of physicians dedicated to the clinical aspects of hyperbaric medicine. Their purpose is to foster ethical growth and development of the science and practice of hyperbaric oxygen therapy. Promotes research and education.

ECH2O2 Newsletter
9845 NE 2nd Avenue
Miami, FL 33138
(305) 758-8710
A public forum for those interested in the oral use of hydrogen peroxide and ozone. Publishes a quarterly newsletter for the public and professionals addressing thousands of uses for hydrogen peroxide and ozone in areas including farming and agriculture, waste and water treatment, industry, bathing, and dentistry.

International Bio-oxidative Medicine Foundation (IBOM)
P.O. Box 13205
Oklahoma City, Oklahoma 73113-1205
(405) 478-IBOM Ext. 4266
The foundation publishes and distributes a newsletter, as well as scientific research data. Supports educational programs that highlight current research and the therapeutic use of oxidative modalities. Encourages basic and clinical research. Membership available.

International Ozone Association
31 Strawberry Hill Avenue
Stamford, Connecticut 06902
(203) 348-3542
A professional scientific organization disseminating information on the use and production of ozone through meetings, synopses, and world congresses. Publishes books and journals on ozone.

Medizone International, Inc.
123 East 54th Street
New York NY 10022
212-421-0303
Developers of ozone-based blood purification systems and treatment for diseases caused by lipid enveloped viruses including AIDS, hepatitis B, and herpes.

North Carolina Bio-Oxidative Health Center
4505 Fair Meadow Lane, Suite 111
Raleigh, North Carolina 27607
(800) 473-9812 (U.S. and Canada)
(407) 967-6466 (Outside North America)
Outpatient facility which focuses on metabolic and intestinal detoxification. Comprehensive and synergistic treatment regimens for each patient are developed utilizing therapies such as colon

hydrotherapy, intravenous therapies (including ozone), and external ozone hydrotherapy. Supportive elements such as acupuncture and lymphatic massage, as well as techniques to address the psychological/emotional components of health and illness are also part of the program.

 # Recommended Reading

Alternative Medicine: The Definitive Guide. The Burton Goldberg Group. Puyallup, WA: Future Medicine Publishing, Inc., 1993.
The most comprehensive reference on alternative medicine ever compiled. Provides in-depth, easily understandable coverage of 43 alternative therapies and over 200 health conditions, with advice from nearly 400 alternative physicians worldwide. See Chapters on "Oxygen Therapy" and "AIDS."

Hydrogen Peroxide Medical Miracle. Douglass, William Campbell. Atlanta, GA: Second Opinion Publishing, 1992. To order, call (800) 728-2288
This book explores the importance of H2O2 in the proper function of the immune system, and in its ability to rid the body of disease and metabolize protein, carbohydrates, fats, vitamins, and minerals.

Oxygen Therapies. McCabe, Ed. Morrisville, NY: Energy Publications, 1988.
Discusses the effects of a low-oxygen environment resulting from sedentary lifestyles, poor food, lack of exercise, and the breathing of polluted air. This book explores how cells in this condition can become breeding grounds for harmful viruses and microbes. Included are methods of increasing cellular oxygenation, medical studies, case histories of former AIDS and other degenerative disease victims, as well as contacts.

Underwater Medicine and Related Sciences: A Guide to the Literature. Shilling, Charles. New York: Plenum Publications, Volume 1, 1973; Volume 2, 1975.
An invaluable book for researching hyperbaric medicine.

The Use of Ozone in Medicine, First English Edition.
Rilling, Siegfried; and Viebahn, Renate. Heidelberg,
Germany: Haug Publishers, 1987.

*A history of ozone/oxygen therapy treatments of lesions, burns, virus
infections such as herpes and hepatitis, circulatory disturbances,
and rheumatic/arthritic complaints. Includes a listing of indications
and applications with exact treatment guide. This book is available
through Medicina Biologica, 2937 N.E. Flanders, Portland, Oregon
97232, or phone (503) 287-6775.*

12 Hyperthermia

Fever is the body's primary, and one of its most powerful, defenses against disease. When the body's temperature is raised above normal, it is a natural physiological attempt to destroy the invading organisms by sweating impurities out of the system.

Hyperthermia artificially induces fever in the patient who is unable to mount a natural fever response to infection, inflammation, or other health challenges. It is used locally or over the entire body to treat diseases ranging from viral infections to cancer, and is an effective self-help treatment for colds and flu.

All viruses and bacteria are heat sensitive to some extent. For this reason a number of different methods of heating the body are used to encourage deactivation or death of viruses, bacteria, and even cancer cells, especially in naturopathic medicine.[1]

Recently, medical research has begun to examine this method.[2] In some clinical settings, most notably in Germany, up to eight hours of immersion in hot water (with frequent cool drinks and cool compresses on the head/neck) are used. This is extremely exhausting for the patient, and less arduous methods are often suggested, especially for home use, which should always be administered under professional guidance.

While hyperthermia treatments may not be able to kill every invading virus (HIV experiences approximately 40 percent inactivation after thirty minutes in a 107.6 degree Fahrenheit bath), they reduce their number, making it easier for the immune system to handle the remaining viruses. Hyperthermia is also a useful technique for detoxification because it releases toxins stored in fat cells.

How Hyperthermia Works

A state of hyperthermia exists when body temperature increases above its normal level of 98.6 degrees Fahrenheit. An increase in body temperature causes many physiological responses to occur. Hyperthermia takes advantage of the fact that many invading organisms tolerate a narrower temperature range than body tissues and are therefore more susceptible to increases in temperature. These organisms may die from over-heating before harm is done to human tissue.

Examples are viruses such as rhinovirus[3] (responsible for one half of all respiratory infections), HIV,[4] and the microorganisms and bacteria that cause syphilis and gonorrhea.[5] Hyperthermia treatments may not be able to kill every invading organism, but can reduce their numbers to a level the immune system can handle.

Hyperthermia additionally stimulates the immune system by increasing the production of antibodies and interferon (a protein substance produced by cells invaded by viruses to prevent the latter from reproducing).

Methods of Inducing Hyperthermia

Body temperature can be swiftly increased by external application of heat. This approach causes peripheral vasodilation (widening of the blood vessels) and initiates perspiration as the body attempts to prevent an increase in temperature. An increase in body temperature may be accomplished by such low-tech methods as immersing the body in hot water, sitting in a sauna or steam bath, or wrapping the body in blankets with a hot water bottle.

Hyperthermia applied locally can be used to treat infections or wounds on the body. For example, upper respiratory infection can be treated using inhalation of steam or by local diathermy (an application of radio frequency electromagnetic energy). Infected wounds in a hand or foot, on the other hand, might respond to immersion in a hot water bath; while an infection in the kidneys might be treated with ultrasound.

Whole-body hyperthermia, by contrast, is used when there is a general infection, when a local application is impractical, or when a general whole body response is desirable. Practitioners normally utilize the methods of full immersion bath, sauna, steam, and blanket packs. In conventional medical settings, whole-body treatment usually involves the more high-tech approaches of diathermy, ultrasound, and radiant and extracorporeal heating.

The HIV Virus and Heat Sensitivity

Laboratory research has proven that the HIV virus is temperature sensitive and suffers greater inactivation per unit time at progressively higher temperatures above 98.6 degrees Fahrenheit. For example, after thirty minutes heating in a water bath at 107.6 degrees Fahrenheit, 40 percent inactivation of HIV virus has been reported, and at 132.8 degrees Fahrenheit, 100 percent inactivation.[6] "I don't believe that hyperthermia is the answer for all HIV patients," says Douglas Lewis, N.D., Chair of Physical Medicine at the Bastyr University Natural Health Clinic in Seattle, Washington, "but I do think it is an appropriate adjunct treatment for all but a few very sick patients." This remarkable way of deactivating the virus continues to attract medical interest and will undoubtedly be more widely employed and refined in the near future.

HIV Infection and Hyperthermia

At the Natural Health Clinic at Bastyr University, hyperthermia is commonly used in the treatment of HIV infection. In 1988 and 1989, the Clinic conducted the Healing AIDS Research Project (HARP) study. The treatment protocol included dietary guidelines, dietary supplements, herbal medicine, homeopathy, counseling, and hyperthermia. Hyperthermia was included in the treatment protocol because of its immune stimulating, detoxifying, and disinfecting properties.

Participants of the study were given a series of hyperthermia baths at 102 degrees Fahrenheit, each for a forty minute period.* These baths were administered twice weekly for three weeks at a time, over the course of a year. According to Leanna Standish, Ph.D., N.D., who oversaw the HARP study, participants reported that hyperthermia was the facet of their treatment that had the greatest impact. There was a decrease in night sweats and in the frequency of secondary infection.

The heat levels suggested by the Bastyr University HARP study are thought best for safety, unless the patient is under constant professional supervision.

Also, many participants reported having a greater sense of well-being after receiving hyperthermia treatments.[7]

Treating Other Viral Infections with Hyperthermia

Dr. Lewis states that a hot immersion bath, if done without raising body temperature and heart rate too quickly or too high, can be used as an adjunctive treatment for a "diverse number of diseases—from upper respiratory infections and sexually transmitted diseases to cancer and AIDS." Hyperthermia in the form of hot baths has also proved useful in the treatment of herpes simplex and herpes zoster (shingles). At first the treatment aggravates the situation, but conditions improve considerably after a short time. It is also useful in treating the common cold and flu, as well as chronic fatigue syndrome.

Dr. Lewis has had good results treating chronic fatigue syndrome with hyperthermia. For certain cases, Dr. Lewis prescribes hyperthermia as a form of self-care. In one instance, he suggested a patient take hot tub treatments at home three to four times weekly. "During the following year," Dr. Lewis reports, "her condition improved wonderfully. While not fully recovered, her energy level is substantially higher, and she credits this to her hot tub routine."

Acute viral infection is another condition Dr. Lewis treats with hyperthermia. In one case, a patient came to him suffering from a combination of pneumonia and bronchitis. His infection had initially been treated with natural remedies, and then antibiotics, both of which produced only minor results. Dr. Lewis prescribed two treatments of hyperthermia forty-eight hours apart, with an additional treatment given at home one week later. The patient began to improve with the first treatment and was significantly better by the time of the final treatment. "In treating acute conditions," Dr. Lewis says, "sometimes the patient will have more difficulty tolerating higher temperatures than those who are suffering from chronic conditions. As the fever response is stimulated, however, usually a higher tolerance follows."

The Controversy Surrounding Extracorporeal Hyperthermia

Despite its proven effectiveness in treating disease, including the HIV virus, hyperthermia has been a controversial topic within the AIDS community. The public debate began in 1990, when the television media publicized the story of a man, Carl Crawford, who claimed he had been cured of AIDS at an Atlanta, Georgia hospital due to hyperthermia treatments. Carl said that his Kaposi's sarcoma lesions had disappeared, his T4 cells had gone up, and that his blood had gone from antigen positive to antigen negative. Today, over four years later, he is living a normal life, and is in remission from KS and AIDS. His doctors say he is on no HIV-related medications and is now symptom-free from AIDS.[8]

Carl's treatment, performed by Kenneth Alonso, M.D., and William D. Logan, M.D., of Atlanta, was the first "high flow" extracorporeal hyperthermia treatment on an AIDS patient in the U.S. (High flow means that the blood that is removed from the body and then heated is processed at rate of three to four liters per minute. This is the equivalent of two-thirds of the blood in one's body.)

A second patient (known only as Tony M.) was selected to go through the procedure, and his treatment was filmed live on CNN. Due to the national media attention on this novel medical procedure, and the ensuing controversy caused by the media's heralding of this as a cure before any lengthy scientific research and evaluation could be done, AIDS activists were calling on Drs. Alonso and Logan to make their findings public.

The National Institutes of Health was contacted and invited by Drs. Alonso and Logan to review the two procedures they had performed. After examining Carl and Tony, the NIH, within one month of their site visit, issued a report which stated that Carl did not have KS but "Cat Scratch Disease" and had been only mildly immunosuppressed.[9] The report further stated that the second patient had no visible improvement. It should be noted that this report was in contradiction to previous verbal discussions between Drs. Alonso and Logan during the site visit investigation. The NIH persuaded the Atlanta hospital to suspend future procedures and discouraged other doctors, who were already doing research with hyperthermia for cancer, from using this procedure for KS or AIDS. The NIH asserted from their own laboratory research that heat caused the HIV virus to multiply.[10] However, most researchers have found the opposite to be true and cannot duplicate the NIH's results.[11]

Dr. Alonso contacted Paolo Pontiggia, M.D., then the President of the European Hyperthermia Society, who arranged for the treatment to be performed at the exclusive European Hospital (part of the University of Rome system) and also at the University of Pavia (outside of Milan). As both hospitals performed this procedure regularly as a cancer treatment, it was believed that the procedure might benefit AIDS patients suffering from Kaposi's sarcoma, and they decided to work with patients and physicians from the United States who believed there would be some benefit.[12]

Two of the first American patients to undergo the hyperthermia treatment in Italy were Chuck DeMarco, Jr., and his partner, Michael; both of them had KS and AIDS and were battling a variety of AIDS symptoms. Chuck had to go on disability in 1989 after collapsing from extreme fatigue. He had lost over thirty-five pounds, and had acyclovir-resistant herpes in his lungs, which caused him on occasion to cough up blood. His blood work indicated that he had extremely high titers to CMV and Epstein Barr virus, a CD4 count of about 200, a CD8 count of 760, was p24 antigen positive with a count of over 100, and was culture positive and PCR positive for HIV. Chuck had Kaposi's sarcoma on his thigh, his gum, and posterior wall of his throat. He was sleeping eighteen to twenty hours per day and infectious disease doctors were recommending that he start on AZT. Michael's condition was not much better. He had a CD4 count of about 200, a CD8 count of 900, oral hairy leukoplakia in his mouth, and extensive Kaposi's sarcoma on his face, scalp, and thigh. Michael also had little energy, and like his partner Chuck, had a p24 antigen count of over 100.

Immediately upon hearing of this treatment, Michael and Chuck were off to Atlanta where they met with Dr. Alonso.

Dr. Alonso examined both of them, took a biopsy from Michael's thigh, and told Chuck to have the lesion on his gum biopsied. (Dr. Alonso was not equipped to do Chuck's biopsy due to its location.) Both biopsies were found to be heat sensitive. Dr. Alonso called their personal physician and gave him the list of medical tests necessary to determine if Michael and Chuck were physically fit enough to go through the hyperthermia procedure. Once all the testing was completed and evaluated, they were told that indeed they were candidates for the procedure.[13]

On March 1, 1991, Michael and Chuck met with the team of doctors at the European Hospital who performed the hyperthermia treatment on them the next day. They were examined, their medical records were reviewed, blood was drawn, and the time was set for the next day for them to have the treatment. Michael was the first American PWA to undergo "low flow" extra-corporeal hyperthermia in Rome. (Unlike the high flow procedure in which two-thirds of a patient's blood is circulated through the machine per minute, only 300 to 400 cc's or approximately one pint of blood is circulated out of the body per minute.) This time the procedure was performed using a special device manufactured just for the treatment. Under general anesthesia, Michael's core body temperature was brought up to above 108 degrees Fahrenheit for almost two hours. Chuck was wheeled into the operating room next. Under general anesthesia, Chuck's core body temperature was brought up by the vascular surgeon, Dr. Christian Nardi, to above 108 degrees Fahrenheit, actually spiking to 112 degrees Fahrenheit for approximately fifteen minutes.

Within twenty-four hours, both Michael and Chuck were on their feet and touring Rome. In a diary they kept of their experiences, they mentioned that their lesions began getting white rings around them and seemed to be healing. Chuck's incessant cough had resolved. Both Michael's and Chuck's hairy leukoplakia vanished almost immediately.

Within ten days, Michael and Chuck were back in New Jersey and went to be examined by Andrew Zablow, M.D. He concurred that their KS lesions were indeed in remission, but only time would tell if all of them would react that way. Blood work was drawn at the end of March, and remarkably, there was an increase in both Michael's and Chuck's CD4 and CD8 levels. Chuck, who had been p24 antigen positive pretreatment, was told he was now p24 antigen negative. Both had extreme amounts of energy and excitedly began to rebuild their private lives. They decided not to announce their treatment, as they were not sure that it would have lasting success.[14]

After approximately 120 days, Michael's KS began to reappear in new areas. Believing in this therapy, and the beneficial effects he previously experienced, Michael returned to Rome in June, 1991 to undergo a second treatment. The second treatment had a beneficial effect on his CD4 level but, ultimately, was not successful in halting the progression of his illness. Over the next six months, as Michael's condition worsened, Chuck's condition continued to improve. With Michael's condition as an example, Chuck fully expected his own KS to return, as well as his cough and other symptoms. Chuck and Michael were together until Michael succumbed to fibrosis of the lungs and extensive KS in November, 1991. After many months of mourning the death of his friend, planning his own future, and checking the mirror daily for signs of KS or other opportunistic infections, Chuck began to be convinced that he would not follow the same fate as his partner, Michael. Chuck was in remission, not only from KS, but also from the HIV virus itself.

In December, 1992, twenty-one months after the treatment, Chuck was informed that indeed he was in "Total Clinical Remission" from HIV. He was on a trip to Rome, where blood samples were taken and thoroughly analyzed. The researchers could not believe what they saw. The tests were repeated three times, and performed at three separate independent research laboratories. Not only was Chuck p24 antigen negative, he was now PCR negative, culture negative, and had an average CD4 count of 800 and a CD8 count of 2,800. After returning to the United States, these tests were performed again to check for errors. At a commercial laboratory in Georgia, his PCR test was indeterminate, and he was still culture negative and p24 antigen negative. At a private laboratory he remained PCR and culture negative for HIV, as he does today. Although he continues to test positive for the HIV antibodies, the HIV virus cannot be grown from his blood. He is not on any anti-retrovirals or HIV-related medications. He takes no medications to prevent opportunistic infections. He has a normal healthy lifestyle with a functioning immune system.

So far, about seventy-five Americans have undergone the treatment in Italy. The Italian doctors, who were originally accommodating the American doctors and patients, are now conducting a formal trial of one hundred Italian HIV patients. Variations of the procedure, determined by the patient's condition, render the data collected on the first seventy patients difficult to correlate. Furthermore, the American patients came from several American doctors and cities, making follow-up very difficult. The only information available is what has been published in the medical journals by Drs. Alonso, Pontiggia, and Nardi, as well as other by doctors who are working on this treatment for HIV, cancer, and other viruses.[15]

Chuck DeMarco, Jr., together with other interested individuals who believe that there is merit in the use of hyperthermia, founded HEAT INFO (Hyperthermia Education and Treatment Information, Inc.). This organization continues to advocate for the use of hyperthermia. Chuck has spoken publicly, written articles, and been interviewed for television, radio, newspapers, and magazines. He and HEAT INFO have set their sights on informing our nation's top health officials as well as the general public of the benefits that can be derived from this treatment. With the help of United States Senator Frank Lautenberg of New Jersey, Chuck and HEAT INFO have started dialogues with the National Institute of Allergy and Infectious Diseases, the NIH, the FDA, the Office of the National AIDS Policy Coordinator, and other public health officials in the hopes of bringing this treatment back to America.

Currently there are several companies that have applied to the FDA for approval to do hyperthermia for AIDS. From information that HEAT INFO and Chuck have obtained, it is believed that Phase I Trials will be happening in the United States in late 1994. Presently, these companies have submitted their protocols and information about their devices for FDA consideration.

Hyperthermia is still being performed in both Rome and Pavia, Italy, in addition to trials being conducted on Italian patients. Researchers have also informed HEAT INFO that the treatment may become available to individuals in Mexico, Germany, and the Bahamas by the fall of 1994. HEAT INFO is optimistic that the use of hyperthermia for AIDS will be approved in the United States sometime in 1994.[16]

Risks Associated with Hyperthermia

Hyperthermia is a safe and effective treatment for many conditions when used knowledgeably and with care. Ill effects of

Hyperthermia at Home

Certain forms of hyperthermia can also be employed as part of a self-care regimen, under the supervision of a qualified health care professional. Hot baths are the simplest method of inducing a fever at home, and for viral infections such as HIV, they can be combined with hot drinks and blanket wrapping to stimulate the immune system. After a hot bath, a person can wrap up in dry blankets, with a hot water bottle over the abdomen, in order to perspire heavily for as long as can be tolerated. This may take several hours and should be followed by a cool shower. It is also possible to produce a mild fever with the hot bath by simply wrapping up in the dry blankets after the bath. Again, allow several hours to perspire heavily and follow with a cool shower.

A wet sheet pack may also be used to raise the body temperature. In this case, the patient wraps in a very cold, wet sheet, followed by several blankets. Like the dry pack, it will take several hours to produce a fever, the cold sheet causing reactions in the body that encourage the production of heat. It is often useful to precede this procedure with some kind of heating such as exercise, a hot bath, or a hot shower.

Local hyperthermia can also be useful at times. Inhalation of steam is useful in the treatment of head colds. Hot packs or hot soaks may also be used to treat local conditions. Treatment for an infection in a hand or foot may include immersion in hot water. A local infection that will not allow immersion might be treated with hot packs applied to the area.

hyperthermia usually appear only when body temperatures exceed 106 degrees Fahrenheit. However, certain individuals are more sensitive to the effects of heat and their conditions should be treated with great care and always under professional guidance. These include people with anemia, heart disease, diabetes, seizure disorders, and tuberculosis.

Other reported risks of hyperthermia include herpes outbreaks,[17] liver toxicity,[18] and nervous system injury.

 Hyperthermia should only be undertaken with proper medical supervision.

 # Where to Find Help

American Association of Naturopathic Physicians
2366 Eastlake Avenue, Suite 322
Seattle, Washington 98102
(206) 323-7610
Provides referrals to a nationwide network of accredited or licensed practitioners. Publishes a quarterly newsletter for both professionals and the general public. Also offers a series of brochures and pamphlets on a variety of subjects.

Bastyr University
Natural Health Clinic
1307 North 45th Street, Suite 200
Seattle, Washington 98103
(206) 632-0354
Bastyr University is an accredited educational institution that offers degree programs in the natural health sciences. These include programs in naturopathic medicine, homeopathy, midwifery, acupuncture, nutrition, Chinese herbal medicine, marriage and family counseling, and applied behavioral sciences. Bastyr also offers a limited number of Distance Learning courses in these areas for students unable to attend classes at its Seattle, Washington facility. The physical medicine department of the Natural Health Clinic of Bastyr University uses hyperthermia treatment for detoxification and for conditions ranging from upper respiratory infection to chronic fatigue syndrome and HIV infection.

HEAT INFO (Hyperthermia Education and Treatment Information, Inc.)
409 Washington Street, Box 108
Hoboken, New Jersey 07030
Office/Fax (201) 865-4483

HEAT INFO is a non-profit organization that advocates the use of Hyperthermia as a medical treatment for HIV/AIDS and other diseases. HEAT's goal is to be a source of information for patients and physicians in making informed decisions about hyperthermia as a medical treatment. HEAT acts as an education center and information exchange providing a resource for study and research in hyperthermia. Information is available upon request for a nominal fee.

National College of Naturopathic Medicine
11231 Southeast Market Street
Portland, Oregon 97216
(503) 255-4860

Offers postgraduate training in naturopathic medicine and supports teaching clinics. The teaching clinic uses hyperthermia for a wide variety of conditions.

 # Recommended Reading

Alternative Medicine: The Definitive Guide. The Burton Goldberg Group. Puyallup, WA: Future Medicine Publishing, Inc., 1993.

The most comprehensive reference on alternative medicine ever compiled. Provides in-depth, easily understandable coverage of 43 alternative therapies and over 200 health conditions, with advice from nearly 400 alternative physicians worldwide. See chapters on "Hyperthermia," "Hydrotherapy," and "AIDS."

Home Remedies. Thrash, Agatha, M.D.; and Thrash, Calvin, M.D. Seale, AL: New Lifestyle Books, 1981.

A helpful book for anyone interested in hydrotherapy and home remedies with useful information on hyperthermia treatment.

Lectures in Naturopathic Hydrotherapy. Boyle, Wade, N.D.; and Saine, Andre, N.D. East Palestine, OH: Buckeye Naturopathic Press, 1991.
A useful book on general hydrotherapy topics, including, but not specific to, hyperthermia.

Water Therapy: How to Use Home Water Treatments for Total Health. Chaitow, Leon, N.D., D.O. London: Thorsons/HarperCollins, 1994.
(Distributed by HarperSanFrancisco)
A laymen's guide to modern hydrotherapy in the home. Includes a section on hyperthermia.

"A cheerful heart is good medicine, but a downcast spirit dries up the bones."

—Proverbs 17:22

13 Massage and Touch Therapies

The therapeutic value of massage has been recognized for centuries, its basic principle being simply that touch is beneficial to the body, mind, and spirit. Massage can also have immense benefits for people with AIDS or HIV. The benefits are physical as well as mental and emotional. Physical benefits include improved blood and lymph circulation and drainage, muscular relaxation, and improved mobility of joints. Mental and emotional benefits include reduced stress and a greater sense of ease and well being.[1]

The reduction of stress derived from massage therapy can also have a powerful immune-enhancing benefit. Research at the Miami School of Medicine, Touch Institute, in Miami, Florida, has shown increased natural killer cell activity and other immune system improvements directly related to massage therapy.[2]

The promise which massage therapy holds for helping to treat HIV positive and AIDS patients was acknowledged by the Office of Alternative Medicine at the National Institutes of Health in September, 1993, when they awarded two out of a total of thirty research grants for the study of the effects of massage on HIV positive patients and HIV-exposed infants.

According to Robert King, L.M.T.,[3] past President of the American Massage Therapy Association and Director of the Chicago School of Massage Therapy, massage creates a nurturing, comforting, supportive, and trusting environment in which emotions relating to issues such as death, dying, and sadness emerge. Massage also acts as a catalyst which reinforces touching and hugging in daily life, improving self-image and self-esteem and breaking down feelings of loneliness.

Yet, despite the obvious advantages of massage therapy for someone who is HIV positive or who has AIDS, it is not always readily available. Due to fear, ignorance, and misinformation about how AIDS is contracted, people with AIDS often suffer from the stigma of being social outcasts. The end result is that touch is one of the first things that leave their lives once they are diagnosed.

The movement among therapists to provide massage to people with AIDS began in 1982, at the hospice of San Francisco General Hospital. Irene Smith, Massage Coordinator of the hospice, is credited with launching the program and her first efforts show that the benefits of massage were substantial. She learned that people who were living and working with persons with AIDS were not contracting any illness and that touch would not put the therapist at risk.

Many alternative practitioners now incorporate massage and other forms of bodywork into their protocol for HIV, AIDS, or other immune-compromising illness, including Subhuti Dharmananda, Ph.D., Director, Institute for Traditional Medicine in Portland, Oregon, who utilizes massage along with Chinese herbs and acupuncture as part of a multifactorial approach to treating AIDS patients and those who are HIV positive. Dr. Dharmananda also regularly augments the acupuncture therapy with shiatsu, and his patients report a greater sense of well being as a result.

The Therapeutic Value of Massage

In theory, massage does the same for people with HIV infection as it does for anyone who may be ill. Massage increases the lymphatic flow (one of the body's primary defenses against infection), addresses muscle aches and neuropathy, counteracts touch deprivation, and stimulates the body's natural ability to heal itself.

Robert King provides the following justification for massage therapy for people with AIDS (PWA's):

- Reduced tension, pain, and stress
- Relief of headaches and improved sleep patterns
- Improved breathing after bouts with pneumocystis carinii pneumonia (PCP)
- Reduced discomfort relating to Kaposi's sarcoma and associated lesions
- Improved superficial circulation and suppleness of skin
- Improved lymphatic drainage
- Better response to acupuncture

According to psychologist Tiffany Fields, Ph.D., Director of the Touch Research Institute at the University of Miami School of Medicine, who has been collaborating with Gail Ironson, M.D., Ph.D., on massage therapy and AIDS studies, massage greatly facilitates the healing process. "We were working with HIV positive and HIV negative men and we gave them one forty-five minute massage a day for four weeks," Dr. Fields reports. "We looked at their anxiety levels, their mood states, how they reacted to the massage, and relaxation levels before and after the massage. We also took blood samples and we found that the level of natural killer cells increased over that period of thirty days. Natural killer cells are very important for warding off infections and viruses."

Further work on massage therapy and HIV is being carried out at the University of Miami School of Medicine by Frank Scafidi, Ph.D., who in September, 1993 was awarded one of the thirty research grants from the Office of Alternative Medicine, National Institutes of Health, in order to study the effects of massage on HIV-exposed infants.

Thomas J. Birk, Ph.D., of Medical College of Ohio, believes that any kind of soothing and relaxing massage-type structural manipulation which reduces anxiety and depression may be beneficial in generating the helpful CD4 and natural killer cells. "When stress hormones are high they tend to reduce effectiveness of the immune system, specifically reducing CD4 levels. This prevents CD4 and natural killer cells from doing what they need to do which is killing any infection which enters the body," he says. Dr. Birk also received one of the original thirty research grants from the Office of Alternative Medicine at the National Institutes of Health in order to study the effects of massage therapy on HIV positive patients.

Many patients also report relief from the side effects of opportunistic infections such as pneumocystis carinii pneumonia (PCP), including improved breathing. "The respiratory process is aided by massage," says King. "The muscles involved in respiration—pectoralis major and minor, serratus anterior, the intercostals, and the diaphragm specifically are sensitive to touch, and free up the respiratory process. This also encourages deeper and fuller breaths which is an immune enhancer. By bringing fresh oxygenated air into the body, it facilitates circulation and helps to battle the virus."

Psychoneurological Benefits

The less tangible psychoneurological benefits, such as enhanced mood, outlook, self-esteem, or even sound sleep, are proving to be every bit as positive for immune function. "Patients report that the benefits from a positive sense of touch are that it significantly reduces the sense of isolation and the pain," says Robert King.

Often, low self-esteem and societal pressures are the most difficult obstacles faced by the person with HIV or AIDS. King remembers **Lou**, a former patient:

"Lou was thirty and had been diagnosed for three years and felt that he was rapidly deteriorating. He had open KS lesions and was very self-conscious about being touched.

"The first visit we didn't do a lot of massage. It was mostly touching, meditating, feeling the pulse, being cognizant of his breath, and just being attentive, palliative, looking to reduce pain on any level just through touch. It's not so much what you do with your hands, it's being present tableside which is often significant.

"After just one session his attitude changed remarkably just because he had felt unclean like a leper in the most profound sense of the word. He said that touch significantly increased the quality of his life for the remaining two years.

"Up to the point when he began massage, he was doing all the other things right but still getting worse. But when your self-esteem is dreadful and you have a deep sense of shame from open lesions on your body, you're not going to feel good no matter what kind of drugs or therapy you're taking. The element of touch breaks down some of the self-inflicted barriers which have such a crippling effect on the immune system."

Massaging People with AIDS

Massage Therapist Beth Winson of Los Angeles explains that it is important to carefully assess the condition of each person with AIDS before beginning a session. "When massaging an HIV positive person, the therapist can use a wide variety of massage techniques, just as they would with any client.

People with AIDS Report the Benefits of Massage

The benefits of massage are as varied as the individual. For many, it is a physical experience, and for others, bodywork meets psychological and emotional needs. The following are just a few of the benefits of massage, as described by people with AIDS:

- "Without being able to exercise, massage is the only thing to loosen me up."
- "You don't know how much this means to me. I haven't been touched since I was diagnosed in August 1984."
- "For the first time in months, I had a really good night's sleep."
- "I'm in pain most of the time, and this was a great break from it."
- "Massage gives me relief from pain, tension, and anxiety from being sick."
- "The physical tightness is gone. The social contact is nice too."
- "Numbness leaves. I'm invigorated and renewed."
- "This massage has an almost healing effect—short of biblical proportions, yet mentally just as effective. These sessions are a godsend."
- "I feel my height has been increased another full inch every time he completes his session."
- "Massage contributes to my positive outlook of myself."

However, when massaging a person with AIDS, it may be necessary to focus on relaxation, comfort, and nurturing, rather than deep tissue or very energetic techniques," Winson notes. "Because massage therapy increases blood circulation and can release toxins into the system, the massage should be conservative. Some people with AIDS have cancer or severe pulmonary problems, and most massage techniques other than gentle holding or rocking are contraindicated."

An attentive therapist will ask many questions about the individual's health and then work accordingly, says Winson. If the massage therapist has any questions about how the patient will best benefit from the massage, the therapist should contact the individual's primary care provider.

It is important to note, however, that if the massage therapist is coughing, sneezing, or is the least bit sick, the session should be postponed, as the therapist's germs can be very dangerous to the PWA.

Specific protocols have been established for applying massage to people with AIDS, which explain how to deal with areas of extreme sensitivity, or where skin lesions exist. For example:

- Pressure should not be put directly on visible lesions.
- Deep tissue work is not advisable due to the possibility of internal lesions.
- Gentle massage and balancing techniques are best for people with advanced AIDS-related illnesses.
- Therapist and patient should maintain communication, as lesions and sensitivities may change from day to day.
- For patients experiencing emotional stress, the practitioner can relax the mind through the use of voice modulation and the suggestion of a calming visualization.
- The vigorousness of each treatment should depend on the vitality of each patient.
- If the practitioner is concerned about any rashes, fungi, or anything else related to the patient's current condition, he or she should ask the patient or his or her primary-care provider for information and guidance.

Anyone with AIDS or who is HIV positive and seeking a licensed massage therapist should ensure that the therapist has some background in dealing with this sensitive emotional area. Contact a local chapter of American Massage Therapy Association for the names of accredited therapists.

In many areas, free massage and even acupuncture treatments are available through outreach programs for anyone who is HIV positive. Many volunteer organizations, such as AIDS Project Los Angeles, also offer on-site walk-in treatments.

Other Beneficial Forms of Touch Therapy
According to Alice Hiatt, R.N., of Berkeley, California, many types of bodywork or touch therapy can be beneficial to the

immune compromised person, including reflexology, shiatsu, acupressure, or Therapeutic Touch.

"Foot reflexology is particularly helpful for aches and pain [as] the whole body can be affected through the feet," says Hiatt. She also uses an acupressure technique called *jin shin*, a method of using acupressure points to reduce swelling that may be occurring in the feet, face, or hands, decrease pain in a joint, or help to clear up the lungs of a patient with pneumocystis carinii pneumonia (PCP).

The *shiatsu* technique is recommended by Hiatt for its emotional healing capabilities. "Shiatsu can be a very gentle kind of a rocking, very rhythmic form of massage that addresses the energy line and helps to calm the spirit, calm the fears," she says. "The person is going through incredible loss, so it helps to strengthen them and helps them to balance. At the same time, shiatsu is really powerful for the immune system, which is ultimately what we're looking for."

The gentle healing of Therapeutic Touch™ is also beneficial to the immune-compromised individual. An energy-based system of bodywork developed by Dolores Krieger, Ph.D., R.N., Professor Emerita at New York University, and Dora Kunz, Therapeutic Touch is a contemporary interpretation of several ancient healing practices. It is one of the few therapies that has been clinically documented, and is practiced and accepted in many hospital situations. Dr. Krieger has taught Therapeutic Touch to over 40,000 nurses and health professionals and it is has been taught in seventy-three countries worldwide. In September 1993, the Office of Alternative Medicine at the National Institutes of Health awarded a research grant to Melodie A. Olson, Ph.D., of the Medical University of South Carolina, to study the effects of Therapeutic Touch upon the immune response to stress.

"The most reliable result we see from Therapeutic Touch is that we can get a relaxation response within two to four minutes," says Dr. Krieger, "which is faster than biofeedback. Secondly, Therapeutic Touch significantly reduces pain, and thirdly, it accelerates the healing process, particularly with pneumocystis carinii pneumonia (PCP) and other opportunistic infections. For this reason, it is considered to have a significant relationship to the immune system.

"We have one fairly well-documented case of the successful use of Therapeutic Touch with Kaposi's sarcoma," continues Dr. Krieger. "The lesions cleared up, although [the treatment] did not affect the underlying AIDS, as they are two different entities."

 # Where to Find Help

Alternative Medicine Yellow Pages. **The Burton Goldberg Group. Puyallup, WA: Future Medicine Publishing, Inc., 1994.**
Lists over 16,000 practitioners of alternative medicine in the United States and Canada. Practitioners are listed by therapy, city, and state. See sections on "Aromatherapy," "Bodywork," "Chiropractic," "Flower Remedies," "Hydrotherapy," "Mind/ Body Medicine," "Osteopathy," "Qigong," and "Yoga."

Massage

American Massage Therapy Association
1130 West North Shore Avenue
Chicago, Illinois 60626-4670
(312) 761-2682
Offers comprehensive information on most areas of massage and bodywork, including an extensive review of scientific research. They also publish the Massage Therapy Journal, *available at many newsstands and health food stores.*

Acupressure and Oriental Body Therapies

Acupressure Institute
1533 Shattuck Avenue
Berkeley, California 94709
(510) 845-1059
For information, career trainings, and mail order catalog.

American Oriental Bodywork Association
6801 Jericho Turnpike
Syosset, New York 11791
(516) 364-5533
For information, professional membership, practitioner directory,
and referrals.

Reflexology

International Institute of Reflexology
P.O. Box 12462
St. Petersburg, Florida 33733
(813) 343-4811
For information, seminars, publications, and referrals.

Therapeutic Touch

Nurse Healers—Professional Associates, Inc.
175 Fifth Avenue, Suite 2755
New York City, New York 10010
(212) 886-3776
Cooperative among health professionals interested in healing.

Recommended Reading

Alternative Medicine: The Definitive Guide. The Burton
Goldberg Group. Puyallup, WA: Future Medicine Publishing,
Inc., 1993.
The most comprehensive reference on alternative medicine ever
compiled. Provides in-depth, easily understandable coverage of 43
alternative therapies and over 200 health conditions, with advice
from nearly 400 alternative physicians worldwide. See chapters on
"Aromatherapy," "Bodywork," "Chiropractic," "Flower
Remedies," "Hydrotherapy," "Mind/Body Medicine,"
"Osteopathy," "Qigong," and "Yoga."

Massage

The Book of Massage. Lidell, Lucinda. New York: Fireside, 1984.
Excellent step-by-step instructional guide with extensive color illustrations on massage, shiatsu, and reflexology techniques.

The Massage Book. Downing, George. New York: Random House, 1972.
Considered the "classic book" on massage.

Massage for Common Ailments. Thomas, Sara. New York: Fireside, 1989.
A simple, comprehensive, step-by-step guide on how to alleviate a range of everyday health problems through massage and shiatsu techniques. Extensive color illustrations.

Acupressure and Oriental Body Therapies

Acupressure's Potent Points. Gach, Michael, R. New York: Bantam Books, 1990.
Written in clear, accessible language with photographs and easy-to-follow line drawings, the book shows how to utilize acupressure on others as well as yourself.

Acu-Yoga: The Acupressure Stress Management Book: Developed to Relieve Stress and Tension. Gach, Michael, R. Tokyo & New York: Japan Publications, 1981.
A comprehensive, highly instructive handbook describing the origin, practice, and benefits of acupressure and yoga, with illustrations, diagrams, exercises, and self-help techniques designed to address a variety of health problems.

The Complete Book of Shiatsu Therapy. Namikoshi, Toru. Tokyo & New York: Japan Publications, 1981.
A thorough scientifically-oriented text and guidebook on shiatsu.

Reflexology

Better Health with Foot Reflexology. Byers, Dwight. St. Petersburg, FL: Ingham Publishing, 1987.
This book is a practical guide that includes an introduction to each anatomical system of the body and step-by-step instructions in applying the tenets of reflexology.

Body Reflexology: Healing at Your Fingertips. Carter, Mildred. West Nyack, NY: Parker Publishing Co., 1986.
The author of several other books on foot and hand reflexology integrates the whole body. Shows safe and easy-to-use methods to relieve pain and discomfort and promote renewed health.

Hand and Foot Reflexology: A Self-Help Guide. Kunz, Kevin; and Kunz, Barbara. New York: Simon and Schuster, 1987.
A comprehensive, hands-on encyclopedia of personal reflexology. Informative, fully illustrated, with step-by-step procedures, including treatment plans for specific ailments from acne to whiplash.

Therapeutic Touch

Accepting Your Power to Heal: Personal Practice of Therapeutic Touch. Krieger, Dolores. Santa Fe: Bear and Company, 1993.
Dr. Krieger's most recent book, especially developed for use by lay people in the home as well as for professionals in health agencies. In-depth details on using Therapeutic Touch in treating over two dozen ailments.

Living the Therapeutic Touch: Healing as Lifestyle. Krieger, Dolores. Wheaton, IL: Quest Books, 1988.
The original book on Therapeutic Touch practice, now in its twenty-seventh edition, has become a classic. This book teaches the reader how to do Therapeutic Touch starting with the simplest beginning steps through the intermediate phase.

Therapeutic Touch: A Practical Guide. McCrae, Janet. New York: Knopf, 1992.
A guide to using graceful, sweeping movements of the hands, a few inches from the body, to scan the patient's energy flow, replenish it where necessary, release congestion, remove obstruction, and generally restore order and balance in the diseased system.

"The greatest discovery of any generation is that human beings can alter their lives by altering the attitudes of their minds."

—*Albert Schweitzer*

Part Three:
Long-Term
Survivors

"The natural force within each one of us is the greatest healer of disease."

—*Hippocrates*

14 Success Stories: The Patient-Physician Partnership

As we have seen, AIDS is not necessarily a fatal disease. It is reasonable to assume that in the near future it will be seen as a chronic, manageable disease because of the many long-term HIV/ARC/AIDS survivors already known across the world. And the numbers of these survivors are increasing daily. Most of them are using a range of alternative treatments coupled with conventional medical approaches. All of these extraordinary individuals see themselves as *living with* AIDS, rather than slowly dying from it.

All successful approaches to treating AIDS and its related illnesses require a true partnership between the patient and physician, as well as a willingness on the part of the patient to do whatever it takes in order to get well. As Dr. George Solomon of the University of San Francisco School of Medicine, who interviewed long-term AIDS survivors, found, "survivors accept the reality of their diagnosis, but refused to see the condition as a death sentence. . . . They thought of their physicians as collaborators and tended to take responsibility for their health. They were inclined to think they could influence their health outcome. . . . They still had a great deal they wanted to do [in the way of] 'unfinished business.'"[1]

This chapter will report upon long-term AIDS survivors and the work of a number of physicians and scientists who have developed successful alternative approaches to AIDS and HIV infection. Many of these approaches, including those of Laurence Badgley, M.D., Jon Kaiser, M.D., Joan Priestley, M.D., and Dr. Gerhard Orth of Germany, have multifactorial protocols that focus on improving nutritional status, strengthening the immune system, combating opportunistic infections, and addressing the patient's emotional and spiritual needs.

Other therapies take a specific therapeutic approach, such as the vitamin C megadose therapy of Robert Cathcart III, M.D., the antineoplaston therapy of Stanislaw Burzynski, M.D., Ph.D., the L-51 therapy of Ignacio Coronel, M.D., and the Somatidian Orthobiology of Gaston Naessens. Vitamin C acts to suppress the symptoms of AIDS and reduce the tendency to secondary infections. Antineoplaston therapy directly acts to reprogram dysfunctioning immune system cells. L-51 therapy interrupts HIV's cycle of replication. Gaston Naessens 714-X helps to fluidify the lymph in order to help in the removal of toxins from the body.

Jon Kaiser, M.D.

Jon Kaiser, M.D., is a primary-care physician based in San Francisco who specializes in natural therapies and mind/body medicine. Dr. Kaiser has been working with AIDS patients for ten years, and he reports that 70 percent of his patients are HIV positive. He has tracked the progress of patients following his treatment protocol over a four-and-one-half-year period and reports a stability rate of 90 percent, meaning that these patients either improved or did not further decline in their diagnosis. The survival rate during that same period was 98 percent. There were only three deaths out of 134 patients, including thirty who had full blown AIDS symptoms.

There are six categories in Dr. Kaiser's AIDS/HIV protocol:

- Diet
- Vitamins and Nutritional Supplements
- Herbs
- Exercise
- Stress Reduction and Positive Attitude
- Medical Therapies

"If somebody comes to me who is asymptomatic but not in any crisis, we examine each of these six categories in order to come up with a set of very thorough and complete recommendations for that individual," Dr. Kaiser explains. "My experience has shown me that by combining these six categories in an integrated protocol, you create a much stronger program for maintaining a healthy immune system than by utilizing only one or any other smaller combination.

"The first five categories form a very strong support for the immune system," Dr. Kaiser continues. "If the first five categories are not 100 percent sufficient for maintaining stability and keeping the viral infection dormant, then the sixth category, medical therapies, can be added. This approach allows you to use less medication, with less side effects, and greater therapeutic effectiveness, than if medication alone was the central pillar of the treatment program, which is the approach of most physicians. I find that when you add medical therapies at this point in the program, whether you are treating HIV, arthritis, or irritable bowel syndrome, the person will need very little medication due to the supporting therapies. This has been the most pleasing and eye opening part of my work."

Diet

Most of the people who come to see Dr. Kaiser have an immune system imbalance. His "Immune Enhancement Diet," detailed in his book *Immune Power: A Comprehensive Treatment Program for HIV*, has both specific and general recommendations for strengthening the immune system.

The diet is 50 percent whole grains, 25 percent vegetables, and 25 percent high quality protein (by volume). Fruits and nuts and seeds are included as snacks, and dairy products are kept to a maximum of 5 percent. Half of the high-quality protein can be derived from vegetarian sources and the other half can be from healthfully-raised animal products such as poultry, fish, and beef. A limited amount of protein will come from dairy products. If the person desires to get all their protein from vegetarian sources, they have to be sure to get adequate amounts. Dr. Kaiser also recommends minimizing the use of processed foods, processed sweeteners, caffeine, and alcohol.

Nutritional Supplements

The second category in Dr. Kaiser's program is nutritional supplements. "The vast majority of nutritional research has shown that even if HIV positive individuals consume excessive amounts of nutrients in their diet, their percentages of nutrient deficiencies are still much higher than is normal," notes Dr. Kaiser. "These deficiencies include vitamin B_2, vitamin B_6, vitamin B_{12}, vitamin E, copper, and zinc. It is my belief that HIV is going to be the first medical condition in which high dose nutrient supplements become the standard of care regarding early treatment."

Dr. Kaiser recommends a high-potency multivitamin with additional antioxidant supplements, including vitamin C, vitamin E, beta-carotene, zinc, and selenium. The daily dosage ranges are as follows:

- Vitamin C (4-12 grams/day)
- Beta-carotene (50-100,000 IU/day)
- Vitamin E (400-1,200 IU/day)
- Zinc (50-75 mg/day)
- Selenium (100-200 mcg/day)
- Co-Enzyme Q-10 (50 mg/two-three times daily)
- NAC (N-Acetyl-l-Cysteine) (500 mg/two-six times daily)

"NAC is a type of amino acid precursor that supplements glutathione, the key amino acid the body uses to support its antioxidant toxin-clearing functions," says Dr. Kaiser. "If you build up too many toxins, HIV activity is enhanced. If you do not have enough glutathione, the 'exhaust system' starts backing up, HIV becomes more active, and you are going to start a whole cascade of increased HIV activity and decline. NAC is stable when taken orally and glutathione is not. For this reason, NAC needs to be a part of the supplement program."

Herbs

The third category in Dr. Kaiser's protocol is herbs. The herbal regime he recommends centers around a product called "Resist,"[2] a Chinese herbal formula comprised of seventeen different herbs that are gentle but effective in supporting the immune system and keeping a person with HIV strong and balanced. The main herbs are astragalus, ligustrum, licorice, atractylodes, and ganoderma mushroom.

Dr. Kaiser uses other herbs to treat symptoms, as well. "If a person is very nervous or anxious, I recommend chamomile and valerian, which are North American herbs," he says. "If a person has upset stomach, I recommend the mints and ginger." The individual herbs allow Dr. Kaiser to create highly individualized programs for his patients rather than having them follow a standardized recipe for health.

"We want patients to understand how these things work and to create a fluid, individualized program," Dr. Kaiser stresses. "By listening to one's body, and giving it what it needs, a person can have the most positive benefit from this type of program. That is why I list categories and give general recommendations, but provide specifics that one individual will focus on more than another based on their particular needs."

Exercise

The fourth category in Dr. Kaiser's protocol is exercise, which he includes in the program because it reduces stress, strengthens immune function, and improves circulation which enhances the body's ability to carry nutrients to the deep recesses of the organs as well as to clean out waste products. He recommends that at least 50 percent of one's regimen be aerobic exercise, as it increases heart rate, promotes sweating, and promotes deep breathing, which all enhance the circulation of the lymphatic system.

"Exercise is very important," notes Dr. Kaiser. "However, it is much easier to over-exercise than to under-exercise, so people need to listen to their bodies, and if they feel tired the day after they exercise, they overdid it. If they feel better, it was just right. The reason over-exercising is bad is because your immune system utilizes your surplus of energy to carry out its activities. The immune system is actually one of the last systems of the body in line for energy. If you deplete your energy through too much exercise, it will take away from the energy that's available to the immune system and the immune system will function at a lower level."

Stress Reduction and Positive Attitude

The fifth category in Dr. Kaiser's protocol is stress reduction and positive attitude. "It is important not only to look outside of yourself for your healing, but also to look within," he says. "The inner work that a person can do on the emotional and spiritual level is of paramount importance in promoting the experience of emotions that enhance immune functions, such as joy, comfort, safety, love, and happiness. The bottom line of this program is that you need to enjoy your life, to grow and to have meaning in your life, as well as to feel like you have positive goals that you are working towards. If these things are not present, one needs to take a very serious look at why they are absent and what changes need to be made to increase these experiences."

The therapy Dr. Kaiser uses is insight-oriented, helping patients "to open up and look inside in order to see why they are or are not happy and how to maximize their enjoyment and fulfillment in life." As a means of helping them get to this point, he has created a set of three relaxation/affirmation tapes that are about fifteen to twenty minutes in length.[3]

"The real challenge is how to accomplish feeling really good about yourself, enjoying your life, and having goals, and growing and that's something that's going to be different for every individual," states Dr. Kaiser.

"It is very heartwarming to talk to patients who have literally transformed their lives," he continues. "Although this might sound strange, many of my patients say that in many ways HIV has actually been a gift to them. When patients look back after five, six, or eight years to examine the quality of their lives when they were first diagnosed and compare it to the joy and fulfillment they are experiencing in their lives right now, they realize it would not have happened unless they were presented with such a challenge."

Medical Therapies

The sixth and final category in Dr. Kaiser's protocol is medical therapies. "Many people will not need medical therapies because the rest of the program is working so well," notes Dr. Kaiser. "They do not need medical therapies if their T-cell tests indicate that they are either stable or improving and are asymptomatic, regardless of their prior condition. However, if a person's T-cell numbers are going in a downward trend despite treatment in the other five categories (never making this decision based on just one test due to their frequent inaccuracy), then I would recommend antivirals to the program without hesitation. I recommend starting at initial dosages which are gentle, and which, when combined with the rest of the program, tend to give a beneficial effect."

Dr. Kaiser's Patients

John is a forty-seven-year-old gay white male who initially tested positive for HIV back in 1985 while living in Los Angeles, although he dates his infection back to 1980. "His initial T-cell count was 757," notes Dr. Kaiser. "As soon as he found out he was HIV positive, he got on a comprehensive healing program." Between 1985 and 1994 his T-cell count fluctuated a bit up and down, but his last test showed that his T-helper cell number was 730. During this time he moved up to San Francisco. He has had to really make several sacrifices to enable him to be on this type of program, and has had some very difficult times emotionally and with regards to his career path, but he's been completely asymptomatic. He has not needed to use any drugs or medications."

Michael, a gay white male, initially came to see Dr. Kaiser in February of 1988, when he was thirty years old. His T-cell number was 234. He did not have any HIV symptoms but he complained of being overweight, of having chronic muscle spasms, and of having chronic anxiety. "When I looked at his nutrition, back in 1988, his diet was heavy on pizza, fast food, processed meats, and fried foods," says Dr. Kaiser. "Although he had recently started taking an herbal formula for HIV, he was not taking any vitamins, was not exercising or doing anything to reduce his stress, and was not happy with his work. He also complained of a lot of intestinal gas, and heartburn.

"We immediately improved his diet, by putting him on the immune enhancement diet, and started a vitamin and herbal regimen," continues Dr. Kaiser. "He began exercising three times a week, listening to the relaxation tapes, and he got very involved in practicing Buddhist meditation. A few years ago he went to live at a Buddhist monastery for six months. He was living on the land, growing and eating organic foods, and was completely vegetarian. While he was there his T-cell count went up to 520, the highest level it had ever been. Getting out of the hectic life-pattern and becoming very connected to the natural rhythm, both externally and internally, really had a good affect on him.

"Michael decided to come back to San Francisco, and was able to find a more rewarding job. As of February 1994, his T-helper cell count was 350, which is still higher than it was six years ago, and he has been asymptomatic the whole time. He has worked very hard to achieve this healing. He quit smoking cigarettes, very rarely drinks alcohol, meditates, and has been able to come back and integrate these elements all together while living in the city and working at a regular job."

Stephen knew he was HIV positive when he first came to see Dr. Kaiser in 1991. He had been following a very strong, natural program, but he had never gotten his T cells tested and assumed that because he was following such a strong natural program and was only experiencing some fatigue, that he was doing fine. "We got his T cells tested and his first T-cell number was 89, which was very low," notes Dr. Kaiser. "By that low number it was clear to me that even though he had not become sick yet, that there was a clear inadequacy in his treatment program up to that point.

"I put Stephen on an antiviral because he was declining even while following a strong natural protocol. We made some adjustments to his natural program, and three months after being on antivirals, his T4s went up from 89 to 141 and his T8s went up from 524 to 869 (ideally, you want both the T4s and T8s to go up), and he reported a large decrease in his fatigue. When antivirals are used by themselves, they usually create an initial rise in T-cell counts and then the decline resumes.

"Over the next four years, Stephen has switched from one antiviral to another to keep the program fresh, and his numbers have now gone up to 173 for the T4s and 786 for the T8s," says Dr. Kaiser. "This is a case in which the program may not have been able to completely rebuild his immune system, but it has kept him healthy and given him measurable improvement over a significant period of time. The most important thing is that he has not been seriously ill one day during the entire four years and has no symptoms."

Frederick dates his HIV exposure back to 1980. Dr. Kaiser started working with him in 1987. "His T-cell count was 621, and he was asymptomatic, working full time at a fairly stressful job that he enjoyed nevertheless," states Dr. Kaiser.

"Frederick made sure several times a day to take these quiet time breaks and do his meditations. His count actually went from 621 in 1987 to 900 in 1991. For the following year and a half, his count went down from 900 to 350.

"During this time we tried everything we could think of to naturally turn around this downward progression," Dr. Kaiser continues. "In April of 1993, when his count was down to 350, I decided we needed to add antivirals. We added ddI and his numbers were up to 569 one month later. Since May of 1993, he has maintained a T-cell count above 500 on the ddI. If he were to decline again on two successive occasions, I would switch to a different antiviral to keep the program fresh."

Dr. Kaiser finds that once a person goes on an antiviral, it is very risky to completely remove the antiviral from the program at a later date. "My experience has been that when people stop the antiviral there seems to be a deficiency in the program and the HIV becomes active again," he says. "Therefore, even though Frederick's count went back up over 500, I have recommended that he keep the antiviral as part of the program, and I think that it has been the right thing for him to do, because fourteen years after he first became exposed he has no symptoms and his T cells still remain over 500. He has been one of those people who have required an antiviral and clearly benefited from it.

"Of course in the future we are going to keep working on all of the levels of the program to make them as strong as possible," Dr. Kaiser concludes. "If the stress from Frederick's job becomes overbearing, I will not hesitate to recommend that he either switch to a different job or that he go on disability or whatever it takes to keep things in balance."

Joan Priestley, M.D.

Joan Priestley, M.D., of Anchorage, Alaska, takes an aggressive approach toward healing with her patients. She reports that her five-part alternative healing program, which works by empowering the individual with vital choices regarding treatment, has resulted in most of her 700 HIV/AIDS patients becoming asymptomatic.

The first point of her program is a lifestyle change which she expects from each of her patients. Those individuals who smoke, drink, or do recreational drugs, must eliminate such practices from their lives. "Even a light-to-moderate smoker or drinker, if HIV positive, is still a person with a death wish in action," Dr. Priestley says. She is also emphatic about the disuse of recreational drugs because they also suppress the immune system.

Diet is the second factor in returning to good health. "AIDS patients need more protein than the general population seems to require," says Dr. Priestley. She recommends a high protein diet of quality foods, and suggests they obtain protein specifically from chicken, fish, eggs, and soybean products such as tofu, tempeh, and soy milk. She tells them to stay away from any other animal meat and all dairy products except for yogurt. Dr. Priestley's diet is largely a fresh, whole foods diet, mostly vegetarian, with a strict avoidance of processed foods.

Vitamin and mineral supplements, the third aspect of the program, figure prominently in Dr. Priestley's protocol. She considers vitamin C, beta-carotene, garlic, and zinc to be the four most important nutrients. "I usually recommend a package of supplements called the Jarrow Pack (from Jarrow Industries in Los Angeles). What's in there is really brilliantly conceived." The supplements are taken once a day, along with a 100 milligram zinc supplement. Her supplement program includes calcium, magnesium, chromium, and vanadium.

Quercetin is another supplement employed by Dr. Priestley. A bioflavinoid found in citrus fruit rind, it appears to be effective in blocking the AIDS virus much in the same way that AZT does, but without the toxic side effects, according to Dr. Priestley. "I have my patients take 1,000 milligrams of quercetin. I use the kind with bromelain, which is a really good combination, so they take 300 milligrams of bromelain with 1,000 milligrams of quercetin."

The fourth part of her program consists of miscellaneous natural compounds, occasionally including drugs such as ddC, Flucongizol, Bactrim, and Peptide-T, which aggressively combat a number of viruses, bacteria, and fungi.

"The AIDS virus today is a more vicious bug than the one we saw in 1980," says Dr. Priestley. "Because there has been so much unrestrained use of AZT, we know that the virus becomes resistant to AZT within about six months. The virus also becomes resistant to ddI and ddC, and with the excessive use of AZT, we have started seeing a multiple drug resistant virus passed around now. In addition, there seems to be millions of strains of the AIDS virus which have evolved, and several major strains which are very deadly to the nervous system. The person infected with that strain quickly deteriorates neurologically. We didn't see that at first.

"It has been my conviction for the longest time that the standard Western medicines used in AIDS cases, specifically, AZT, and to some extent ddI, will simply shorten life rather than extend it." continues Dr. Priestley. "AZT, for instance, has been found to deplete T8 cells within two years. When I heard that, I said, 'Oh, I got it!' That's the missing link. That's why people live for two years and then they die. T8 cells are very important for survival."

The drug ddC has appeared to be the least toxic of the three drugs approved by the FDA to date. But Dr. Priestley does not recommend any of them. "Often, patients insist on taking one of those deadly poisons," Dr. Priestley says. She then suggests they use ddC because it is the most benign.

There is also an impending change in the way that T cells are evaluated. "We used to think that the T4 cell, also called the helper cell, was the key marker for disease progression: low T cells equals severe AIDS. Now we know that the T8 cell is more important," Dr. Priestley says. "The level of the T8 cells and the quality of the person's life are the two things I believe are most important."

Dr. Priestley also uses another diagnostic test called the CBC, which measures red cells, white cells, and cell fragments called platelets. "The white cells are significant because when the type of white cell called the T cell goes down, the total white cell count goes down also, so you want to see what the white cell count is. The red cells are significant because many patients develop anemia for one reason or another during this infection and the anemia needs to be corrected," says

Dr. Priestley, noting that anemia all by itself appears to suppress the immune system and can be easily treated.

In her protocol, Dr. Priestley also uses herbs to enhance the immune system. She considers garlic to be very effective and suggests that patients avoid the deodorized version. St. John's Wort is another immune-enhancing herb. She also recommends several Japanese herbs, using all of the mushrooms: *shiitake*, *maitake*, *lentinan*, and *reishi*, both separately and in combination with each other. "I am involved with a *maitake* study and I am involved in a special *lentinan* study right now, and they are both very good as immune modulators," she says.

Peptide T, a little known protein developed by Candace Pert, Ph.D. (former Chief of the Section on Brain Biochemistry of the Clinical Neuroscience Branch at the National Institute of Mental Health), has been quite effective in treating AIDS, despite the difficulty in obtaining it, reports Dr. Priestley. "Peptide T prevents the virus from getting inside the cells," she says. "It is like a floating key that 'leaves a key broken off in the lock' on the cell surface. When the virus tries to penetrate a cell it can't get in."

Dr. Priestley considers the fifth point of her protocol, the spiritual aspect, to be the most important point. "If you have a crummy attitude you will sabotage the other parts of the therapy program, so attitude adjustment is definitely necessary," she says. "Some of these people have horrible experiences in their past that still color their outlook. They need to handle these issues."

She also includes acupuncture, exercise, and massage, as well as getting out and contributing to the community, as other parts of the fifth point of her program. "We have men who are thirty years old with Ph.D.'s who are on disability because they lost their jobs, and they are sitting around watching soap operas all day long. They are not expressing their creativity, and they are not empowering themselves. You can see how absurd it is, in light of this, for a doctor to say, 'Here, take AZT five times a day, and ignore all this other stuff. You'll do fine,'" she says.

She also encourages individuals to be mindful of their thoughts. "Stop yourself if you are thinking things that scare you. Don't ever say things like, 'This weather's killing me.'

Your unconscious hears it, and doesn't understand that you don't really mean it," she explains.

Doctor Priestley believes that the combination of diet, supplements, and spirituality create the most noticeable results in the shortest period of time. She says that within thirty days her patients usually report how improved they feel. To help this process, she recommends that patients read supportive books such as *Living In The Light* by Shakti Gawain, *Creating Money* by Sanaya Roman and Duane Packer, and *Beyond AIDS* by George Melton.

Dr. Priestley's Patients

"**Mark** is truly an extraordinary success story," Dr. Priestley relates. "When he came to me in April of 1991, he weighed 115 pounds, having lost forty pounds or so gradually. He had relentless diarrhea, and anyone with diarrhea is suffering from malabsorption. They have to be fed through a vein. Mark was making all sorts of noise because his parents were coming in two weeks and he didn't want to be involved with catheters, and bags of fluid hanging from him. I said, 'Mark, you have to let me insert a catheter to feed you, and you must let me do it to you now.' I am usually not that adamant, but he had at that point about a three month life expectancy just because of his crummy labs and his diarrhea, his chronic dehydration, and his weight loss. No one can continue that and live, so you have to cut that cycle off by doing something very aggressive. His other doctors didn't recognize that. Fortunately, Mark decided to start a program of intravenous feeding."

Mark was placed on a program of total parenteral nutrition (TPN), a standard medical process that has been developed over the last twenty years, and involves a twelve-hour intravenous drip at home when the patient cannot eat or digest food, or has serious diarrhea. TPN is not used sufficiently or appropriately in AIDS patients, Dr. Priestley feels. "This is really a very standard medical procedure," she says. "It's just that doctors don't recognize that when someone loses weight drastically, like Mark had, that there is a high risk of developing a fatal infection. Weight loss suppresses the immune system, and doctors don't recognize how important it is for people to maintain their weight.

"Mark was the winner. Doctors tell you that once people lose weight to that extent you can't replace it. That is an absolute myth! Mark went from 115 pounds, gradually over the next six months or so, up to 155 pounds. TPN saved his life, obviously. It increases muscle mass; it increases stamina and energy. The company I was working with let me put vitamins right into the TPN formula, including fifty grams of vitamin C every day. That turned him around. Mark is a medical miracle and because of his case his other doctors have recognized the value of feeding someone by whatever means necessary. He really should have been dead two years ago, maybe three years ago actually."

Mark describes himself as a long-term survivor. He was diagnosed six years ago as HIV positive and has had AIDS for five years. At one point he had almost no T cells, and now he's up to twenty-six. He also takes a "3-pack," a clay supplement that dissolves in water, which he drinks twice a day. He previously suffered from Crohn's disease. At this time, his MAI (Mycobacterium avium intracellulare) infection has left his system, and he often has no symptoms despite his very low T-cell count. All the medicines he is currently taking are preventative to guard against infection.

Mark walks daily and uses an exercise machine for toning. He's been using acupuncture and herbs for over a year and practices Buddhist chanting twice a day. He affirms, "I think of myself in HIV recovery, not destined to die. It's a chronic disability. I read and correspond with people, shop for the house a lot, take naps, go to movies, and enjoy my life. My wife is my rock.

"After the fear, anger, and denial has passed, if you can look at AIDS as a challenge and understand that it came into your life for a reason, it doesn't mean that you have to die or that your expectancy is just a few years," says Mark. "You can learn from it. I'm thankful I became HIV positive. It forced me to look at so many parts of my life. Half of HIV and AIDS is physical, the other half is psychological and filled with guilt and denial. If you address those things, that's half the battle. Don't feel victimized. Look at it as a challenge that can be overcome. You have to take responsibility for your disease and your life. Once you realize you don't have to hide from being HIV positive, you can take control and decide your own fate."

Michael was tested six years ago when he had a case of hepatitis which caused his lymph glands to become swollen. When he was diagnosed as HIV positive, his only symptom was swollen glands. He explains, "The conventional medical doctor wanted me to take AZT, but according to everything I'd read, I did not want to put such a highly toxic drug into my body. Then I went to a seminar about holistic medicine and HIV. The speakers were Will Garcia, George Melton, and Dr. Laurence Badgley. These men got rid of serious symptoms through alternative medicine and meditation. Hearing them speak was the beginning of empowerment in my life. After that, I started with Dr. Priestley's protocol. Since then, my lymph gland swellings have gone down. Blood tests are stable and dramatically improved (T4s were 400, now 600-750; ratio .34, now .72). I'm diabetic too, but have had no symptoms for the past four years."

To abet his recovery, Michael receives acupuncture and chiropractic treatments once a week, as well as seeing a naturopathic doctor once every three months, all as part of his approach towards dealing with the spiritual and emotional aspects of HIV and healing.

Laurence Badgley, M.D.

There is no perfect regimen, perfect protocol, or perfect group of vitamins, minerals, and nutrients for an immune compromised person to take, according to Laurence E. Badgley, M.D.,[4] of Foster City, California. "I suggest that the individual familiarize him- or herself with as much as is out there— review all the literature, and then construct his or her own program, in order to empower his- or herself to take control. By creating something that has a positive quality, something one will do everyday, one sends positive messages to the brain that their intention is to heal. This attitude alone will feed back to the brain and arouse positive changes in functioning of the immune system," says Dr. Badgley.

"The goal when choosing the natural approach to boosting immune system function is to create a balance in the body. The patient must put enough good things in and take enough bad things out. They don't have to create a so-called 'perfect combination,' but they have to do enough," Dr. Badgley continues. "Dietary changes, certain vitamins and minerals, herbal medicines, meditation, some mind/body work, and exercise can comprise many types of different programs for many different types of bodies. Different people come to natural therapies programs from many different backgrounds. One person might come from his hot dog world. In his case, you start by inducing him to go from hot dogs to soy beans, for example."

Dr. Badgley believes that the ultimate goal of natural therapists is to alter the course of the disease process by boosting the immune system and to teach patients how to avoid negative co-factors. "Nutrition is the foundation of natural therapy," he says. "Broad segments of the American population have been proven to be deficient in specific vitamins and minerals, which are critical to immune system function. For example, persons with AIDS have been discovered to be deficient in folic acid, selenium, zinc, and iron."

In Dr. Badgley's study of thirty-six HIV positive individuals, each was encouraged to "take charge" of their situation. This was implemented through dietary changes, nutritional supplementation, meditation, exercise, and a positive outlook. Many participants used homeopathic remedies and/or acupuncture, as well.

The results of the six month study are as follows:

- Eighty-three percent of participants said their health improved.
- T-4 cell count increased 13 percent, from an average of 378 to 427.
- Average body weight increased.

The study participants took an average of 35 percent of their diet as uncooked "live" foods, and an average of 9.6 glasses of freshly squeezed vegetable and fruit juices per week.

Each day, most of the participants ingested a mixture of carotenoid pigments derived from algae. "Recently, certain algae pigments have been discovered to enhance immune system function," Dr. Badgley notes. About 80 percent of the participants used supplementary vitamins and minerals. Fifty-six percent of the study participants used medicinal herbs and mushrooms. Eighty-five percent of the participants reported that their orthodox physicians supported their nutritional programs. The average yearly expense per person for nutritional supplements and herbal preparations was $1,582.

Seventy-two percent of the participants exercised three times a week, including walking, weight lifting, and calisthenics. The two highest T-cell counts were found in persons who were long distance runners. Additionally, 82 percent of the participants used acupuncture, 25 percent did weekly sweats via sauna or steam bath, and 81 percent took homeopathic remedies. Almost everyone in the study believed that they could "control their health." Dr. Badgley reports that 47 percent of the participants were in a supportive love relationship, and 72 percent meditated an average of 4.2 hours per week.

According to Dr. Badgley, the brain has been discovered to be a giant immune system gland, responding positively to hope, joy, love, and low stress. He believes that doctors who give their patients death sentences are inhibiting immune system function, programming their patients to die, and may be performing malpractice. He states that a total program of natural therapies improves the quality of life of persons with AIDS, and most powerfully in persons who are early on in the disease process.

"Since 1985 I've watched these individuals make the hard choices: 'I'm not going to do AZT ever; I'm going to do other things.' These people are still around, enjoying life—they've plateaued. Their immune systems are not diminishing. Whereas their peers, who had the same status in the mid- to late 1980s, but instead jumped over and got into the whole drug regimen, are long gone. I think other doctors have made the same empirical observations," notes Dr. Badgley. "The Emperor doesn't have any clothes, but who wants to hear it?"

Dr. Badgley's Patients
Jon was diagnosed in 1984 with Kaposi's sarcoma. Nine years later, he works two full time jobs as an airport shuttle

driver, and a Certified Hypnotherapist. As a hypnotherapist, he works with AIDS and cancer patients and also uses general behavior modification.

Like many of Dr. Badgley's patients, Jon researched the information and treatment options and empowered himself by creating his own program. His protocol includes herbs, vitamins, and a macrobiotic diet when possible.

Jon explains, "Before I took action for myself, I had hepatitis for a year. I was thin and weak. My former doctors wanted me to go for chemotherapy, but I refused. Instead, I started on lots of vitamin C. Then I read the book, *Natural Healing With Herbs*, and started experimenting with herbs and began feeling better and stronger."

Jon mixes a spoonful of echinacea, red clover tops, chaparral, dandelion, sarsaparilla, and pau d'arco and brews the herbs as a tea. "It contributes a great deal to my health and stimulates my appetite. I keep weight on and feel strong," he says.

Hypnosis is also an integral part of Jon's protocol. Once he is in a relaxed hypnotic state, this is the imagery he suggests to himself: "I see myself on a tropical island, feeling very healthy. My lungs are pink and healthy. I see a mirror in front of a palm tree. When I look into it, I see myself exactly as I'd like to look. I'm healthy, my skin is clear and free of any lesions. There's a healthy glow in my eyes. I imagine myself jumping into the ocean. It's a healing, cleansing water. When I come out, the beads of water represent the virus leaving my body. I shake the beads of water off my body, like a dog. And I walk away, into a brand new world, free of a life-threatening illness."

Jon is very active in his own health care, stating, "I haven't taken any official medicines, and I won't. I believe state-of-mind has the greatest impact on the state of health. I think that the emotional impact of people saying negative things to you can have a profound impact on your health. As a child, my family teased me about my hands and feet. When I developed Kaposi's sarcoma it appeared *only* on my hands and feet. Saying negative things can wound your subconscious and your immune system."

Lynn has been HIV positive for at least eight years. He explains, "I was diagnosed with AIDS three years ago, but I don't have any symptoms now. Two years ago I just got so disgusted with the established medical community, the V.A., and Social Security, that I decided to just get rid of all my medications and vitamins. I attribute my good health to research. I got my system cleaned out so that it will heal by itself.

"The first step was to change my diet. I do not eat any cooked food. Instead I have raw organic fruits and vegetables. I grow my own sprouts, and make my own cheeses from nuts and seeds. I have lots of wheat grass, and other fresh juices. Moderation and variety in food are very important. Your body and mind get tired of the same thing all the time. You have to nudge it along and shock it. That's what keeps you going."

Lynn also utilized a fair amount of enemas to help rid his system of toxins (and medications) and to cleanse the colon (because that's one place where the virus is harbored). He avoids any foods that are mucus forming (dairy products, etc.). The cheeses he makes from sunflower seeds and pumpkin seeds are very time consuming, but as Lynn says, "It depends on how badly you want to live. My whole life has changed, but I've never felt better. My blood counts are very high."

Lynn's T-cell ranges from 1,100 to 958. When he was first diagnosed, the T-cell count was 382. His liver disease—for which he was advised to get a transplant a few years ago, but declined—is now in remission too. One doctor said, "I can't believe you're HIV positive, your (blood) counts are higher than most healthy people."

Lynn adds, "I believe in positive attitude and exercise, reiki [a form of energy healing], meditation, massage, and acupuncture. I'm convinced Baroque music has a healthful effect. I've stopped taking B_{12} injections. I sit in a sauna frequently and take very hot baths. I have wheat grass juice, orally as well as in enema form."

Lynn believes that it is imperative for AIDS and HIV positive patients to start cleaning out their bodies and to have a positive attitude. Ridding your systems of toxins and mucus can create emotional changes and upheavals in many cases, and for this reason, he strongly recommends getting into a support system where people are going through the same experience. "That will give you strength because talking to someone who's had the same experience and understands what you're going through is very important," he says.

"When you start to eliminate prescribed medications, alcohol, and recreational drugs from the system, your body will heal itself naturally," adds Lynn. "But the healing process is slow. It takes about a year for the effects to show. Either the virus will be completely gone or your immune system will be strong enough to work for you. You have to give yourself a lot of support and a lot of love. Things can be very frustrating. You can't give up."

Dr. Gerhard Orth (Germany)

Dr. Gerhard Orth of Leutkirch, Germany, uses a combination of naturopathic methods to treat AIDS.[5] He believes AIDS is a group of conditions which involves the whole body and has very little to do with the HIV organism. After treating over one hundred cases of AIDS, Dr. Orth has proven to his own satisfaction that it is not HIV which creates the environment in which damage occurs, but, instead, it is the result of the patient and everything that has happened to him/her to date. When this "terrain" (the field in which the virus operates) is modified, HIV can be eradicated, he says.

Dr. Orth maintains the following:

- HIV is a weak organism which can only survive, let alone thrive, in specific environmental conditions.
- Effective AIDS therapy requires that a combined antiviral, antibacterial, and antiyeast treatment, which also supports immune function, be followed.
- The acidity of the body fluids needs to be altered towards a more alkaline state because fungal infection increases and HIV thrives in an acidic environment.

Dr. Orth explains, "I have found in almost every case that the individual's immune system had been suppressed (by drug and/or medicine misuse, inappropriate lifestyle, or faulty diet, etc.) before the acquisition of the virus, which seems to creep in after the earlier immune suppression. This damage is augmented by the medical treatment given to AIDS patients."

Dr. Orth's protocol includes:

- Herbs to fight the viral activity
- Altering blood and tissue acidity levels
- Specific fungal treatment
- Eliminating allergens
- Normalizing the bowel flora
- Dietary changes to a more alkaline balance
- Limiting toxic medication
- Restructuring lifestyle

Herbs to Fight the Viral Activity

A combination of fourteen essential oils from plants is mixed with olive oil in a ratio of 40:60 and massaged into the skin. Research has shown these oils to have specific antiviral, antibacterial, and antifungal properties. The oils come from tree barks as well as a number of seeds and fruits (including cinnamon oil, ginger oil, and juniper berry oil).

Altering Blood and Tissue Acidity Levels

Bicarbonate of soda and magnesium bicarbonate are included in the various herbal preparations in order to reduce the acidity of blood and tissues, since as these become more alkaline, there is inhibition of the activity of fungi in the body. It has been found that the more fungal infection, the further advanced is the decline in immune function.

Medication used in this phase is "Multiplasen H33" tablets for the blood and, if necessary, "Alkala-N"[6] powder for balancing the acidity of the digestive tract (along with diet). This process is further helped by the drinking of a combination of organic vegetable juices (Austrian "Breuss" juice) or organic beetroot juice.

Specific Fungal Treatment

Mycosis in the blood is treated using medicinal herbs and alkaline trace elements as well as Nystatin. The herbal formulas utilized include "Pefrkehl," "D5" drops, "D4" capsules, and "D3" suppositories.[7] Diet at this stage must be alkaline, including a wide range of vegetable-based foods, as well as avoiding sugar and refined products of any kind. Dr. Orth is strongly against the use of broad-spectrum antibiotics unless absolutely vital, as these allow the development of an environment in which fungi flourish.

Eliminating Allergens
Damage to the bowel flora (through infection, antibiotic use, fungal overgrowth, etc.) leads to the easy passage of proteins from the bowel through the bowel mucous membrane. Once these enter the circulation they provide allergic reactions, including skin eruptions and many unpleasant symptoms.

When diarrhea is a problem, Dr. Orth states, "It has been possible to show in all cases of HIV positive patients that by stopping milk, yogurt, cheese, egg, and yeast preparations, diarrhea and skin lesions soon abated and disappeared." Patients then began to gain weight. If antibiotics were being used, these were stopped and the plant nasturtium was used instead.

Normalizing the Bowel Flora
Medicinal herbs are used to treat the digestive system for toxicity. "Multiplasen GL17"[8] is prescribed for this purpose, at the same time as antifungal medicines. Dr. Orth also prescribes "friendly bacterial cultures" (such as *Lactobacillus acidophilus*), since he believes that an appropriate diet, aided by probiotic supplementation, resettles the bowel flora.

Dietary Changes to a More Alkaline Balance
Dr. Orth prescribes the use of apple cider vinegar to appropriately and effectively control acidity. This can be taken in a glass of purified water. Fruits and vegetables (including grains and legumes) are suggested to comprise 75 percent of the total food intake (of which 25 percent is eaten raw and the rest cooked). If there are no allergic problems, the rest of the diet comprises cheese, eggs, fish, and meat.

The aim of the diet is to achieve an acidity of blood of pH 7.4, urine between 6.7 and 6.8, and stools of 5.5 to 5.6, and the diet is modified until this is achieved.

Limiting Toxic Medication
A step-by-step approach is made to eliminate all medications, while carefully monitoring the effects. Where necessary, these are replaced with herbal medicines.

Restructuring Lifestyle
A daily "ordered lifestyle" routine is introduced, including exercise, breathing techniques, body care, and a balanced eating pattern—largely based on traditional German "nature cure" principles dating back to the 19th Century and the work of Father Kneipp, a well-known figure in the annals of German lore.

Results of Dr. Orth's Protocol
Approximately 100 patients (97 percent male) have followed this approach to AIDS. Average age is thirty. Patients were in all four stages of AIDS illness as defined by the Centers for Disease Control. The time elapsed between HIV positive diagnosis and entering the Orth program varied from two to ten years.

In all cases, there were improvements unless complete destruction had taken place in the ecology of the bowel, reports Dr. Orth. Of these patients, five died (one by suicide). The majority of the others, he says, have returned to productive lives. After treatment, some patients remained HIV positive, while others had become HIV negative. Dr. Orth himself has no explanation for this, calling the result incomprehensible, since, "the antibody [to HIV] should normally always be detectable."

Using Dark Field Microscopy (the use of a special type of microscope which allows physicians to discern the status of a patient by viewing a live blood specimen), Dr. Orth found that when a "cure" had been achieved, the blood pictures were "completely in order." What was not always curable was the fungal problem. He explained, "It was only possible to curb the Candida mycosis, not to fully heal it. The diet of the patient was decisive. The intestinal mucosa damaged by the Candida is seen as the main reason for the reduction in T4 cells, since they are required as defense against allergens and microbes in this area."

Dr. Hulda Regehr Clark

A bold theory on the role of parasites and solvents in the onset of AIDS has been put forward by an independent research scientist Hulda Regehr Clark, Ph.D., N.D., in her book *The Cure for HIV and AIDS.*[9] Dr. Clark reports that her research shows that a parasite, the human intestinal fluke *(Fasciolopsis buskii)*, normally found only in the intestine, can establish itself in the thymus gland if benzene (a solvent) has accumulated there, and cause a destruction of T cells in the thymus. This situation, she reports, is essential for HIV to gain a foothold in the body.

According to Dr. Clark, the secret to eliminating HIV is to first eliminate the intestinal fluke parasite from the thymus with a five-day protocol that includes herbs (black walnut hull tincture, wormwood combination, and cloves). This is followed by a three-week anti-parasitic program and a tapeworm treatment to rid the body of most other parasites. Through electronic resonance scanning (a method of screening that tests the electrical properties of internal organs), she reports that HIV will completely leave the body within twenty-four hours after the intestinal fluke parasite has been eliminated from the thymus.

After HIV is no longer in the body, says Dr. Clark, it is then essential to rid the body of benzene. Benzene is a highly toxic solvent which Dr. Clark finds facilitates cloning of the intestinal fluke parasites resulting in a population burst. Dr. Clark reports that she finds traces of benzene in many common household products, including flavored foods, hand creams and moisturizers, petroleum jelly products, toothpaste, cold cereals, chewing gum, ice cream, and cooking oil. She counsels HIV positive individuals and those with AIDS to first stop using all products that may contain benzene and then to take at least 50 milligrams of vitamin B_2 (riboflavin) to help detoxify benzopyrenes which slow down benzene detoxification.

After the intestinal fluke parasite, HIV, and benzene have been eliminated from the body, Dr. Clark recommends a maintenance program to build the health of the thymus gland which includes removing unwanted unnatural chemicals from your mouth (amalgam and most other metals used in dental work), removing unnatural chemicals from your diet, removing all unnatural chemicals from your body, and removing all unnatural chemicals from your home.

Dr. Clark cites seventy case studies in her book of individuals who she tested as being HIV positive or having AIDS, the vast majority of which, she says, markedly improved by following her protocol.

 If Dr. Clark's findings as to the role of the intestinal fluke parasite and benzene in the AIDS and AIDS-like conditions are accurate, it is imperative that a well-funded research effort be immediately undertaken in this area. Her treatment protocol is inexpensive and could potentially bring about a significant improvement in the health status of individuals who are HIV positive or suffering from AIDS.

Dr. Burzynski and Antineoplaston AS2-1

Stanislaw Burzynski, M.D., Ph.D.,[10] is a graduate of the Lublin Medical Academy in Poland, where he graduated first in his class in 1967. A year later, at the age of twenty-five, he earned his Ph.D. in biochemistry. Dr. Burzynski has performed three preliminary studies on AIDS patients at his medical center in Houston, using AS2-1, a type of unorthodox medicine he has synthesized called *antineoplastons*. The results have been encouraging. Of twenty-seven patients who had AIDS resistant to standard antiviral therapy, sixteen have significantly increased their T4 counts as a result of receiving treatment. In addition, twelve patients out of twenty-seven increased their T4/T8 ratios, and seventeen out of twenty-seven gained weight during an eight-to-twelve week period. "A number of patients," Dr. Burzynski states of the second study, "had marked improvement in their physical condition [with] the disappearance of recurrent viral infections such as herpes simplex."[11]

Dr. Burzynski's treatment method reflects his theory that the body has a parallel defense system independent of the immune system. He refers to this system as the Biochemical Defense System (BDS) and is credited with its discovery. Whereas the immune system operates by destroying invading pathogens, according to Dr. Burzynski, the role of the BDS is to reprogram defective cells in the body. Instead of killing the defective cells, the BDS changes their programming so that they once again begin to function normally. In the case of people whose health has been compromised, however, the ability of the BDS to reprogram defective cells becomes diminished due to the deficiency of antineoplastons, enabling the cells to proliferate unchecked to the point where illness can become severe, if not fatal.

The agents responsible for proper function of the BDS are the antineoplastons, according to Dr. Burzynski, which he describes as "nontoxic, naturally-occurring peptides and amino acid derivatives that are part of the body's natural defense system, and which were originally isolated from human blood, and then urine." Although these chemicals are produced naturally by the body (principally the liver), Dr. Burzynski finds that it is more effective to reproduce them synthetically.

The antineoplastons have antiviral activity and assist in reprogramming immune system cells which are not functioning properly. AS2-1 specifically, Dr. Burzynski feels, may help B cells to abandon what is called an autoimmune response. "Suppose the B cells are making antibodies which attack the person's own T4 cells," he says. "This would be very damaging. My hypothesis is that this process, during treatment [with AS2-1], stops."

As of this writing, the status of antineoplastons is formally as an "Investigational New Drug" (IND), and as a result, Dr. Burzynski's treatment is available only in Texas because the Food and Drug Administration sets limitations on the transportation of experimental drugs over state lines. Antineoplaston therapy has been approved by the FDA for investigational use as a treatment for breast cancer and malignant brain tumors only. In Europe, Japan, and other areas of the world, however, Dr. Burzynski's work is heralded as an important breakthrough.

Dr. Burzynski's Patients
Paul was diagnosed in 1989 with AIDS after a serious bout of pneumonia. "I was walking around with pneumonia," he says. "Of course I didn't know it. I went to several doctors, and

couldn't find out what it was. Once, I couldn't breathe, so my partner took me to the hospital. I spent two and a half weeks in intensive care, and another two and a half months in the hospital. They were ready to write me off. I developed diabetes and liver problems.

"Two years later, I went to Dr. Burzynski. I had a T-cell count of 5 at the time. I had been able to maintain my weight but the diabetes was horrible. My blood sugar went up and down, all over the place. After three months of Dr. Burzynski's treatment, I was no longer diabetic. My doctor at home is amazed. I don't need any more insulin. There's no more fear of losing my sight. No more herpes, either. No more opportunistic infections at all.

"Of course I know I'm not out of the woods yet, because my T cells have stayed low, but the best part is how I feel now. A week before I went to see Dr. Burzynski, I was stuck in my house with an antibiotic IV in my arm. My muscles were sagging. I felt I was losing cells faster than I could replace them. I could smell death in my room. Now there's no more of that. It's turned around. I work out at the gym. I weigh a hundred and seventy pounds. If you saw this tanned guy with solid muscles on the street, you'd never imagine the situation I had been in. I'm out of the house now, I talk to people, I feel better and look better."

Mike, another patient, says, "About two years ago I went to visit Dr. Burzynski in Houston, Texas. I showed good results six months after the protocol started. He gives you a checkup and looks over your lab work and then gives you three months worth of antineoplaston. Then he schedules to see you three months later. It's all a matter of when you can go to Houston. I usually go for an overnight visit. The treatment is in capsule form. I take three of the capsules four times a day. The main reason to go to Houston is pick up the antineoplaston and so that he can discuss what is happening in your lab work and what he expects your body to be doing in the next three to four months.

"With regards to lab results, the benefits were immense. For someone who is asymptomatic, the antigen will be very low (the virus will be dormant). The antibodies (which fight viral activity) will be very high. What the treatment does for asymptomatic people is to make the antigens stay negative (keeping the virus in check), while the antibodies increase dramatically. This all means that the virus is being eliminated from your body.

"I think this treatment could benefit a lot of people, but not people who are expecting immediate results in two or three months. When that doesn't happen, they become impatient and move on to something else. I believe if you stay on it a year it will eliminate HIV from your body. You have to be patient and trusting. You have to realize it's not an overnight cure. It's something that goes down to the RNA and DNA levels of every HIV infected cell. Every cell is literally being reprogrammed into a healthy cell. That's what antineoplastons do. It takes time; it varies from person to person."

Robert Cathcart III, M.D., and Vitamin C

There are a number of doctors who treat AIDS patients with supplements. Robert Cathcart III, M.D., of Los Altos, California,[12] employs megadoses of vitamin C, plus other relevant vitamins and minerals. He also puts his patients on a program of better nutrition.

In 1984, Dr. Cathcart published a study, "Vitamin C in the Treatment of AIDS." In it he writes, "Preliminary clinical evidence is that massive doses of ascorbate (vitamin C) . . . can suppress the symptoms of the disease and can markedly reduce the tendency for secondary infections."[13] Working from an anecdotal group of 102 patients, most of whom were taking vitamin C on their own, Dr. Cathcart reports "considerable improvement" in most of the patients' conditions. Examples of change included a marked reduction of a case of diseased lymph glands, and the disappearance of a case of Kaposi sarcoma lesions.

Jeff, a patient of Dr. Cathcart's, comments on his improvement since starting the doctor's regimen a year and three months ago: "I had been diagnosed as HIV positive. My T-cell count was dropping, which means my immune system wasn't doing too well. I was starting to feel weak and faint at work. I had night sweats and fever, which now I only have very rarely. With Dr. Cathcart, my T cells went from just under 300 up to

600. There are no side effects from the vitamin C. I get sixty grams of C from Dr. Cathcart three times a month, by IV. He's had me cut out all sugar and junk food [after] he explained to me what they were doing to my immune system. I've had no colds or flu this year, for the first time in my life. I do meditation as well. It isn't just the treatments. I'm around positive people; I drink good filtered water at home. It's important to me that I'm on a spiritual path."

Ignacio Coronel, M.D., and L-51 (Mexico)

Ignacio Coronel, M.D., of Mexico City,[14] is completing the paperwork on a clinical study on two hundred people who, as volunteers, have been treated with his own medication, L-51, the base of which is sodium borate.

"L-51," says Dr. Coronel, "blocks the calcium channels in T cell surfaces, so the virus can't make copies of itself and kill cells."

The study began in 1987, and the first patient who received treatment "has now gone five years without medication, which is excellent," Dr. Coronel says. "We've taken people in various stages. HIV positive and no symptoms, HIV positive with some early symptoms, and full-blown AIDS cases. If the T4s are below 150, I haven't been able to help."

Of the 200 patients in this long-term study, seventy-five percent are still alive, states Dr. Coronel. Those who died had T cells under 200 when they began treatment. Patients with T-cell counts above that level have done well. The treatment period ranges from three months to one year. The medication is, for the most part, administered orally, so the patient does not have to stay in Mexico City for a long period.

"We want to establish a real basis for treatment, not that it works on just a few people, but that it is truly effective," says Dr. Coronel. "Some people have been recovering fast. If their T cells are 400, they usually only need three months of treatment. People ask me when they should start and I say right away, the earlier the better. The longer the person waits, the more damage has been done. If the illness gets down to the bone marrow and does serious harm there (where immune cells are manufactured), this is very, very serious. Start treatment early."

Dr. Coronel states that T-cell numbers have gone up slowly in all surviving patients, "and in some, they reach normal levels. All symptoms disappear, they gain weight, regain appetite, and if they have diarrhea, that slowly improves. Of course, we are separately treating certain conditions, such as opportunistic infections, with proper medication, too."

Dr. Coronel is forwarding his as yet unpublished study to the Mexican government, seeking approval for L-51 to be used anywhere in Mexico.

Gaston Naessens and Somatidian Orthobiology (Canada)

Gaston Naessens, a French-born biologist, has devoted the past forty years of his life to research in the field of hematology. C.E.R.B.E., Mr. Naessens's private laboratory, has served as the basis for the fundamental research in the field of Somatidian Orthobiology.

Mr. Naessens became known mostly as a result of the historical court case in Canada, which he won in December 1989. This court case involved the criminal accusations directed against Mr. Naessens and his product, 714-X, a compound of his own formulation, by the Quebec Medical Corporation. An historical account of these events are related in the book *The Persecution and Trial of Gaston Naessens*.[15]

Mr. Naessens not only won his case against the Quebec Medical Corporation, but some of those who testified in his behalf were important Canadian and international business leaders and officials whom he had previously treated. Shortly after Mr. Naessens's acquittal, 714-X was made legally available to Canadian patients when authorized by the Chief Doctor of the Health Protection Branch of the Health and Welfare Department of Canada (after application to the Emergency Drug Release program by the treating physician).

Although Mr. Naessens is known primarily for his work in the cancer field, he has also oriented his research towards AIDS and HIV, always preoccupied with immune-enhancing treatments.

Mr. Naessens work appears to be a natural continuation of Antoine Bechamp's controversial discoveries of pleomorphism[16] in the 19th century, although, curiously enough, Mr. Naessens learned of this contemporary competitor of Pasteur only in the early 1980s, after having recorded all his own observations and his own theory. Since Mr. Naessens's discovery of the somatid, pleomorphism has gained more serious consideration by the scientific community. Conventional medicine, on the other hand, supported by the medical establishment, promotes only monomorphism in conformity with Louis Pasteur's proposals.

The major breakthrough introduced by Gaston Naessens in the late 1940s in France was the development of a home-built, highly sophisticated optic microscope capable of an astonishingly high resolution (150 Angstrom). This research tool, called a "somatoscope," makes the observation of tiny particles within live tissue or blood possible.

Upon observing these unknown particles, he named them "somatids"—Latin for "tiny bodies." Mr. Naessens states, "These tiny particles, seen in live blood, are the smallest unit of life, probably the precursor of DNA, and undoubtedly capable of transforming energy into matter." Mr. Naessens also observed that these tiny somatids move without ever binding together since they bear an electrical charge. Their nuclei are positive while their membranes are negative. Consequently, whenever two somatids come near each other, automatic repulsion takes place much in the same way two magnets repulse when joined at negative poles.

Mr. Naessens devoted over a decade investigating the somatid; his observations enabled him to record the existence of the somatid's pleomorphic cycle. According to Naessens, the somatid is created within the red blood cells. First, it bears a liquid form, then its density increases as it is expulsed into the plasma. His research reveals that within healthy organisms somatids progress normally through a three-stage microcycle: somatid, spore, and double spore.

Mr. Naessens's observations also show that this microcycle produces a proliferation hormone necessary for normal cellular division. He also observed that under certain conditions the microcycle is no longer blocked (stages 4–16) by blood

228

The Somatidian Cycle

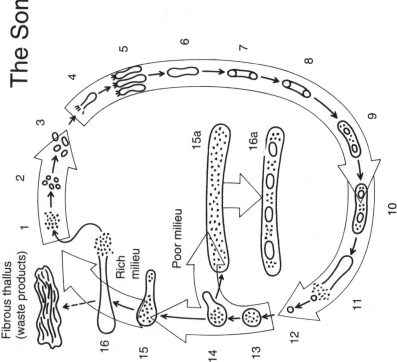

1. Somatids
2. Spores
3. Double spores
4. Bacterial form
5. Double bacterial form
6. Rod form
7. Bacterial form with double spores
8. Bacterial form with granular double spores
9. & 10. Microbial globular forms
11. Bursting
12. Yeast form
13. Ascopore form
14. & 15. Mycelial forms
15a. & 16a. Resistant mycelial

Fibrous thallus (waste products)

Rich milieu

Poor milieu

inhibitors which permits the somatid to pursue a macrocycle consisting of thirteen additional stages (see illustration). When this macrocycle occurs, the blood characteristically demonstrates the presence of these polymorphic forms. This puts additional stress on the immune system, creating symptoms such as fatigue, depression, muscular weakness, and pain. This macrocycle (allowed by the absence of blood inhibitors) can be triggered in a variety of ways, including pollution, sickness, and/or emotional shock or distress. In all types of degenerative diseases, including AIDS and cancer, the complete macrocycle or certain of its components are observable within the live blood.

Although the components of the macrocycle are not the cause of disease, their presence is evidence of the progressive weakening of the body's natural defenses. To detect their presence in the blood is certainly not a diagnosis but rather a concrete observation of biological parameters clearly indicating that the body is becoming vulnerable to invasion. Medically speaking, all the people within whom the macrocycle is observed are not yet diagnosed with a degenerative disease. Nevertheless, if the cycle is not brought under control (returning to the three-stage microcycle) within twelve to eighteen months, a more serious health condition will most likely occur. 714-X was originally conceived to reestablish the healthy microcycle of the somatid before disease gains a stronghold.

HIV/AIDS and 714-X
Basic treatment with 714-X for HIV/AIDS consists of three rounds of twenty-one consecutive days of injections. Because of its composition, and the way it is administered, via the lymph system, 714-X helps fluidify the lymph and promotes a healthier lymphatic circulation, which in turn allows for the elimination of toxins through natural routes. Naessens is quick to point out that 714-X is not designed for a specific disease, and therefore has no direct effect on abnormal cells. All 714-X does is reinstate the equilibrium necessary for the body's normal blood inhibitors to resume their function of restricting the somatid to its healthy three-stage microcycle.

Knowing that 714-X also has an important antiviral action, Mr. Naessens believes it might be of great benefit to people with AIDS or HIV. In fact, he asserts that after three consecutive cycles of 714-X, one can expect to notice an abatement of preliminary symptoms such as diarrhea, fatigue, sweating, fever, etc.

Despite these various improvements, Mr. Naessens points out that such patients remain carriers of the HIV virus. Many people with AIDS or people with HIV, treated with 714-X over the last few years, appear in good health and are leading normal lives (see case histories).

Commenting on the fact that 714-X has not been officially approved by the Canadian government (714-X is an investigational drug), Mr. Naessens points to the urgent need to release 714-X because of the tragic phenomena of AIDS. "You certainly would not let someone drown just because you had to walk on private property in order to rescue him or her. Neither can I. In good conscience, I cannot hold back 714-X treatment which has shown significant clinical results since its first human use in 1976. Such treatments cannot be indefinitely withheld because those who would regulate such compounds insist upon further testing of the product's toxicity."

At this point it is important to underline that Mr. Naessens is not a physician and does not directly treat patients afflicted with cancer, HIV, AIDS, or any other disease. Many consenting physicians worldwide are reportedly prescribing 714-X for such conditions upon the request of their patients.

Mr. Naessens insists that potential patients with HIV or AIDS be informed that 714-X is not a vaccine against AIDS, and does not protect from the possibility of contracting or transmitting the virus.[17]

What Expectations Can Those With AIDS or Who Are HIV Positive Have of Somatidian Orthobiology?

- A new hopeful vision: the pleomorphic vision of the HIV virus considers its presence as a reversible condition that can be mastered without full-blown AIDS necessarily developing.
- Interest is increasing in somatidian orthobiology. Perhaps, as Mr. Naessens's theory becomes widely known, more

and more health care practitioners will be able to accomo-
date patients by providing access to 714-X, clinical fol-
low-ups, and somatidian blood assessments.
- Hopefully, in the next few years, if research conditions
remain as good as they are now, a new product specific to
HIV/AIDS will be made available to doctors. This product, called ANA-10, is presently being clinically tested in
various private clinics.

This report of an upcoming treatment (ANA-10) is not to
create false hope, nor unnecessary pressures, but rather to
inform HIV positive people and people with AIDS that within
the biological research field, private-funded laboratories are
also highly committed to the realities of HIV/AIDS and the
urgency of this situation.

Anecdotes of People Using 714-X

Barry discovered that he had AIDS in 1984 while he was
working abroad in Paris. Prior to his diagnosis, he had suffered from chronic colds for two years. In cold weather, he
experienced croup-like symptoms and had difficulty breathing. "The doctor I saw in Paris told me to return to Canada
since AIDS was still very much misunderstood and feared at
that time. Besides, there was not much he could do for me,"
Barry relates.

Once back in his homeland, Barry consulted with a friend
of his, a conventional M.D. It was discovered that his condition had manifested as Kaposi's sarcoma. Also, toxoplasmosis
was affecting his eyesight. "In addition, I had cyotomegla-
virus, severe oral thrush, and I had lost forty-five pounds,"
Barry says. "And my T-cell count had dropped to 200. My
doctor friend admitted there was no known conventional treatment for AIDS, at least nothing worth investigating. He then
estimated that, unless something changed, I had about two to
three months to live. But he suggested to me that I consult
with Mr. Naessens, because he was impressed with reports he
had heard of Naessens's treatment methods."

Barry himself had little idea who Mr. Naessens was. At the
same time, however, he had already witnessed the deaths of
friends who had received treatments of AZT and interferon, so

he knew that he needed to try something different. "I was resolved to help myself in anyway possible," Barry says. "I knew that AZT was not right for me, and also knew that it had already been rejected as a cure for leukemia, so it made me wonder why it was being touted as a treatment for AIDS. Rather than admit that it doesn't work, I'm convinced that the pharmaceutical companies promoted it simply as another way for them to make money."

Barry met with Mr. Naessens with the belief that physicians are only a part of the solution toward health, "not people you have to give your life over to." "I believe that every citizen has the right to choose his or her method of health care, and that, in order to do so, they must be made properly aware of how each treatment works. I was impressed with Mr. Naessens in this regard, because one of the first things that he told me was that his treatment method was not a miracle cure, and that he would make no promises as to what results it would have with me. He also recommended that I take full responsibility for my life, and to not simply rely on his compounds for help."

As a result, Barry underwent a series of colonic irrigations to detoxify his system of waste products. He then adopted a vegetarian diet, eliminating sugar and all dairy products. "I also supplemented my diet with vitamins A, C, and E, as well as a mineral complex, and I grew wheat grass which I juiced and drank daily," he says. "I stopped exposing myself to television, radio, and newspapers since I wanted to protect myself from the negative influences of the media. Also, I stopped working to help the recuperative processes, and to avoid the stresses associated with my job."

After becoming aware of Mr. Naessens's protocol, and after consenting to it, Barry undertook his treatment with 714-X. "I began receiving three series of 714-X injections," he recounts. "During those first series, my energy level greatly improved and I regained my appetite. By the end of those first three weeks, my KS lesions, toxoplasmosis, cytomegalovirus, and the oral thrush all began to disappear as my lymph was being cleared out. After the second series, I felt close to full health, and was actually shocked by how much my health had taken a turn for the better. By the final series, I was completely well again. I didn't even have the croup or breathing problems during cold weather. Although I had experienced these problems all of my life, they went away after the first treatment and never returned. I could hardly believe what had happened, and I recall doubting that the treatments would withstand the test of time."

Following these three series of 714-X, Barry was part of a limited clinical trial testing of ANA-10, the product developed by Mr. Naessens, and specifically designed for combating HIV.

Barry has remained in good health ever since. Not only did he recover the weight he had initially lost, but today he jokes about being a few pounds overweight. As a precautionary measure, he continues to receive 714-X treatments at regular intervals to maintain the circulation of his lymph. He also has no idea what his T-cell count is and is not concerned by this. "It's not important to me," he says. "People can have a T-cell count of 1,000 and still die, while others have counts of almost zero and live very well. For me, getting tested all the time would only create added stress that I do not need. What is important is that I am living proof that people with AIDS can live without AZT, ddI, and/or interferon."

Barry's appreciation of life has also deepened as a result of his experience. "Life is a gift which occurs in really just a moment," he says, "and we need to greet it with some humor and be willing to enjoy and learn from our experiences." Recognizing this, Barry, who describes himself as previously being "a hard-working capitalistic businessman," has simplified his lifestyle considerably, and now devotes time each week as a volunteer helping others. "I'm enjoying myself more than ever," he says. "I now take my life day by day, and for the first time I have a positive sense of having a future."

In summation, Barry is critical of the way most AIDS research is currently being conducted. "The primary problem surrounding AIDS is that so much of the research is focused in only one direction," he points out. "Everybody wants to find a drug that will kill the disease, without paying attention to the chemical imbalances these drugs can cause, and the further damage they can do as a result. If we are going to help people, we need to have research into many directions, so that patients can be well-informed of all of the options available to them. As citizens of our governments, this freedom to choose is not only necessary, it is our right."

(The patient in the following case history underwent treatment only with 714-X since he was not included in the limited clinical tests with ANA-10.)

Fred discovered he had a brain mass in 1983, probably a symptom of his "GRID" diagnosis. He refused a biopsy for it, and refused surgery as well. "My whole family has always been involved in natural healing," he explains. "So I changed my diet for eight months, did self-hypnosis, went to a chiropractor, and eventually the mass went away.

"In spite of my improved lifestyle, in 1987, I realized my health was once again declining. I developed diarrhea, and was in bed constantly. I probably had pneumonia, although it was never officially diagnosed. After the inconclusive lymph-node-biopsy performed in 1982, under local anesthesia, I've remained cautious when dealing with doctors; I know of their tendencies to treat PWA's as test subjects for sometimes dangerous substances and I strive to avoid that at any cost.

"In addition, I had been told, in 1984, when my ELISA test came out, that I was HIV positive," Fred continues. "I got over the pneumonia, but began looking for a way to fully deal with my condition. In January 1988, through a friend, I found out about 714-X. I received a series of injections, and learned how to administer them myself. After one series, there was a greatly noticeable improvement. After the three recommended series, my T-cell count went from 150 up to 350, and there were no side effects. Since then my T-cell count has declined somewhat. However, I am much better than before I began taking 714-X. I am able to lead a quasi-normal lifestyle, help my family, and hold a full-time job. I've also had no major infections or diarrhea, and my energy level is pretty good. It's been six years, and still counting, since I started using 714-X at regular intervals, and I honestly attribute these essentially borrowed years to Mr. Naessens' product, 714-X. I just hope that everyone will eventually be allowed to benefit from this man's discoveries, and that medicine will use his fundamental discoveries as a new solid basis for what researchers are now calling the 'post-antibiotic era.'"

Qingcai Zhang, M.D., and Chinese Bitter Melon

Qingcai Zhang, M.D. (China), Lic. Ac., of New York City,[18] reports a certain amount of success in using the antiviral herb, Chinese Bitter Melon (*Momordica charantia*), to treat HIV positive individuals and AIDS patients. Bitter melon is a plant commonly used by Asians, particularly Filipinos, as part of their diet and as a medicinal folk herb for a wide variety of ailments. Traditionally, it is believed that eating bitter melon regularly will clean and purify blood and ward off a variety of infections. The herb has also been used therapeutically for treatment of malaria, asthma, diabetes, stomach aches, insect bites, and numerous blood-related illnesses.

Since the early 1980s, bitter melon fruits and seeds have been tested *in vitro* (in a glass such as a test tube) and *in vivo* (in a living body) for its effectiveness as a treatment for cancer, tumors, and HIV infection. According to Dr. Zhang, research shows bitter melon to have the following therapeutic qualities:

- **Anti-HIV Effects:** Bitter melon contains three anti-HIV proteins (alpha- and beta-momocharin, and MAP-30). These proteins have been tested in vitro and found to possess inhibitory effects on HIV-infected macrophages and T cells, and to inhibit cell to cell infection. By inactivating the functions of ribosome in HIV-infected cells, the proteins also stop protein synthesis and kill infected cells. Significantly, these proteins do not appear to be toxic to uninfected cells.[19]
- **Antiviral Effects:** The proteins isolated from extracts of bitter melon have been found to inhibit replication of Herpes simplex (HSV-1) and poliovirus.[20]
- **Anti-tumor Effects:** The in vivo anti-tumor activity of a crude extract from bitter melon was shown to inhibit tumor formation in mice. Its enhancement of immune function in vivo further indicates that bitter melon may possess anti-tumor effects.[21]
- **Stimulation of Insulin Release:** An aqueous extract of bitter melon was found to be a potent stimulator of insulin

release in vivo, thereby improving glucose tolerance and reducing blood sugar levels.[22]

Dr. Zhang also reports very low clinical toxicity with bitter melon extract. Hundreds of patients have used it daily for more than one year and there were no obvious side effects reported, he notes. He is currently initiating the pilot program for gathering data for bitter melon programs in New York, and reports that the Free University of Berlin is initiating a study on bitter melon for treating HIV, as well.

In 1990, Sylvia Lee-Huang of New York University's School of Medicine reported that her research team had isolated a purified protein taken from the seeds and fruit of bitter melon, called MAP-30 (Momordica Anti-HIV Protein). In lab studies, MAP-30 blocked the reverse transcriptase enzyme activity necessary in order for HIV to overpower a cell. It reduced cell release of p24 antigens (HIV particles that spread the infection to other cells), and it lowered syncytis formation (large cell-massing and cell death that occurs in AIDS).[23]

At the Amsterdam International Conference on AIDS in July of 1992, Dr. Zhang presented his data on the use of bitter melon with HIV positive individuals and AIDS patients. He reported that those who took bitter melon for four months to three years had a CD4 count increase of between 33 percent to 285 percent. His impression was that in most cases bitter melon normalized CD4/CD8 ratios, raised CD4 counts over time, and increased energy and one's sense of well-being. He also noted that bitter melon blocks HIV-infected macrophage (which AZT does not), as well as infected lymphocytes, such as CD4 cells.[24]

But the true pioneer of bitter melon therapy is Stanley Rebultan, a Filipino-American who is HIV positive, and who took bitter melon liquid extract for over four years as his sole antiviral treatment. Rebultan was raised in the Philippines where bitter melon is an accepted food supplement and medicinal remedy for many conditions, including leukemia. As leukemia and HIV share many clinical aspects, he concluded that perhaps bitter melon might have some benefit in treating his HIV infection.

Rebultan saw his CDA (T4) cell count increase by 121 percent (480 to 1,060), his CDA/CDS ratio improve by 68 percent (.91 to 1.53), and his CD4 percentage rise by 77 percent (26 percent to 46 percent). Today, Rebultan's only method of treatment is bitter melon. He speaks to various doctors and AIDS groups about its use and benefits. His current T-cell count is 1,060.

Rebultan says, "You should supplement a doctor's therapy with bitter melon therapy, especially if your T-cell count is in the higher levels. Once you are down, based on statistics, the health and well-being is maintained or enhanced, but the T-cell count may take time to raise. People with HIV or AIDS focus so much attention on time and numbers."

Bitter melon can be administered orally or rectally. A rectal retention enema is recommended, though, because boiled decoctions of the plant are very bitter and unpleasant to drink, and may cause nausea. Using the retention enema also avoids the breakdown of the bitter melon proteins in the stomach acid, allowing them to instead be absorbed directly into the bloodstream through the colon and large intestines.

The therapy is also affordable. The fruit leaves and stems, purchased in Asian markets, cost about $10 to $20 a month. Dr. Zhang's freeze dried extract from whole bitter melon from China, in packets or capsules, costs about $60 a month (plus the cost of office visits). It can be prepared and taken effectively at home.

While bitter melon has shown remarkable results for those who stick with it, many people quit before the therapy can take effect. Rebultan admits that it took three months before he felt comfortable with the treatment procedure, but explains, "It's a long-term therapy. You won't gain results overnight. It takes at least six months to see results. If I have to do this my entire life to maintain a normal sense of well-being, then I will. Herbal therapy takes a long time. It's not like the overnight miracles of pill popping that American medicine feels so entitled to."

Conclusion

As the treatments and case histories discussed in this chapter show, the issue of AIDS is not without hope. Despite the majority consensus which continues to be reinforced by both federal AIDS research agencies and most of the media that AIDS is invariably fatal, the truth of the matter is that growing numbers of people with the illness are restoring themselves to health or, at the very least, reducing their condition to something that is manageable and does not interfere with their day to day lives. And the vast majority of these cases are achieving their successes using options common to the field of alternative medicine.

In light of this fact, one has to wonder why, after having already spent as much as 10 billion dollars on researching AIDS and HIV with only poor results, our government research agencies are not investigating these alternative methods with equal attention and enthusiasm. At the same time, however, as the genuinely inspiring cases histories above make clear, to wait until outside agencies—be they private or public—come up with a solution to the AIDS crisis is unwise. We also need to look to those physicians who are on the front-line working with alternative medicine for solutions.

The patients and physicians that we have profiled in this book are testaments to the fact that health is an individual responsibility and that, once that responsibility is wholly accepted, the seemingly miraculous can actually become possible. With that thought in mind, we encourage those readers out there who are either afflicted with AIDS and its satellite conditions, or who have loved ones who are, to follow up on the information provided above and in the accompanying endnotes. Investigate the choices which are available to you and make your own informed decisions after you have done so. As you do, you will be joining others who are helping to build a growing wave of hope and empowerment. And as this wave grows, federal agencies will be more likely to recognize at last the proper direction in which their energies must be directed.

Recommended Reading

Alternative Medicine: The Definitive Guide. The Burton Goldberg Group. Puyallup, WA: Future Medicine Publishing, Inc., 1993.

The most comprehensive reference on alternative medicine ever compiled. Provides in-depth, easily understandable coverage of 43 alternative therapies and over 200 health conditions, with advice from nearly 400 alternative physicians worldwide. See chapters on "Diet," "Nutritional Supplements," "Orthomolecular Medicine," "Herbal Medicine," "AIDS," "Cancer" (for more information on Dr. Burzynski and Mr. Naessens), and "Mind/Body Medicine."

The Cure for HIV and AIDS. Clark, Hulda R., Ph.D., N.D. San Diego, CA: ProMotion Publishing, 1993.

Dr. Clark, a research scientist, explains how a human intestinal fluke parasite affects the thymus gland and T cells. This book also demonstrates how chemicals, such as benzene, unknowingly put into the body promote this condition. Most importantly, she reveals three simple things one must do to clear the body of HIV and prevent AIDS from occurring. Over seventy case studies are reviewed. [To order, call (800) 249-8500.]

Healing AIDS Naturally. Badgley, Laurence, M.D. Foster City, CA: Healing Energy Press, 1987.

Outlines Dr. Badgley's protocol for treating AIDS using alternative medicine.

Immune Power: A Comprehensive Treatment Program for HIV. Kaiser, Jon D., M.D. New York: St. Martin's Press, 1993.

Dr. Kaiser has been on the front lines of those treating people with HIV/AIDS. His book offers a ground-breaking treatment program of great use to people who are HIV positive, their medical caregivers, and anyone interested in a successful, comprehensive approach to treating HIV infection and AIDS. By utilizing a comprehensive clinical approach, 90 percent of his patients have remained stable in their diagnosis or improved the strength of their immune systems. These results are startlingly dramatic when compared to those commonly seen and reported.

The Persecution and Trial of Gaston Naessens. Bird,
Christopher. Tiburon, CA: H.J. Kramer, 1991.
*Highlights the work of Gaston Naessens in the field of cancer and
other illnesses, including 714-X, and the trial he faced because of
his discoveries.*

15 A Woman's Journey: Sharon Lund

Sharon Lund has dedicated her life to helping men, women, and children living with HIV/AIDS, to improve their quality of life.[1] In 1985, she became active in the Los Angeles AIDS Community. Through the use of visualization, meditation, stress reduction, emotional clearing, and body dialogue, she taught gay men (who at that time were considered to be the primary focus of the virus) techniques to heal their bodies, minds, and spirits.

For the past seven years, Sharon has traveled nationally and internationally, educating youth and adults about the myths and reality of HIV/AIDS, including prevention, transmission, and issues surrounding women infected with this condition. Through her presentations, she hopes to save people from infecting themselves and others with HIV.

Little did Sharon know that the work she was doing in the AIDS community would prepare her to face her own personal challenge of living with HIV. As she recalls, "It was a few days before Christmas in 1986, when my life changed right before my eyes. My parents were visiting with my daughter Jeaneen and I from Hawaii. Aware of the work I was doing in the AIDS Community, they had videotaped several television programs on AIDS for me. We decided to watch one of the AIDS specials hosted by Dan Rather. Within a matter of a few minutes after I'd turned on the video, I saw and heard my ex-husband Bill saying he was dying of AIDS. Shocked and confused, I screamed and threw something. I felt so faint and weak that I thought I was going to pass out.

"My parents didn't recognize Bill because they had only met him one time during our brief six-month marriage in 1984. They tried to reassure me it wasn't Bill, and for a brief moment, I wanted to believe them. But feeling sick inside, I knew it was him. Even with his face being somewhat screened out, I could still see his mustache, his hair, and the sweater I had given him two years before for Christmas. I continued to scream, 'I know it's Bill, I know it's him!'"

Sharon called her ex-husband, who denied he was on the show. "It was not until a few years later, when he was on his death bed, that Bill called me to confess that it was him on the AIDS special, and that he was aware of his infection prior to our marriage."

Upon seeing the AIDS special, Sharon knew she had to be tested for the HIV antibodies. Back then, there were very few anonymous test sites available in Los Angeles and to her horror she was told it would take three months before she could be tested.

"I will never forget the day I received my test results," Sharon says. "The counselor walked into the room with his head down and as he looked up at me I could see tears in his eyes. He told me I was infected with HIV. My body became numb as he gave me a handful of brochures with different support groups, and resources available for gay men. He told me he was sorry he didn't have any information for heterosexual woman.

"When I got to my car, tears flooded my eyes. The reality of the words 'you are infected with HIV' sunk in. I thought to myself, 'how could this be, I had never heard of a women becoming infected through her husband or partner.' In shock, I glanced through the brochures and I immediately stuck them in my glove compartment, where they remained for years."

At that time, Sharon was feeling fine and had no symptoms associated with HIV or AIDS. Allowing herself to go into denial, at first she admitted she was infected only to her minister, boyfriend, and her sister, Joyce.

A little over a year later, however, Sharon began to experience the symptoms associated with HIV/AIDS. "I'll never forget waking up in the middle of the night with drenching night sweats. The top part of my body, night clothes, and sheets were soaking wet. Occasionally, my hair was so wet, that it felt like I could actually wring the sweat out of it. My daughter Jeaneen, then twelve, would help me change the bedding, sometimes two or three times a night. She would often crawl into bed with me. As we embraced one another, we would take a moment to pray. The moment seemed everlasting, as I was able to experience inner peace.

"It wasn't long before I began to notice swollen lymph nodes. Then I started getting severe diarrhea, and lost about twenty-three pounds. I experienced memory loss and had difficulty comprehending things. Chronic fatigue set in and some days I found it hard just to get out of bed. It was at that point that my daughter Jeaneen became the mother and I became the child."

Sharon found a doctor who treated infectious diseases, who told her that, given her poor condition, she had about six months to live. Sharon went home and began to get her affairs in order. She put together a will and a living power of attorney, and even called her parents to ask them to care for Jeaneen after she died.

Sharon recalls, "Then I realized through a meditation that I had bought into the doctor's death sentence and I had made him God. I immediately called my doctor and stated, 'You are not God. You don't know how or when anyone is going to die, and I'm not going to buy into this death sentence.' He said something like, 'So you are going to continue to live in denial?' I responded with a feeling of inner strength, 'No, from this day forward I am going to start doing all I can to build up my immune system. I'm going to stop taking life for granted and live my life to its fullest.'"

Sharon realized that she had to start practicing the techniques that she had been teaching to people who were infected with HIV and AIDS. She says, "The day I came out of denial about being infected with HIV was the day my healing really began."

At a friend's suggestion, Sharon checked herself into a holistic clinic. She didn't say she was HIV positive because at that time they would not have taken her as a patient. Instead, she went in for chronic fatigue.

"The main thing I had to change was my eating habits. Before entering the clinic, my main diet consisted of candy bars throughout the day, sodas, and hamburgers with extra pickles. I lived, or shall I say survived, off of junk food." The clinic put her on a whole foods diet with plenty of raw vegetables and wheat grass juice. Colon therapy and acupuncture were also included in the regimen, as well as exercise and guided imagery.

"When I walked into the clinic, I was really weak and pale. In a matter of four to five days people were saying, 'You're getting your color back, and you look healthier.' I realized through the clinic that in order for me to really heal, I had to not only heal my mind and spirit, but also my body." Aware that she had neglected the importance proper diet and exercise played in her life, she knew that changes would have to be made.

Shortly after Sharon returned home from the clinic, she searched for a doctor who could help treat her for any possible symptoms associated with HIV/AIDS. She began interviewing several physicians, taking notes on their thoughts about the virus and asking questions. "Was he/she open to alternative therapies? Was he/she willing to spend that extra bit of time answering all my questions, instead of looking at his/her watch every few minutes? Was he/she educated on women's health issues around HIV/AIDS? I knew, when it came to my healing, that I needed to find a doctor I could trust and work in partnership with."

Several months later, Sharon met with Dr. Joan Priestley in Los Angeles, California. "Joan took me in with a deep understanding of my needs. She immediately put me on a protocol of herbs, vitamins, antioxidants, and amino acids. She then introduced me to Dr. Stanislaw Burzynski in Houston, Texas, who put me on his treatment of a natural substance called antineoplastons AS2-1, which is a naturally-occurring amino acid derivative. After I started his program, along with Dr. Priestley's, my T cells went back up into the 500s." Sharon also started using acupuncture, reflexology, massage, Chinese herbs, and energy work on a regular basis.

For the past seven years, Sharon has continued to follow an alternative/natural treatment regimen. She has never taken any of the Western drugs such as AZT, ddI, or ddC. "I have chosen to use only holistic therapies," she explains. "I am not willing to use conventional therapies or drugs because of their side effects. I believe the drugs disturb the natural balance of my body."

Sharon continues, "I recommend that individuals faced with a life-challenging illness, such as HIV/AIDS, educate themselves on all of the conventional and alternative therapies which are available. The person is then able to make a conscious decision on which treatments would feel comfortable for him or her. It's important to know that there are many choices available and what works for one person may not work for another." As part of her on-going self-education about HIV/AIDS, Sharon has spent hours at the World Research Foundation in Sherman Oaks, California, exploring its library for records of treatments for her condition from throughout the world.

Sharon now actively practices in her life the same techniques that she has been teaching people faced with disease. To help heal the body she uses such methods as exercise, proper diet, stress reduction, body dialogue, and visualization. "I find visualization to be immensely healing," she explains, sharing one of her techniques. "When I take a shower, instead of seeing the water going on the outside of my body, I visualize it going inside of me and flushing the virus out. Sometimes I close my eyes and visualize the virus as black dots inside my body and I see a Pac-Man eating up the black dots. Body dialogue is also extremely important. It allows me to get in touch with my body and listen to what it needs."

To reduce the inevitable stress that accompanies life, Sharon recommends journal writing, yoga, exercise, deep breathing, being in nature, hot baths with soft music and candle light, confronting the situation, or just walking away from it. "It doesn't matter how you release the stress, what's important is to reduce it in your life," she says. "I quit my job and broke off an engagement in order to reduce stress in my life. I wasn't willing to sacrifice my health for the job or the relationship. I searched and could not find another solution for reducing the stress.

"For the mind, I use affirmations, positive thoughts, emotional clearing, a positive attitude, inner child work, and support," Sharon continues. "It is extremely important to have support when faced with any life-challenging illness. Your support might come from your family, friends, clergy, the

AIDS community, support groups, or a therapist. Support is vital to your health. Find that special person or persons who show you compassion, love, and understanding. I feel very fortunate, because I have found my support in my daughter, mom, dad, sister, friends, and God."

Sharon also concentrates on her spiritual healing. "A strong focal point in my healing is prayer and meditation. I believe that spirituality also includes forgiveness (of self and of others), giving thanks for all the blessings in our life and for all that mother earth has offered us. Traditionally, it's not acceptable to ask others for what we want or for help, but I feel that asking for what we believe we need is important. Also, there comes a time in which an individual needs to take care of themselves, and realize not only that this is okay, but that it is necessary. Learning to set limits is also extremely important. I find some people are givers, and others are receivers. In healing, I believe that there has to be an open channel of giving and receiving back to one another."

It's been seven years since Sharon was told she had six months to live and she remains active and healthy. "I believe my journey to health was due to my Higher Power and the use of treatments such as acupuncture, applied kinesiology, Ayurvedic medicine, biofeedback, bodywork, chi energy, colon therapy, craniosacral therapy, detox therapy, diet, energy medicine, enzyme therapy, fasting, flower remedies, guided imagery, herbal medicine, homeopathy, hypnotherapy, juice therapy, light therapy, magnetic field therapy, meditation, mind/body medicine, naturopathic medicine, network chiropractic, Neuro-Linguistic Programming, nutritional supplements, oxygen therapy, qigong (a Chinese healing pratice), sound therapy, Traditional Chinese Medicine, and yoga," she states.

Sharon daily maintains a positive state of mind and confidence in her regime. "While in my meditation, I ask my body what it needs and I change my treatments accordingly," she says. "In a way, I am my own physician. The virus has empowered me to become responsible for my life. As a result of my healing process, I have learned to love and appreciate life, people, and myself."

Sharon credits her longevity to her state of mind and confidence in her health regimen. "If I deviate from my program, I know it," she explains, "The night sweats return and the swollen lymph nodes soon begin to re-emerge. In 1992, I had difficulty accessing my doctors' services, vitamins, and herbs, because I didn't have much money and I had lost my health insurance." In a matter of seven months, her health plummeted and many of her HIV/AIDS symptoms resurfaced.

Sharon encourages others to take better care of themselves. "When people find out they are infected with HIV/AIDS, sometimes I hear 'woe, is me, I'm dying' and they give up on life and stop living. Others take the virus and allow it to empower them. They see it as an opportunity to live." She continues, "My whole life has changed. My commitment to life has changed. I live life to the fullest and I appreciate every moment. When I wake up in the morning the first thoughts in my mind are, 'Thank you, God. I'm happy to be alive.' I have found that inner peace . . . within myself."

Special Challenges for Women with HIV/AIDS

One of the hardest times in Sharon's life was when she learned that she had HIV and she had not met another woman who was infected. "I knew if I was infected, I couldn't be the only woman with HIV or AIDS," Sharon remembers. "I knew that there had to be other women who felt alone and lost just like I was." She felt that if she could unite women faced with similar situations and problems, there would be hope, so she started the first Women's HIV/AIDS Support Group in Los Angeles. She recalls, "At first there were only two women that came to the support group, but as the months went by, and the word got out, we ended up having about eight women coming on a regular basis. It was a wonderful feeling to know that we were not alone. We came together in a safe and healing environment, which allowed us to share from our heart our own personal experiences and needs. Through our compassion, love, and understanding, we were able to give one another the encouragement and support we needed.

"Traditionally, women are the caregivers in their families and relationships. A lot of times I see that coping with this

virus can be harder for an infected women, who has the
responsibilities of children and a husband or lover. Infected
women usually feel more isolated than gay men, who tend to
form strong communities. Women may believe that there is
little that can be done for them.

"Women also have many unique challenges. Their
child(ren) might be infected. It can be harder for women to
access services then men. Many women are single parents and
therefore are faced with financial difficulties. And many doctors are not educated in women's issues and health problems
when it comes to HIV and AIDS."

Sharon goes on to say, "Infected women are also faced
with other issues, such as: how and when to disclose their
HIV/AIDS status to their partner and child(ren); the decision
to have or not to have children; the concerns about who will
care for their child(ren) when they are sick, or have passed
away; and the fact that women have had a harder time getting
disability benefits. Overall, infected women feel more isolated
than gay men do. Unfortunately, early intervention is not a
reality for most women infected with HIV or AIDS."

When Sharon became ill, she knew she had to go on disability and apply for Social Security benefits. She turned to
AIDS Project Los Angeles (APLA) for support and guidance.
"When I needed to keep going, when every moment seemed
like eternity, APLA was my strength and my spirit.

"The staff at APLA told me before I filed for my benefits
that my chances of qualifying for Social Security didn't look
good because I hadn't acquired any of the opportunistic infections listed in the AIDS definition."

But Sharon determinedly fought the system by document-
ing over thirty pages of additional information. She recalls, "It
took me hours upon hours, relentless days upon relentless
nights, to document every detail of what I was capable, and no
longer capable, of doing since becoming HIV-symptomatic."
Her efforts were rewarded, however, as she became one of the
first HIV positive women to qualify for Social Security
Disability Benefits in Los Angeles. This was an important
accomplishment, not only for herself, but for all other women
infected with HIV and AIDS, because it has subsequently
made it easier for such women to qualify for the benefits that

they are properly entitled to. And for the past few years, Sharon's documentation has been used by APLA's Public Benefits Department to assist other women infected with HIV/AIDS in qualifying for Social Security Benefits.

Sharon states, "One of the biggest problems that face infected women is that this virus manifests itself differently in our bodies. We are not only experiencing the usual opportunistic infections, we are also experiencing problems such as pelvic inflammatory disease (PID), cervical cancer caused by the human papilloma virus (HPV), recurrent bacterial pneumonia, abnormal pap smears, irregular menstrual cycle, and recurrent yeast infections."

In September 1992, Sharon and three other women infected with HIV/AIDS were invited by the Centers for Disease Control (CDC) in Atlanta, Georgia to testify on behalf of the expansion of the AIDS Surveillance Definition, with the hope of including women's symptoms. Since January 1993, the AIDS definition has added cervical cancer, recurrent bacterial pneumonia, and any infected person with a T-cell count of 200 or less.

Sharon continues to make a difference on a global scale. In 1992, one week prior to the VIII International Conference on AIDS in Amsterdam, fifty-nine women throughout the world were chosen to gather for the First International Pre-Conference for Women Living with HIV/AIDS. Sharon was one of those chosen to participate. The group assembled a list of global issues concerning infected women and their loved ones. They also learned techniques to empower their lives, and to take back their spirit.

Sharon recalls, "Common issues were identified, and we formulated twelve needs statements to improve the situation of women living with HIV/AIDS throughout the world. We made the following needs known at the VIII International Conference on AIDS, in Amsterdam."

1) We need encouragement, support, and funding for the development of self-help groups, local and international networks of women living with HIV/AIDS.
2) We need the media to realistically portray us, not to stigmatize us.

3) We need equitable, accessible, and affordable treatments for, and research into, how the virus affects women (psychosocial and medical aspects, complementary and allopathic treatments).

4) We need funding for services and support for women living with HIV/AIDS, to alleviate our isolation and meet our basic needs. All funding directed to us needs to be evaluated and monitored to ensure that we get it.

5) We need the right to make our own choices about reproduction and to be respected and supported in those choices, and the right to have children.

6) We need recognition of the right of our children/orphans to be cared for and the importance of our role as parents.

7) We need education and training of health care providers and the community at large about women's risks and needs; up to date, accurate information concerning all issues about women living with HIV/AIDS should be readily available.

8) We need the gynecological manifestation of women's symptoms to be included whenever the AIDS definition is considered.

9) We need recognition of the fundamental human rights of all women living with HIV/AIDS, with special consideration for women in prison, drug users, and sex workers.

10) We need research about woman to woman transmission, recognition of and support for lesbians living with HIV/AIDS.

11) We need decision making power and consultation on all levels of policies and programs affecting women with HIV/AIDS.

12) We need to provide economic support for women living with HIV/AIDS in developing countries to help them to be self-sufficient and independent.

Sharon smiles as she remembers these fifty-nine women from all over the world, with their different backgrounds and their different issues, who came from various cultures, religions, and lifestyles, and yet were all committed to the betterment of all women living with HIV/AIDS. In Sharon's eyes, although they were all women who are infected by HIV or AIDS, they are also women who have become empowered by their very condition.

Taking what she learned from the conference, Sharon counsels, "It doesn't matter where you live, if your needs are not being met, make it known to your community, the media, and the government. In whatever way you can, demand that they be met. Remember, whatever you are feeling or experiencing, there are other women going through similar situations. Unfortunately, women are just now beginning to be recognized as part of the AIDS pandemic. As women infected and affected by HIV/AIDS, we need to join together effectively to make sure that our special needs are met. You may be the one in your community that needs to start up a women's program. I really support you in taking an active role, not only for yourself, but for those who are not able to do so. Our voices must be heard!"

Sharon has assisted AIDS organizations in putting together brochures and programs that are specially designed for women who are infected with HIV/AIDS. She was also a key player in helping to set up the first women's HIV/AIDS clinic in Los Angeles. Through her educational AIDS Programs, which she teaches at high schools, colleges, businesses, churches, clubs, women's groups, and conferences, Sharon has dedicated her life to saving people from infecting themselves or others with HIV. She talks openly to her audience about the myths and reality of HIV/AIDS, including transmission and prevention, as well as drugs and alcohol, discrimination, and AIDS in the work place, and shares from her heart her own personal experiences since becoming infected. She also continues to enjoy teaching healing techniques to people faced with any life-challenging illness. Additionally, Sharon and Jeaneen travel worldwide educating health care providers, laypersons, teachers, and persons with AIDS in such far-off locales as Canada, Russia, and Korea.

In 1992, Sharon and Jeaneen were invited by the International Center for Better Health, now administrated through the International AIDS Project, to become part of their educational AIDS Program in Russia. Sharon addressed health issues around women and children infected with HIV, alternative therapies, AIDS and intimacy, and AIDS and spirituality. She was also asked by the women from the former Soviet Union to lead a seminar on self-esteem and empowerment. As a teen AIDS Educator, Jeaneen was able to teach issues on AIDS to her peers in Russia. Sharon recalls, "We provided HIV/AIDS education to two hundred and fifty health care providers, teachers, clergy people, lay-persons, and people with AIDS throughout the former Soviet Union. Through our educational programs, the Russian people were able to go back to their communities and educate their peers. We were also able to help the Russian people develop and set up their own grassroots AIDS programs in Moscow and St. Petersburg. The importance of these groups goes well beyond those of manmade borders; it's humanity that is in desperate need of healing. The work we did in Russia wasn't really about HIV or AIDS, it was about love."

Sharon continues her international work in Vilnius, Lithuania, Moscow, St. Petersburg (Russia), and Korea, while contributing to positive changes in people's perceptions about women and AIDS, and maintaining an active, visible presence.

As a pioneer in women's issues regarding HIV/AIDS, Sharon was the first HIV-infected woman elected to the Los Angeles Health Service HIV Planning Council as well as the first HIV-infected woman elected to the Board of Directors of the following organizations: AIDS Project Los Angeles; AIDS, Medicine, and Miracles; and the International AIDS Program—a testament to the profound difference she has made in the AIDS community at large.

Throughout all of her activities, Sharon takes time for herself, enjoying nature, visiting with her family and friends, writing poetry, and working on three books which are the natural outgrowth of her experiences and realizations garnered over the past seven years. She also continues to ensure her health with her varied regimen of alternative therapies, and believes that if it were not for her treatments, she probably would not be alive today. She still feels fatigue is a constant barrier, yet she continues to see each day as a new opportunity. "I live each day to its fullest," she says. "HIV/AIDS is about living, not about dying."

Resources

"The next major advance in the health of the American people will be determined by what the individual is willing to do for himself."

—John Knowles,
Former President of the
Rockefeller Foundation

Where to Find Help

AIDS Organizations

The following groups provide information about the various aspects of dealing with AIDS and HIV.

United States

AIDS Alternative Health Project
3223 N. Sheffield Avenue
Chicago, Illinois 60657
(312) 327-6437

An organization staffed by professional volunteers who offer chiropractic, acupuncture, bodywork, nutritional and herbal counseling, and massage therapy to HIV positive individuals. Services are available for a nominal fee, which can be waived for people who are unemployed, or receiving unemployment, social security, or disability benefits.

AIDS Medicine & Miracles
P.O. Box 9130
Maxwell Building
311 Mapleton
Boulder, CO 80301-9130
(303) 447-8777

A non-profit organization which strives to educate, nurture, and empower all people confronting AIDS. In a supportive retreat setting, national conferences explore medical and complementary therapies, as well as psychosocial and spiritual opportunities. This organization also serves the loved ones and caregivers of those living with HIV/AIDS by promoting health, growth, and social action.

AIDS Project Los Angeles
1313 N. Vine Street
Los Angeles, California 90028
(213) 962-1600

AIDS Project Los Angeles (APLA), the nation's second largest AIDS service organization, responds to the educational needs of the public and of people with HIV/AIDS as well as providing public policy/ advocacy in California and Washington, D.C. APLA provides a wide range of client services—from Southern California's only HIV-dedicated dental clinic, to case management, mental health, a food pantry, counseling for addictive behaviors, and others.

C.A.R.E. Program
(Comprehensive AIDS Resource Education)
411 East 10th St., Suite 202
Long Beach, CA 90813
(310) 491-9905
(310) 491-9867 (FAX)

C.A.R.E. is a community-based, non-profit organization whose purpose is to assist and empower HIV/AIDS-infected individuals by identifying and accessing needed social and healthcare resources. Their program offers a comprehensive continuum of non-emergency health and human services for people with HIV-spectrum disease and supportive counseling for their families and significant others.

Cure Now
P.O. Box 29386
Los Angeles, California 90029
(213) 660-7563

Cure Now is a group formed to educate people on positive healing alternatives, and to improve the psychological and spiritual attitudes surrounding AIDS and HIV.

Gay Men's Health Crisis (GMHC)
129 West 20th Street
New York, NY 10011-0022
Hotline Phone: (212) 807-6655

Gay Men's Health Crisis (GMHC) is the nation's oldest and largest AIDS organization, providing direct services to more than 5,000 men, women, and children with HIV illness and serving tens of thousands more through its education and advocacy programs.

Group for the Scientific Reappraisal
of the HIV/AIDS Hypothesis
2040 Polk Street, Suite 321
San Francisco, CA 94109
(415) 775-1984 (FAX)

The Group for the Scientific Reappraisal of the HIV Hypothesis is comprised of over four hundred scientists and physicians worldwide. Publishes a monthly newsletter called Rethinking AIDS. *The group came into existence as a result of its efforts to get the following four sentence letter published in a number of prominent scientific journals. All have refused to do so.*

"It is widely believed by the general public that a retrovirus called HIV causes the group of diseases called AIDS. Many biomedical scientists now question this hypothesis. We propose that thorough reappraisal of the existing evidence for and against this hypothesis be conducted by a suitable independent group. We further propose that critical epidemiological studies be devised and undertaken."

HEAL (Health Education AIDS Liaison)
16 East 16th Street
New York, New York 10003
(212) 674-HOPE

Offers information to people seeking to strengthen their health and immune systems. Provides information on an alternative approach to health that "precludes toxic, immunosuppressive drugs, but includes physical, emotional, psychological, and spiritual efforts." Also provides referrals to hypnotherapists trained to deal with the fears of an HIV diagnosis.

Project AIDS International
8033 Sunset Boulevard, #2640
Los Angeles, California 90046-2427
(213) 857-0809

A division of People's International Health Project, Project AIDS International performs research into the causation of AIDS, as well as various treatments for opportunistic infections—both conventional and alternative. They perform a wide range of services for the AIDS community, operating a hotline for referrals, conducting lectures and public information forums, educating health care workers, and delivering medical supplies such as hospital beds, syringes, and medicines. These activities are supported by donations. Publishes the Journal of International Health Research, *whose main purpose is to offer international exposure for peer-review of science papers dealing with AIDS, cancer, chronic fatigue immune deficiency syndrome (CFIDS), hemophilia, and matters of general health that may not be published elsewhere. It also serves as an international communications link between organizations, carries new treatment reviews as well as listings and updates from around the world.*

Project Inform
1965 Market Street, Suite 220
San Francisco, CA 94103
(415) 558-8669
(415) 558-0684 FAX
Hotline: (800) 822-7422 (Mon–Sat. 10 A.M.–4 P.M. PST)

Project Inform is a national treatment information and advocacy organization based in San Francisco dedicated to the goals of accelerating research into and access to effective treatments for HIV/AIDS. Project Inform conducts informational Town Meetings, seeks to affect public policy through the Treatment Action Network, produces two HIV treatment information journals, and offers one of the nation's most widely used HIV treatment hotlines.

The San Francisco Center for Living
4054 18th St.
San Francisco, CA 94114
(415) 252-1666
(415) 252-1568 FAX

The San Francisco Center for Living is an organization of volunteers dedicated to helping those experiencing a life-challenging illness as well as their families, friends, or caregivers. The Center creates a supportive environment where people do not have to face their diagnosis, fear, or grief alone. The Center offers workshops and support groups, psychological and spiritual counseling, bodywork, healthy communal meals, and classes in living, healing, and dying.

SEARCH Alliance
7481 Beverly Boulevard, Suite 304
Los Angeles, CA 90036
(213) 930-8820

SEARCH Alliance is a private, non-profit AIDS research organization dedicated to finding more effective treatments and, ultimately, a cure for AIDS. SEARCH conducts fast-track research & human clinical trials on promising new HIV/AIDS therapeutics. SEARCH focuses its research on therapies which have the potential of having a significant impact on the course of HIV disease, including anti-retrovirals, immuno-modulators, gene therapy, and O.I. treatments. SEARCH works with over seventy HIV-specialist physicians and scientists to facilitate its efforts. SEARCH Alliance is entirely funded through private donations.

United Kingdom

Continuum
P.O. Box 2754
London NW10 8UF
011 4481 961 1170
011 4481 961 2330 (FAX)

An organization for long-term survivors of HIV and AIDS. Publishes the magazine Continuum. *Excellent source of information about alternative treatments for HIV/AIDS and the latest developments in AIDS research from Europe and around the world.*

Immune Development Trust
Gatesden, Cromer Street
King's Cross, London, WC1H 8EA
011 4471-837-2151
011 4471-837-7742 (FAX)

The Trust accepts without charge anyone who is HIV positive, and provides a range of alternative treatments, including acupuncture, herbal medicine, massage therapy, and other types of bodywork.

Buyer's Clubs

There are a number of independent buyer's clubs around the United States. They make preparations available that are used by people with AIDS. Items often are offered at a savings.

The Healing Alternatives Foundation
1748 Market Street, Suite 204
San Francisco, CA 94102

Non-profit buyers club organized to assist people with AIDS in obtaining medications. Alternative treatments available. Mail orders accepted.

PWA Health Group
150 West 26th Street, Suite 201
New York, New York 10001
(212) 255-0520

Non-profit buyers club organized to assist people with AIDS in obtaining medications. Alternative treatments available. Mail orders accepted. Updates on experimental treatments in bi-monthly newsletter.

Recommended Reading

AIDS and Syphilis—The Hidden Link. Coulter, Harris.
Berkeley, California: North Atlantic Books, and Washington,
DC: Wehawken Book Company, 1987.
*According to Dr. Coulter, "The AIDS virus is probably another
'opportunistic' infection of an already destroyed immune system ...
the search should be for factors which undermine the immune
system and thus predispose to infection with the AIDS virus and
others which may otherwise be quite innocuous."*

AIDS: The HIV Myth. Adams, Jad. New York: St. Martin's
Press, 1989.
*An exploration of Peter Duesberg's HIV hypothesis that debunks the
theory that the virus causes AIDS.*

AIDS INC.: Scandal of the Century. Rappoport, Jon. Foster
City, California: Human Energy Press, 1988.
*Investigative reporter Jon Rappoport uncovers the shocking truth
about AIDS: Thousands are dying needlessly as the medical world
and media pull off one of the biggest scandals of our time—all for
the love of power and money. AIDS INC. takes you on a behind-the-
scenes tour of laboratories, newsrooms, and even the White House
to expose the real killers behind the disease and to propose a multifactorial model for the causation of AIDS. The author proposes that
AIDS represents the confluence of many different factors within the
"modern" lifestyle such as historically unprecedented sexual
promiscuity, drug abuse, promiscuous use of pharmaceuticals,
rampant sexually transmitted diseases, widespread malnutrition
(even in the U.S. where processed foods are common), and massive
vaccination campaigns.*

AIDS: Passageway to Transformation. Shealy, C. Norman;
and Myss, Caroline M. Walpole, NH: Stillpoint Publishing,
1991.
*To understand AIDS, the authors have placed this much-feared
disease in a larger perspective where one sees the parallel between
AIDS on the personal level and the breakdown of the Earth's
immune system; and between "victim consciousness" and the
threat of nuclear devastation. A fascinating book expands what you
already know about AIDS with an insightful global perspective.*

Includes a recommended holistic regimen people can use for effective prevention and treatment.

The AIDS War: Propaganda, Profiteering, and Genocide from the Medical-Industrial Complex. Lauritson, John. New York: Asklepios, 1993.

A leading AIDS dissident journalist debunks the HIV-AIDS hypotheses and AZT therapy. Contains the latest information regarding the dangers of using AZT to treat AIDS, as well as the censure Peter Duesberg received from the conventional medical establishment for his theory that HIV does not cause AIDS. (Available from Asklepios, 26 Saint Marks Place, New York City 10003.)

Alternative Medicine: The Definitive Guide. The Burton Goldberg Group. Puyallup, WA: Future Medicine Publishing, Inc., 1993.

The most comprehensive reference on alternative medicine ever compiled. Provides in-depth, easily understandable coverage of 43 alternative therapies and over 200 health conditions, with advice from nearly 400 alternative physicians worldwide. See chapter on "AIDS."

Healing into Immortality. Epstein, Gerald. New York: Bantam Books, 1994.

"The ultimate aim is to attain not only a state of healing, but eventually to bring ourselves to a state of incredible longevity. We might even reach the point of defeating death itself." With this bold statement, Gerald Epstein, M.D., a leading pioneer in the field of mind-body medicine, introduces a breakthrough book that can quite literally save—and perhaps indefinitely extend—your life.

How to Live Between Office Visits: A Guide to Life, Love and Health. Siegel, Bernard. HarperCollins, 1993.

In this inspirational book, Dr. Siegel shows us how to look into our hearts, listen to ourselves, draw on our strength and that of our loved ones, and confront our difficulties in a healthy way—whether they be illness or any other of life's serious problems. He talks with us about handling the fear of recurrent illness, asking for help, dealing with anger and pain, becoming open, confronting destructive images of ourselves, understanding the gift of hope and unconditional love, and learning how to live.

Poison By Prescription: The AZT Story. Lauritson, John. New York: Asklepios, 1990.

An expose of the politics involved in AIDS research and how AZT, a known toxic substance, became the conventional medical establish-

ment's drug of choice for dealing with AIDS and HIV. (Available from Asklepios, 26 Saint Marks Place, New York City 10003.)

Rethinking AIDS. Root-Bernstein, Robert. New York: The Free Press, 1993.
A thorough investigation which indicates that HIV alone does not cause AIDS.

Surviving AIDS. Callen, Michael. New York: Harper Collins, 1990.
Outlines the alternative medicine approach to health taken by the author, one of the longest survivors of AIDS.

A World Without AIDS. Chaitow, Leon, D.O., N.D.; and Martin, Simon. London, England: Thorsons Publishing Group, 1988. [Available only from Nutri Centre, 7 Park Crescent, London W1 (FAX 011-4471-436-5171)]
A convincing argument that conventional medicine approaches do not "cure" disease, which outlines how AIDS can be treated using methods of naturopathic medicine. Also includes an appendix outlining twenty-one ways to strengthen the immune system.

Newsletters

Rethinking AIDS
2040 Polk Street, Suite 321
San Francisco, CA 94109
FAX (415) 775-1984
A monthly newsletter published by the Group for the Scientific Reappraisal of the HIV Hypothesis, comprised of over four hundred scientists and physicians worldwide.

Choosing an Alternative Health Professional

The choice to explore alternative medicine can be a crucial turning point in the life of a person with HIV infection or with AIDS, affecting physical as well as mental and emotional health. With the help of an alternative health professional, it may be possible to take control of one's personal health, eliminating the sense of frustration and helplessness many feel when dealing with conventional medicine.

"It is extremely important for anyone who is newly diagnosed or looking for a new doctor to interview several doctors or get recommendations from other people who are infected," says Sharon Lund, an International AIDS educator and activist, who has been HIV positive for ten years. "Ask, 'Who are your doctors? What kind of treatments do they use? Do you feel comfortable with your doctor? Are they open to alternatives and are they willing to spend quality time with you to discuss these options and explain what is going on with your health and your treatments? Are they well informed on the latest treatments and issues surrounding HIV and AIDS?'"

Not surprisingly, many of the same criteria used to choose a conventional doctor are important in seeking out an expert in alternative medicine. Yet, because the very nature of the alternative approach is far more encompassing than the conventional one, there are a number of other critical factors that should be taken into account in the selection process.

The following suggestions offer basic guidelines for choosing an alternative practitioner:

- **Educate yourself about the general principles of alternative health care.** The success of alternative care is as dependent upon an informed patient as it is on a knowledgeable practitioner. Even after selecting a practitioner, the education process must continue, becoming an ongoing aspect of a person's approach to alternative care. As Garry F. Gordon, M.D., co-founder of the American

College of Advancement in Medicine, notes, "I encourage people to learn to become their own doctor, and use health practitioners as 'educators,' realizing that we can learn something from everyone."

- **If you are selecting a general practitioner, choose someone with a diverse background and expertise in a wide variety of disciplines.** "I think you want to find someone who has a relatively eclectic background," says Elson Haas, M.D., Director of the Center for Preventive Medicine in San Rafael, California. "A great limitation of conventional medicine is that the only choice is really drugs or surgery. Ideally, you want someone who can use both natural approaches as well as pharmaceutical ones, someone who can balance their rational approach with a more intuitive approach, so that they are not just operating from their own bias."

- **Find a practitioner with whom you can communicate openly and with whom you have a good rapport.** The relationship between patient and doctor is perhaps the most crucial difference between conventional and alternative medicine. "The dictatorship of the physician is the foundation of standard medical practice," notes Jay Holder, M.D., D.C., Ph.D., Director of the Exodus, a treatment center for addiction in Miami, Florida. "In alternative health care, however, the tradition is just the opposite: the patient dictates and the doctor serves."

"If you do not have a doctor who will sit back and listen to what you have to say for twenty minutes to a half hour," says John R. Lee, M.D., of Sebastopol, California, "you do not have a doctor who is going to find the cause."

Dr. Gordon takes this point one step farther: "If you don't feel you can communicate adequately and get your questions answered, you need to shop some more, because any anxiety over the doctor-patient selection puts a real negative damper on the healing process."

Sharon Lund concurs: "You don't owe your doctor anything. This is your life, so you can walk away at any point when you do not feel in control of your treatment or your doctor is not providing you with what you need. Walk away, find someone else."

- Select a physician who is sensitive to your particular needs and circumstances. Dr. Haas stresses the importance of what he calls "patient-centered" health care. "This means you really take the person as the primary mode and really work around what their needs are," he says.
- **Choose an alternative approach in which you have confidence.** In natural medicine, the mental and emotional aspects of healing cannot be separated from the physical. It is vital, therefore, that one believe in the alternative method one has chosen. As Dr. Gordon explains, "If I could show you stacks of evidence about homeopathy, but you tell me that you will never understand how it works, I'm going to get half the effect from you than I would from a person that had a neighbor whose life was saved by homeopathy, was well-informed about therapy, and was ready to take a homeopathic remedy when they walked in the door."

There are numerous ways to locate alternative practitioners. In the "Where to Find Help" sections at the back of the chapters in Part Two, you will find listings of organizations that can provide nationwide referrals. Another valuable resource is the *Alternative Medicine Yellow Pages* (Future Medicine Publishing, Inc., 1994).

"Great spirits have always encountered violent opposition from mediocre minds."

—*Albert Einstein*

Scientific Appendix: Human Immunodeficiency Virus

Robert Jacobs, N.M.D., D.Hom. (Med)

To date, the World Health Organization estimates that 14 million people in the world are infected with the HIV virus.[1] By the year 2000, it is forecasted that this figure will grow to 40 million people.[2] New regions of the world continue to be drawn into the orbit of the virus, as its spread seems to continue unchecked.

Pathogenesis

HIV is spread by sexual contact, exposure to infected blood or blood products, and perinatal transmission from mother to child. Sixty percent of all cases of HIV are the result of heterosexual contact.[3]

HIV is a retrovirus, a member of the *Lentivirnae* subfamily of retroviruses affecting humans. Lentiviruses cause infections of the nervous system, including demyelinating encephalomyelitis, interstitial pneumonia in sheep, and simian immunodeficiency virus (an AIDS type of disease in Asian monkeys). The lentivirus family also includes caprine arthritis-encephalitis virus, equine infectious anemia virus, visna virus, maedi ciruses virus, and feline immunodeficiency virus. Lentiviral infections have long periods of latency and characteristically have weak humoral immune responses mounted against them. They also show a persistent viremia. Other known retroviral infections cause leukemia, Kawasaki disease, and tropical spastic paraparesis.[4]

The HIV virus has a twenty-sided outer coat containing seventy-two external spikes. These spikes are formed by the two major viral-envelope proteins, gp120 and gp41. The core of the virus contains four nucleocapsid proteins, p24, p17, p9, and p7.[5]

The major target of the HIV virus is the CD4+ T-lymphocytes, macrophages, and monocytes. The CD4 receptor on
these cell surfaces has a high affinity for the virus.
Specifically the gp120 envelope protein of HIV binds with the
CD4 receptor.[6]

Once the gp120 envelope protein binds with the CD4
receptor, the gp41 envelope protein fuses with the cell membrane which permits HIV to enter the cell. The virus then
uncoats and begins the process of converting the virus's RNA
to a double strand of DNA which can invade the host nucleus.
This process, called "reverse transcription," is accomplished
by the enzyme "reverse transcriptase" which is manufactured
by the virus "pol" gene. The viral DNA is then inserted into
the host DNA by the enzyme "integrase," another product of
the "pol" gene.[7]

One method of slowing down the viral invasion of the body
is to block the reverse transcription process. This prevents the
viral RNA from being converted to DNA, and stops the replication of the viral particle. The class of drugs that inhibit
reverse transcription are called *dideoxynucleosides*. The three
already in general use are AZT, ddI, and ddC. They have a significant impact on viral replication, but each one has strong
side effects that can ultimately prevent their continued use.
AZT causes bone marrow suppression, ddC causes peripheral
neuropathy, and ddI can cause pancreatitis. Furthermore, HIV
mutates into strains of the virus which are resistant to these
drugs and continues on with the destruction of the immune system. These shortcomings will probably prevent the dideoxynucleosides from becoming a main weapon against HIV.

Once the viral DNA is integrated into the host DNA, the
viral DNA begins the manufacture of new viral components,
including RNA and viral structural proteins. The new viral
particles are assembled in a step-wise manner, initially involving aggregation of the ribonucleoprotein core in the cytoplasm
of the infected cell. These retroviral cores are composed of the
HIV-1 RNA, "Gag" gene proteins, and the various enzymes
encoded by the "pol" gene, such as reverse transcriptase and
integrase. Once assembled, these cores move to the surface
and bud through the plasma membrane, where they acquire
their lipid membranes, complete with the two protein products

of the HIV-1 "env" gene. The new virions are released into the extracellular fluid by viral budding and they continue the spread of the infection.

The most critical effect of the HIV-1 virus is to kill the CD4+ T-lymphocytes and inactivate the CD8+ cytotoxic lymphocytes. A significant reduction of the CD4+ T-cell population causes immunodeficiency and can ultimately lead to the disease picture which is known as AIDS. The CD8+ cytotoxic lymphocytes kill virus-infected cells and prevent the increase in the HIV infection. They represent one of the body's primary methods of killing HIV. Antibodies which would be the normal method of clearing virus infection from the body are not as effective with HIV. In fact, the antibodies may increase the virulence of the viral infection because of their involvement with programmed cell death (apoptosis) through the formation of superantigens. When the body produces antibodies to the virus's gp120 envelope protein, the anti-gp120 antibody and the gp120 envelope protein crosslink. If the gp120 viral particle is bound to the CD4+ receptor of the T cell when the crosslinking occurs, a superantigen is created and programmed cell death is triggered. Programmed cell death or "apoptosis" is a process inherent in the cells where cell death occurs when enzymes that naturally occur in the cell break down the cell's DNA. A concentration of 10 ng/ml of gp120 is all that is needed to trigger the programmed cell death. AIDS patients typically have 12-92 ng/ml of circulating gp120.[8]

Monocytes, also infected by HIV-1, are not killed to nearly the same degree as the CD4+ T cells. The monocytes in fact may be a reservoir for HIV-1, carrying the infection to the brain and other organs. During the course of infection with HIV-1, many different strains of HIV-1 mutate, and the various strains have different affinities for different cells. Some strains of the virus preferentially infect monocytes, some CD4+ T cells, some gut epithelium, glial cells of the brain, and bone marrow cells. The different locations of the virus are responsible for the various problems associated with AIDS such as dementia, diarrhea, blood abnormalities, and the wasting syndrome. There are as many as twenty different strains of HIV in an infected person during the course of the disease.

Once HIV enters the CD4+ T cell, it may become latent or continue onto a persistent form of infection. Information to date suggests that the virus will not replicate in resting T cells.[9] Some activation or trigger must start an immune response for the virus to begin replication. These triggers can include antigens, mitogens, various gene products of Human T-cell Leukemia Virus Type 1, Herpes Simplex Virus, Epstein Barr Virus, Cytomegalic Virus, Hepatitis B Virus, Human Herpes Virus Type 6, bacteria, mycobacteria, and various cytokines. The cytokines which most activate HIV are TNF-alpha and Interleukin 1 and 6.[10]

When these are present, the virus becomes very active and the infection proceeds rapidly. This knowledge gives another possible method of preventing the virus activation. Keep the body healthy and free from any major infections which happen independently of HIV. This requires an awareness of life style and stopping habits which detract from health. Natural forms of health care are best suited to assist at this point. If there are no activating factors, the virus can remain latent for an extremely long period of time.[11]

The progression of HIV infection is in three stages. The first stage, the acute, lasts for weeks. The primary infection causes an acute self-limited viral syndrome. Six to fifteen days after the onset of symptoms, high titres of infectious HIV and viral p24 antigen are detected. These titres fall precipitately after day twenty-seven and the decline coincides with an increase in the levels of antiviral antibodies. The next phase is the chronic phase lasting years and characterized by minimal measurable pathologic changes. Viral replication does continue during this phase however. The final phase is ARC (AIDS-Related Complex) or full blown AIDS which can last from months to years. All stages involve active replication of HIV. The acute phase is characterized by high levels of virus, the chronic phase by low levels of virus, and the third phase by a resurgence of active virus in the plasma and renewed infection in the cells.[12]

During a fully active HIV infection, only 1/100 CD4+ T cells are infected with HIV. Only 1/1,000 peripheral blood CD4+ T cells are infected. The question of how such a small amount of virus can cause such damage has been elucidated by recent research, which has shown that the virus has many ways of killing the body's CD4+ T cells and doesn't need to infect the cells to kill them. One such method is called programmed cell death or apoptosis as mentioned above.[13] Viremia in plasma is now thought to be a better indicator of the stage of illness and viral activity than the level of p24 antigen or antibody. This gives a better way to test the efficacy of new drugs and natural therapies before the disease progresses beyond the level in which these therapies can be effective.[14]

Another method of cellular killing is by cell fusion and syncytium formation. A syncytia is an aggregate of cells fused together forming one large multinucleated body. This fusion is mediated by the gp41 protein after the gp120 protein interacts with the CD4 receptor. Actual viral infection of the cell is not necessary for it to form a syncytia. Large numbers of cells are bound together forming multinucleated syncytia. These multinucleated syncytia ultimately lead to the death of many T cells.

Additionally, autoimmune destruction of CD4+ T cells occurs by the following mechanism. HIV infection causes CD4+ T cells to behave aberrantly as if they were encountering non-self tissues (alloantigens). The CD4+ T cells respond to the viral induced alloantigen phenomenon and become activated. The activation increases the viral replication within the CD4+ T cells and the activated CD4+ T cells cause cytotoxic CD8+ T cells to be generated. The CD8+ cytotoxic T cells destroy CD4+ T cells with viral markers on their surface regardless of whether or not they are infected with the virus, and there are many uninfected CD4+ T cells with viral markers on the surface.[15] Thus a wide spread destruction of CD4+ T cells occurs without the cells ever being infected. The body is tricked into destroying itself.

The monocytes and macrophages are not affected by most of these methods of cell death and thus contain the virus within them and are not killed by the virus. The chemotactic response of the monocyte-macrophage population is, however, impaired even at in infection rate of only 1/1,000-1/100,000.[16]

There are different strains of the HIV-1 virus and these different strains show different levels of cytopathic effects. Three main groups have been classified according to replication rate, syncytium-inducing capacity, and host range of HIV isolates. The most rapid progression to AIDS and the lowest survival rate were observed in individuals with high-replicating, syncytium-inducing HIV isolates. The next were the high-replicating, non-syncytium-inducing isolates, and the best survival is with low-replicating, non-syncytium-inducing HIV isolates. The HIV can mutate into more virulent strains over time.[17]

Dr. Luc Montagnier, of the Pasteur Institute, feels that AIDS pathogenesis depends upon the interplay of three variables: HIV, the immune system of the infected individual, and co-factors. He suggests that these co-factors are superantigens such as bacterial toxins that can cause an exaggerated immune response (autoimmune) which attacks the body's own T cells and causes the depletion of large portions of the T cells.[18]

Montagnier feels that the HIV gp120 envelope glycoprotein causes abnormal activation of CD4+ T cells, making them vulnerable to superantigen-induced apoptosis. "If at the early stage [of HIV infection] we can diminish the extent of immune activation, we can limit the extent of CD4 cell depletion," Montagnier suggested.[19]

Why doesn't the initial infection with HIV get eliminated like most other viral infections? The virus is not totally cleared at the sites of entry from the initial immune response. However, HIV infection is controlled for long periods of time due to what appears to be effective immunity. Once in the body the virus rapidly mutates its outer coat to stave off attack by antibodies and T cells. HIV then begins its degradation of immune function which goes beyond the infection of the CD4+ T cells. Cells that are not infected with HIV have functional defects. B-cell lymphocytes, natural killer cells, and CD8+ cytotoxic lymphocytes show profound functional defects.[20]

Several places to break the HIV life cycle have been identified. These include attachment and internalization of the virion, reverse transcription, integration, viral transcription, viral RNA-splicing and transport, and virus assembly and budding. This is the basis for new medicines being developed.

A strong immune system at the time of infection is the best chance to prevent AIDS from developing. Finding ways to strengthen the immune system remains one of the great hopes for the current state of HIV disease. Until a vaccine or drug is developed that can improve immune response, natural therapies such as homeopathy, herbology, acupuncture, and others are the only ways of actually strengthening the immune system. It is essential to have a positive attitude as well. Studies have shown that people with HIV who are depressed do worse than those who remain positive.[21]

Vaccines

Recent experiments have shown that a protective immune response against lentiviral-induced disease is possible. Two research groups successfully immunized monkeys from simian immunodeficiency virus and they resisted a challenge from the active virus after immunization. It also appears that a vaccine can bolster protective immunity in already infected people.[22]

It is now felt that a successful vaccine will have to stimulate the CD8+ cytotoxic T lymphocytes. These appear to be the body's strongest defense against HIV. Antibodies do not seem to be effective in clearing the virus and possibly can contribute to the programmed cell death associated with HIV. The gp120 envelope protein cross-linked with anti-gp120 antibodies and attached to the cell surface of CD4+ T cells cause the cells to die. Increasing the number of antibodies may only increase the speed at which the apoptosis occurs. Dr. Jonas Salk feels that the most effective vaccine would stimulate only the killer T cells and not antibodies. He feels that antibodies work best when the invading agent is outside the cell. In the case of HIV, the virus is inside the cell as well as outside.[23]

To date, there are many vaccines being researched. Some target viral envelope proteins; others target viral core nucleoproteins. There are vaccines against the conserved parts of the virus, and others against combinations of many viral particles. No one knows which will work. We are a long way from an effective vaccine to prevent infection with HIV. We may be closer to a vaccine which will boost immunity in people already infected with HIV. This is a new idea pioneered since the HIV infection and such vaccines are already being tested on infected people.

Drug Therapies

There are three main drugs being used to fight HIV at this time, and dozens more are being researched at different phases of the testing process. The three currently being used are AZT, ddI, and ddC. These drugs are all reverse transcriptase inhibitors. They have a proven ability to slow down the viral replication, and in some cases to increase life span. However, several studies have shed doubt upon the efficacy of AZT. In a Veterans Administration study of HIV positive healthy individuals, the researchers found that there was "no statistical difference in progression to AIDS," between the AZT group and the placebo group. In addition, *The Lancet* recently published the final findings of the Anglo-French Concorde study, reporting that "the results of Concorde do not encourage the early use of zidovudine (AZT) in symptom-free, HIV-infected adults."[24]

There are also several problems with these drugs. First of all, HIV develops resistance to them over time by mutating into different viral strains. Secondly, the ability to block the reverse transcription does not occur in all the cells that the virus resides in. Thirdly, these drugs have serious side effects which in the long term can be dangerous. AZT, for example, suppresses the bone marrow. Without proper bone marrow function, the entire immune system will collapse regardless of the virus or not. The drug ddC is associated with peripheral neuropathies, and ddI can lead to fatal pancreatitis.[25]

If these medications really did stop the spread of the virus within a person, or greatly added to the life span, or even increased the quality of life, perhaps these side effects would be worthwhile. In a recent three-year study in Europe and Australia, it was found that the difference in HIV disease progression in the group using AZT and controls over three years was 12 percent.

That means that 12 percent fewer people progressed using AZT. This is of benefit, but after three years the use of AZT has diminishing returns. The virus mutates into resistant strains, and the suppression of the bone marrow and other toxic effects mount up and suppress the body's ability to continue to fight. In a sense, the toxicity ensures that in the long term the patient will die, but in the short term there may be an increase in CD4+ T-cell numbers and short term health gains. Because these problems are acknowledged by the medical community, trials are underway to combine AZT with ddI and ddC to be able to reduce the dosage of each and have a better effect. Even so, the breakthrough in HIV will probably come in a different area. The antiretrovirals are helpful if other methods of self help are not used.

HIV Testing

The current tests for HIV infection, Western Blot and the ELISA test, use the method of antibody detection. This method shows the presence of antibodies to HIV. It is believed that the antibodies will show up within six months of infection with HIV. Newer methods of testing are being licensed now that can test HIV from the urine, and even home tests are being developed. However, there are false negative and false positive results from both the Western Blot and the ELISA tests. When questionable results are obtained from these tests, a Polymerase Chain Reaction test (PCR) and viral culture can be performed for confirmation. The Western Blot and the ELISA are good screening tests, but for absolute confirmation, PCR and viral culture tests are utilized. Even with these methods, it is possible to have some uncertainty because of the many strains of the virus. Some cases that show all of the signs of HIV infection have failed to be confirmed by any of these methods. Are those cases caused by a new virus or is a lack of detection caused by flaws in our current methods of testing?

AIDS without HIV

Recently a new disease has appeared that has AIDS-like symptoms of low CD4+ count and sustained immunodeficiency, however no HIV can be found in any of these cases. The total number of cases to date is extremely small. Dr. Luc Montagnier has found some evidence of a virus in the urine of these patients, and electron microscopy has revealed the

Ed. Note: Evidence exists that indicates that HIV, of itself, may not be enough to trigger the Acquired Immune Deficiency Syndrome (AIDS). For further details, see Chapter One.

presence of a virus with a defective coat. It is unclear if a new strain of HIV has been found, or if this is another disease all together. Fifty-four percent of the cases reported have no risk factors for HIV, and risk factors were found in 96 percent of the AIDS cases.

The CDC (Center for Disease Control) feels that this is not another AIDS virus. The illness has been given the name Idiopathic T-Lymphocytopenia (ITL). It is not clear whether this can be transmitted by blood, and studies are currently underway. The small number of cases of ITL does not invalidate the current methods of HIV testing or make them inaccurate, and does not herald a new AIDS virus. Blood banks are still considered as safe, with the risk of contracting HIV less than one-in-225,000.[26]

Lifestyle

One major area of self help is in lifestyle. Changing to a lifestyle that is health supportive has definite immune-enhancing effects. The cessation of cigarettes, alcohol, and drugs will help the body get stronger. Improving nutrition and supplementing the diet have been shown to be of great help to people with HIV.[27]

Changing from negative to positive mental attitudes has a proven health-enhancing effect. Avoiding sexually transmitted diseases, and other illnesses that can be prevented may increase the life span enormously. The long-term survivors of HIV all speak of these lifestyle changes, and they have not used AZT. They stand as a symbol of a positive fight against this disease.

Prophylactic Drug Therapy

The most significant breakthrough in treatment of HIV has been in the development of effective drugs to treat the opportunistic infections that ultimately take the life of an AIDS patient. This has been the real breakthrough that medicine can be proud of. Pneumocystis Carinii Pneumonia (PCP) can be prevented by the use of Bactrim or aerosol pentamidine. PCP is responsible for 60 percent of all cases progressing from HIV to AIDS. The ability to prevent this illness has saved countless lives. There are drugs for toxoplasmosis, cryptosporidium, mycobacterium avium complex, and many other complications of AIDS. These drugs do not have the toxic effects of the antiretroviral drugs, and they stop real dangers from occurring. That is why today's survival time has increased so dramatically. When AIDS was first identified, survival was as little as a few months. Now patients with diagnosed AIDS can live five to ten more years. The prophylactic drugs are so helpful and even people with very low CD4+ counts can be free of opportunistic infection for years.

Co-factors for Disease Progression

It is clear that HIV needs co-factors to become the deadly disease AIDS. These co-factors can be other infections, stress (causing immune suppression), herpes infection, hepatitis infection, toxic substances, and a toxic lifestyle. HIV cannot activate in resting CD4+ T cells. The virus needs the activation of the cytokine pathways to turn into an active infection. This gives one important chance to slow down or stop the progression of HIV infection to the disease AIDS.

Natural Therapies

There are many natural therapies which have proven to be of great interest and of enormous help to sufferers with HIV. Unfortunately these therapies have not been as well studied because the funding has not been available. However, there are community-based trials in the U.S. that do give these natural methods fair tests. Such methods have been with Chinese herbs, such as Compound Q, and bitter melon. Other studies have been with oral interferon at homeopathic dilutions, hypericin, ozone, hyperthermia, N-acetyl-cysteine, and aloe vera extract. Each of these studies has shown some benefit to AIDS patients, and patients with HIV.

The most well documented studies have been done with nutrition. It has been proven that oral nutritional supplementation is beneficial and health enhancing to patients with HIV infection. Malnutrition, an effect of the viral infection, can be offset by oral supplementation and the wasting syndrome can be forestalled if not totally prevented. When a person is initially infected with HIV, the condition of their immune system makes all the difference in the world. Immune-strengthening therapies are one of the major weapons that people have to protect themselves from AIDS. If infection occurs, maintaining health is even more important. The virus can become latent or active based upon the condition of the immune system, and how activated the immune system becomes fighting other immune-assaulting factors.[28]

Stress is another area that can hurt the immune system function. It has been proven by the science of psychoneuroimmunology that stress can suppress the immune function by up to 60 percent. Controlling or eliminating stress is one of the greatest anchors of health. Educating people in these self-empowering methods is one of the functions of natural healing, and can lead the way to a person becoming a long-term survivor of HIV. Why be a long term survivor? Because new methods are being researched and tested that will increase the function of the immune system and may even remove the virus from an infected person. The key is to fight as hard as you can to stay well. Live a healthy life style, remove toxic inputs from the body, and hope for a breakthrough in medicine.

Glossary

Abscess: a swollen or inflamed area of body tissue in which pus gathers.

Acid/Alkaline balance: (See pH balance.)

Acid pH: (See pH balance.)

Acidosis: an excessive acidity of body fluids due to either an accumulation of acids or a loss of bicarbonate (the hydrogen ion concentration is increased and thus the pH is decreased). See pH balance.

Acupoints: acupuncture points throughout the body, along the meridians, which correspond to specific organs. See Meridian.

Acute: (in medicine) having rapid onset, severe symptoms, and short duration. Opposite of chronic.

Adaptogen: a substance with qualities which increase resistance and resilience to stress, enabling the body to adapt around the problem and to avoid reaching collapse. Adaptogens work through support of the adrenal glands.

Alkaline pH: (See pH balance.)

Allergens: substances that cause manifestations of allergy (these may or may not be antigens). See Antigen.

Alterative: a substance with properties that gradually restore proper functioning of the body, increasing health and vitality.

Amino acids: the building blocks of which proteins are constructed, and the end product of protein digestion.

Anaerobic: pertaining to an organism, the ability to live without oxygen.

Analgesic: a pain-relieving substance.

Anthelmintic: a substance with the property to destroy or expel intestinal worms.

Antibacterial: a substance which has the property of destroying or stopping the growth of bacteria.

Antibiotics: any of a variety of natural or synthetic substances that inhibit the growth of, or destroy, microorganisms.

Antigen: a protein, carbohydrate, or fat carbohydrate complex with the ability to identify cells as harmless and belonging to the body, or as foreign cells to be destroyed. Antigens stimulate the production of antibodies which can neutralize or destroy invading organisms. Antigens on the body's own cells are called autoantigens. Antigens on all other cells are called foreign antigens.

Anti-inflammatory: a substance which soothes inflammation or reduces the inflammatory response of the tissue directly. Anti-inflammatories work in a number of different ways, but rarely inhibit the natural inflammatory reaction.

Antimicrobial: antimicrobials help the body destroy or resist pathogenic (disease-causing) microorganisms by helping the body strengthen its own resistance to infective organisms.

Antiviral: any substance which bears the properties of opposing the action of a virus.

ARC (AIDS-Related Complex): the term "ARC," not officially defined or recognized by the Centers for Disease Control, is intended to describe patients with some HIV-related symptoms but no AIDS-defining diagnosis. Symptoms may include unexplained weight loss, swollen lymph nodes, recurrent fevers, and fungal infection of the mouth and throat. ARC is also commonly described as symptomatic HIV infection.

Astringent: astringents have a binding action on mucous membranes, skin, and other tissue. They reduce irritation and inflammation, and create a barrier against infection that is helpful to wounds and burns.

Autoimmune disease: a disease produced when the body's normal tolerance of its own antigenic markers on cells disappears. Autoantibodies are produced by B lymphocytes and attack normal cells, whose surface contains a "self" antigen or autoantigen, causing destruction of tissue.

Autonomic nervous system: the part of the nervous system that is concerned with the control of involuntary bodily functions. It regulates the function of glands, especially the salivary, gastric, and sweat glands, and the adrenal medulla; smooth muscle tissue, and the heart. The autonomic nervous system may act on these tissues to reduce or slow activity or to initiate their function.

AZT (Zidovudine): the most commonly used drug against AIDS, AZT is a reverse transcriptase inhibitor. The reverse transcriptase enzyme is used by HIV to help it in the process of converting its RNA into DNA, by entering the genetic material of the healthy T cell.

B Cells (B-lymphocytes): one of two major classes of lymphocytes. Derived from the bone marrow (hence "B" cells). During infections, these cells are transformed into plasma cells which produce large quantities of antibodies directed at a specific pathogen. This transformation occurs through interactions with various types of T cells and other components of the immune system.

Bifidobacteria (*Bifidobacterium bifidum and bifidobacterium-longum*): these are the main inhabitants of the large intestine. *Bifidobacterium bifidum* is also found in the vagina and the lower part of the small intestine. The bacteria produce a number of specialized acids and use these to prevent colonization of the large intestine by invading bacteria, yeasts, and some viruses. They also produce some B vitamins. The numbers and efficient working of these bacteria decline with any compromising of our health status.

Bile: stored in both the liver and gallbladder, it is important as a digestive juice due to its emulsifying action which facilitates the digestion of fats in the intestines, as well as stimulating peristalsis.

Bioaccumulation: a buildup in the body of foreign substances.

Blood clotting: (See Platelet aggregation.)

Blood sugar: sugar in the form of glucose present in the blood, normally 60 to 100 milligrams/100 milliliters of blood. It rises after a meal to as much as 150 milligrams/100 milliliters of blood, but this may vary.

Bowel dysbiosis: toxic and unhealthy intestinal tract with consequent malabsorption and toxic problems.

Bowel tolerance: the maximum amount a person can take in of a substance before experiencing loose stools or diarrhea.

Bowel toxemia: a condition in which poisonous products of bacteria growing in the bowels produce severe virus-like symptoms such as fever, diarrhea, and vomiting.

Bronchioles: a subdivision of the bronchial tubes.

Bronchodilators: chemicals that relax or open the air passages in the lungs.

Candida albicans: small, oval-budding fungus or yeast that is the primary disease-causing organism of the infection moniliasis candidiasis, commonly referred to as candida.

Capillaries: any of the minute blood vessels, averaging 0.008 millimeter in diameter, carrying blood and forming the capillary system. Capillaries connect the ends of the smallest arteries with the beginnings of the smallest veins.

Carbohydrate: a chemical compound that contains only carbon, hydrogen, and oxygen. Found in plants, carbohydrates—which include all sugars, starches, and celluloses—constitute a major class of animal food and are a basic source of human energy.

Carcinogens: cancer-producing agents.

Cardiac arrhythmia: irregular beating of the heart.

Cardiovascular: relating to or involving the heart and blood vessels.

Carminative: plants that are rich in aromatic volatile oils. They stimulate the digestive system to work properly and with ease, soothe the gut wall, reduce any inflammation that might be present, ease gripping pains, and help with the removal of gas from the digestive tract.

CD4: a protein marker embedded on the surface of helper T-lymphocytes (T4 cells); also found to a lesser degree on the surface of monocyte/macrophage and other immune cells. HIV invades cells by first attaching to the CD4 molecule (CD4 receptor).

CD8: a protein marker embedded in the cell surface of suppressor T-lymphocytes (T8 cells).

Cell membranes: the membrane that encloses the cell. Composed of proteins, lipids, and carbohydrates.

Cervical cancer: cancer of the cervix. Often found in women who have AIDS. According to the new guidelines from the Centers for Disease Control, any woman with cervical cancer who is also HIV positive will be diagnosed with AIDS.

Chi: (See Qi.)

Chronic: pertaining to a disease or illness of long duration showing little change or of slow progression. Opposite of acute.

Circadian rhythm: pertains to events that occur at approximately twenty-four-hour intervals, such as certain physiological phenomena.

Circulating Immune Complexes (CIC): also known as antigen-antibody complexes.

Cortisol: an adrenocortical hormone, usually referred to pharmaceutically as hydrocortisone. Closely related to cortisone in physiological effects.

Coxsackievirus: a group of viruses first isolated in 1948 from two children in Coxsackie, NY. Most coxsackievirus infections in humans are mild, but the viruses do produce a variety of illnesses, including aseptic meningitis (inflammation of the meninges not due to microorganisms), herpangina (a benign infectious disease of children), epidemic pleurodynia (disease characterized by pain of sharp intensity in the chest accompanied by fever), acute upper respiratory infection, and myocarditis of the newborn (inflammation of the middle layer of the walls of the heart), among others. It is possible that infection during the first trimester of pregnancy can cause increased incidence of congenital heart lesions in newborns.

Cyanosis: a bluish discoloration of the skin due to abnormal amounts of reduced hemoglobin in the blood.

Cyst: a closed sac or pouch with a definite wall, that contains fluid, semifluid, or solid material.

Cytokines: chemical messengers that are involved in the regulation of almost every system in the body and are important in controlling local and systemic inflammatory response.

Cytomegalovirus (CMV): a member of the herpes family of viruses that inhabits the salivary glands. Often suspected as a co-factor for AIDS. See Herpes virus.

Cytotoxin: any substance with properties which harm or destroy cells.

ddC (dideooxycytidine): ddC and ddI are both reverse transcriptase inhibitors and, next to AZT, are the most widely used drugs to combat HIV infection.

ddI (dideoxynosine): (See ddC.)

Demulcent: an herb that is rich in mucilage and soothes and protects irritated or inflamed tissue. Demulcent herbs reduce irritation along the whole length of the bowel, reduce sensitivity to potentially corrosive gastric acids, help prevent diarrhea, and reduce the muscle spasms that cause colic.

Dental amalgam: an alloy containing mercury, tin, silver, and copper that is used in dentistry to restore teeth.

Dermatitis: inflammation of the skin with itching, redness, and various skin lesions.

Detoxification: the process of removing toxins from the body.

Diuretic: a substance which increases the production and elimination of urine.

Doshas: the three basic types of biological humors in Ayurvedic medicine, which determine an individual's constitution.

Edema: retention of excessive amounts of fluid by the body tissues.

Electroacupuncture biofeedback: measurement of the electrical properties of acupuncture points.

ELISA (Enzyme Linked ImmunoSorbent Assay): most commonly used test to check for the presence of HIV antibodies. Known to give a high rate of false positive results.

Endocrine gland: a gland that secretes directly into the bloodstream.

Endorphins: natural opiates produced in the brain which function as the body's own natural painkillers.

Enkephalin: a chemical substance produced by the brain which acts as an opiate and produces analgesia to increase the threshold for pain.

Enzyme: any one of the numerous complex proteins that are produced by living cells and catalyze specific biochemical reactions.

Epidemiology: a branch of medical science that deals with the incidence, distribution, and control of disease in a population.

Epstein-Barr virus (EBV): a member of the herpes family of viruses. Causes mononucleosis and is involved in some forms of chronic fatigue syndrome. Present in a large percentage of the population, this virus, along with other members of the herpes family of viruses, usually remains inactive unless immune function declines. Extremely common in people who are HIV positive or who have AIDS. See Herpes virus.

Essential fatty acids (EFA): unsaturated fatty acids (linoleic, linolenic, and arachidonic) which cannot by synthesized in the body and are considered essential for maintaining health.

Expectorant: a substance that stimulates removal of mucus from the lungs. Stimulating expectorants "irritate" the bronchioles (a smaller subdivision of the bronchial tubes) causing expulsion of material. Relaxing expectorants soothe bronchial spasm and loosen mucus secretions, and are helpful in treating dry, irritating coughs.

Fat: adipose tissue of the body which serves as an energy reserve. Also, in chemistry, a term used to describe one of a group of organic compounds or fatty acids. See Essential fatty acids.

Fluid retention: failure to eliminate fluids from the body because of a high level of salt in the body. Can also be caused by a renal, cardiac, or metabolic disease.

Free radicals: molecules containing an odd number of electrons resulting in an open bond or half bond, making them highly reactive and, as a result, potentially destructive.

Fungus: a cellular organism that subsists on organic matter.

Giardia lamblia: a parasitic infection transmitted by an ingestion of cysts in fecally contaminated water or food.

Gastroenteritis: inflammation of the stomach and intestinal tract.

Gastrointestinal system: pertaining to the stomach and intestines.

Genitourinary system: pertaining to the genitals and urinary organs.

Geopathic stress: stress to the human body caused by harmful radiation from the earth.

Glucose: blood sugar, an intermediate in the metabolism of carbohydrates in the body.

Hemoglobin: the iron-containing pigment of the red blood cells.

Hemophilia: a serious disease in which the body's natural blood-clotting capacity is impaired.

Hemorrhage: heavy or uncontrollable bleeding.

Hepatic: hepatics aid the liver by toning and strengthening it, and in some cases, by increasing the flow of bile. They are fundamental in maintaining health because of the important role the liver plays by not only facilitating digestion but also by removing toxins from the body.

Hepatitis B virus (HBV): a strain of the hepatitis virus. Spread by blood and serum-derived fluids, and by direct contact with body fluids.

Hepatotoxic: any substance which is toxic to the liver.

Herpes virus: a family of viruses which belongs to the herpes group and includes herpes simplex (HSV-1, HSV-2), herpes zoster virus, Epstein-Barr virus, cytomegalovirus (CMV), and human herpes virus 6. Most adults harbor three or more of these viruses, which usually remain inactive unless immune function declines. Extremely common in people who are HIV positive or who have AIDS.

Herpes simplex virus: a member of the herpes family of viruses. Includes HSV-1 (causes cold sores) and HSV-2 (genital herpes). See Herpes virus.

Herpes zoster virus: a member of the herpes family of viruses. Causes chicken pox and shingles. See Herpes virus.

HIV (Human Immunodeficiency Virus): a retrovirus believed to be a contributing cause of AIDS.

Homeostasis: a relatively stable state of equilibrium between the interdependent elements of an organism or group.

Hydrochloric acid (HCl): a strong corrosive irritating acid, normally present in dilute form in gastric juice.

Hyperthermia: unusually high fever often artificially induced for therapeutic purposes.

Hypothalamus: a gland which contains neurosecretions that are of importance in the control of certain metabolic activities, such as water balance, sugar and fat metabolism, regulation of body temperature, and secretion of releasing and inhibiting hormones.

Iatrogenic: treatment-induced.

IgA: an antibody in the colon that binds food and bacterial antigens.

Immune reaction: antibody production.

Immunosuppressive: a substance which suppresses the body's natural immune response to an antigen.

Inflammation: an immune reaction that occurs in response to any type of bodily injury. Can include redness, heat, swelling, or pain.

Insulin: a hormone secreted by the pancreas essential for the metabolism of carbohydrates and used in the treatment and control of diabetes.

Interferon: a group of proteins released by the white blood cells that combat a virus.

Interleukin-1: a compound produced by the body in response to infection, inflammation, or other immunologic challenges.

Intra-arterially: introduced (usually injected) within an artery.

Intra-articularly: introduced (usually injected) into the joint.

Intradermally: introduced (usually injected) within the substance of the skin.

Intramuscularly: introduced (usually injected) within the muscle.

Intravenously: introduced (usually injected) into a vein.

Kapha: a dosha in Ayurvedic medicine which determines an individual's constitution.

Kaposi's sarcoma: a commonly-associated illness of AIDS. Involves a tumor on the walls of blood vessels or in the lymphatic system resulting in multiple pink to purple lesions on the skin. It may also occur internally in addition to, or independent of, lesions.

Lactobacillus acidophilus: the principal friendly bacteria inhabiting the small intestine in humans and animals. It is also found in the mouth and vagina. Acidophilus manufactures lactase to digest milk and sugar, and produces lactic acid which suppresses undesirable bacteria and yeasts. Some strains produce natural antibiotics. They also kill candida yeasts and are very susceptible to poor diet, stress conditions, pollution, and antibiotics such as penicillin.

Lactobacillus bulgaricus: a transient but very important bacteria. Some strains produce antibiotics which kill harmful bacteria. By manufacturing lactic acid, it helps encourage a good environment for the resident bacteria such as acidophilus and bifidobacteria.

Lactose intolerant: an intolerance to milk and some dairy products, characterized by gastrointestinal symptoms.

Laxative: a substance which promotes bowel movements. Laxatives are divided into those that work by providing bulk, those that stimulate the production of bile in the liver and its release from the gallbladder, and those which directly trigger peristalsis.

Legumes: chickpeas, mung beans, lentils, kidney beans, or any other sort of beans.

Lesion: an injury, wound, or single infected patch in a skin disease.

Leukocytes: white blood cells.

Leukocytosis: an increased white blood cell count, usually caused by the presence of an infection.

Leukosis: abnormal growth of white blood cells.

Limbic system: a group of brain structures that influences the endocrine and autonomic motor systems.

Lymphatic system: a system of vessels and nodes throughout the body which carry the lymph fluid and help to remove toxins from the body.

Lymphocytes: cells produced chiefly by the lymphoid tissue which are the cellular mediators of immunity. See T Cells and B Cells.

Macrophage: scavenger cells that have the ability to recognize and ingest all foreign antigens, especially harmful bacteria, as well as cell debris and other waste in the blood. The macrophage may be a reservoir for HIV.

MAI (Mycobacterium avium intracellulare): a myco-bacterial organism that causes a common opportunistic infection, Mycobacterium avium complex (MAC).

Meridian: a channel in the body through which *qi* flows. Acupuncture diagnoses illness by seeking blockages in the body's twelve major meridians.

Metabolism: the transformation in the body of the chemical energy of foodstuffs to mechanical energy or heat.

Metastasis: the spreading of tumor cells from their site of origin to distant sites, usually through the bloodstream or the lymphatic system.

Monocyte: a large white blood cell which acts as a scavenger, capable of destroying invading bacteria or other foreign material. Precursor to the macrophage.

Musculoskeletal system: pertaining to the muscles and the skeleton.

Mycobacterium avium intracellulare: (See MAI.)

Mycoplasma: a microscopic organism proposed by Luc Montagnier of the Pasteur Institute in Paris as being the co-factor that works in conjunction with HIV to cause AIDS.

Natural killer cells (NK cells): large granular lymphocytes that attack and destroy tumor cells and infected body cells. They are known as "natural" killers because they attack without first having to recognize specific antigens (a substance which, when introduced into the body, is capable of inducing the production of a specific antibody).

Nervine: nervines help the nervous system and can be subdivided into three groups. Nervine tonics strengthen and restore the nervous system. Nervine relaxants ease anxiety and tension by soothing both body and mind. Nervine stimulants directly stimulate nerve activity.

Neurological: pertaining to the study of nervous diseases.

Neuromuscular: concerning both the nerves and muscles.

Neurotoxicity: having the capability of harming nerve tissue.

Neurotransmitters: substances that transmit nerve impulses to the brain.

Oxygenation: to supply or combine with oxygen.

p24 antigen: one of four nucleocapsid proteins contained on the core of the HIV virus.

Parasites: (internal) an organism such as a protozoon or worm that lives within the body of the host, occupying the digestive tract or body cavities, or living within body organs, blood, tissues, or even cells.

Parasympathetic nervous system: the craniosacral division of the autonomic nervous system. Effects of parasympathetic stimulation are the constriction of the pupils, contraction of the smooth muscle of the alimentary canal, constriction of bronchioles, slowing of heart rate, and increased secretion by glands, except sweat glands.

Pathogens: disease-producing microorganisms and toxins.

PCP (Pneumocystis carinii pneumonia): a common illness associated with AIDS.

PCR (Polymerase Chain Reaction): a test for the presence of HIV virus developed by Nobel laureate, Dr. Karry Mullis.

Peptide: a substance formed by two or more amino acids.

Peripheral nervous system: connects the central nervous system to all body tissues and voluntary muscles.

pH balance: a method of measurement used in chemistry to express the degree of acidity or alkalinity of a solution. A pH of 7 represents the neutral point where the solution is neither acid nor alkaline. Any higher alkalinity is expressed by a number greater than 7, and higher acidity, by a number less than 7. The calculations of these numbers are based on logarithms.

Pitta: a dosha in Ayurvedic medicine which determines an individual's constitution.

Placebo: substances having no pharmacological effect.

Plasma: the liquid part of the lymph and of the blood.

Platelet aggregation: the clustering of disks found in human blood that facilitate blood coagulation.

Pneumocystis carinii pneumonia: (See PCP.)

Polypeptide: a molecule resulting from the union of two or more amino acids.

Postacute: the period after the rapid and severe onset of symptoms.

Probiotics: substances that promote the growth of beneficial bacteria in the intestines.

Protein: complex nitrogenous compounds that occur naturally in plants and animals and yield amino acids. Essential for the growth and repair of animal tissue.

Qi: (also chi) referred to in Chinese medicine as the vital life energy which circulates throughout the body.

Qi stagnation: any blockage of energy in the body that interrupts the body's natural functions or the healing process.

Qigong: a Chinese healing practice.

Renal insufficiency: the reduced capacity of the kidney to perform its functions.

Retrovirus: a class of viruses which copy genetic material using RNA as a template for making DNA. HIV is a retrovirus.

Reverse transcriptase enzyme: the reverse transcriptase enzyme is used by HIV to help it enter the genetic material of the healthy T cell in order to convert its RNA into DNA.

Secretory IgA: promoting secretion or secreting immunoglobulin gamma A.

Sperm: the male reproductive cell carried in the seminal discharge.

Stimulant: a substance which quickens and enlivens the physiological and metabolic activity of the body.

Subacute: a state between acute and chronic when symptoms have lessened in severity or duration.

T Cells (T-lymphocytes): a thymus derived white blood cell that participates in a variety of cell-mediated immune reactions. Three fundamentally different types of T cells are recognized: helper (T4), killer (NK), and suppressor (T8). According to conventional wisdom, the ratio of T4 (helper) to T8 (suppressor) cells should be 2:1. In AIDS, this ratio is usually reverse (1:2 or less).

- **T4 cells (T-Helper lymphocytes):** immune cells called helper cells which activate themselves in response to an antigen (cloning to produce large numbers) and bringing into action B cells, both of which target the enemy in different ways. Derived from the thymus gland (hence "T" cells). T4 cells produce lymphokines (proteins) which stimulate macrophage activity, targeting the invading organism.

- **T8 cells (T-Suppressor lymphocytes):** immune cells called T-suppressor cells that halt antibody production and other immune responses. T8 cells are there to modify and calm activity of T4 and B cells in order to prevent overreaction by the immune system. When the ratio of T4 to T8 cells alters in dominance of the latter, as in AIDS, the ability to neutralize invading organisms diminishes dramatically, or vanishes altogether.

- **Natural killer cells (NK cells):** (See Natural killer cells.)

Thoracic: pertaining to the chest or thorax.

Thymus: a glandular structure of largely lymphoid tissue that functions in the development of the body's immune system, located in the upper chest or at the base of the neck.

Tonic: often used in Traditional Chinese Medicine and Ayurvedic medicine, tonics are often taken as a preventative measure to nurture and enliven.

Toxoplasmosis: disease caused by protozoa that damages the central nervous system.

Tuberculosis: an infectious disease caused by the tubercle bacillus, *Mycobacterium tuberculosis*, and characterized pathologically by inflammatory infiltrations, formation of tubercles, necrosis, abscesses, fibroisis, and calicificaton. It most commonly affects the respiratory system, but other parts of the body may become infected as well. Commonly associated with AIDS.

Tumor: an abnormal mass of tissue that is not inflammatory, arises without obvious cause from cells, and possesses no physiologic function.

Vascular system: includes the heart, blood vessels, lymphatic, pulmonary, and portal systems.

Vasodilator: a substance which causes the blood vessels to widen.

Vata: a dosha in Ayurvedic medicine which determines an individual's constitution.

Veins: the tubular branching vessels that carry blood from the capillaries toward the heart.

Western Blot Test: a more sophisticated form of testing for HIV antibodies than the ELISA test, but it also suffers from a lack of accuracy.

Yang deficiency: because yang cannot function properly without yin, an imbalance in the energy systems of the body can create a yang deficiency, causing the yang organs to become stagnant. See Qi.

Yang organs: yang organs are hollow, surface organs such as the intestines, spleen, gallblader, and the skin.

Yeast: unicellular fungi of the genus which reproduce by budding, and can cause infections.

Yin deficiency: because yin cannot function properly without yang, an imbalance in the energy systems of the body can create a yin deficiency, causing the yin organs to become stagnant. See Qi.

Yin organs: yin organs are dense, internal organs such as the kidneys, lungs, heart, liver, and bones.

Notes

Introduction

1 Duesberg, P. H. "AIDS Acquired by Drug Consumption and Other Noncontagious Risk Factors." *Pharmac. Ther.* vol. 55 (1992): 201–277.
2 Evans, A. S. "Does HIV Cause AIDS? An Historical Perspective." *Journal of AIDS* 2 (1989): 107–113.
Dufoort, G.; et al. "No Clinical Signs Fourteen Years After HIV-2 Transmission Via Blood Transfusion." *The Lancet* (Aug 27, 1988): 510.
3 Maver, R. *Rethinking AIDS* (Newsletter) vol. 1, Number 7 (July, 1993): 3.
Sheer R. "AIDS Threat to All—How Serious?" *LA Times* (Aug 14, 1987): pt 1, p 1.
4 Root-Bernstein, R. *Rethinking AIDS.* New York: Macmillan Free Press, 1992, 40.

PART ONE: UNDERSTANDING AIDS

Chapter One

1 Duesberg, P. H. "AIDS Acquired by Drug Consumption and Other Noncontagious Risk Factors." *Pharmac. Ther.* vol. 55 (1992): 201–277.
2 Barnes, D. M. "Losing AIDS Antibodies." *Science* (June 10, 1988) 240 (4858): 1407.
3 Corbitt, G.; et al. "HIV Infection in Manchester in 1959." *The Lancet* (July 7, 1990) 336 (8706): 51.
Froland, S.; et al. "HIV Infection in Norwegian Family Before 1970." *The Lancet* (June 11, 1988) 1 (8598): 1344–5.
Garry, R.; et al. "Documentation of an AIDS Virus Infection in the US in 1968." *Journal of the American Medical Association* 260: 2085–2087 (1988).
4 Breimer, L. "Did Moritz Kaposi Describe AIDS in 1872?" *Clio Medica* 19: 156–159 (1984).
Huminer, D.; et al. "AIDS in the Pre-AIDS Era." *Review of Infectious Diseases* 9: 1102–1108 (1987).
5 Root-Bernstein, R. *The Wall Street Journal* (Dec 2, 1993).
6 Duesberg, P. H. "AIDS Acquired by Drug Consumption and Other Noncontagious Risk Factors." *Pharmac. Ther.* vol. 55 (1992): 201–277.
7 Hodgkinson, N. "Report AIDS." *The Sunday Times* London (Dec 12, 1993).
8 France, A. J. "Changing Case-Definition for AIDS." *The Lancet* (Dec 5, 1992) 340(8832): 1414.
Stewart, G. T. "Changing Case-Definition for AIDS." *The Lancet* (Dec 5, 1992) 340(8832): 1414.
9 Duesberg, P. H. "AIDS Acquired by Drug Consumption and Other Noncontagious Risk

Factors. "*Pharmac. Ther.* vol. 55, (1992): 209.
10 Duesberg, P. H. "AIDS Acquired by Drug Consumption and Other Noncontagious Risk Factors. "*Pharmac. Ther.* vol. 55 (1992): 210.
11 Chen, Edwin. "U.S. Admits French Role in HIV Test Kit." *Los Angeles Times.* (July 12, 1994): A12.
12 Farber, C. "Fatal Distraction." *SPIN Magazine* 8 no. 3 (May, 1992): 36.
13 Farber, C. "Fatal Distraction." *SPIN Magazine* 8 no. 3 (May, 1992): 73.
14 Friedman-Kein, Q. A.; et al. "Kaposi's Sarcoma in HIV Negative Homosexual Men" *The Lancet* (Jan 20, 1990) 335(8682): 168–9.
Garcia-Muret, M.; et al. "AIDS and Kaposi's Sarcoma in HIV Negative Bisexual Men." *The Lancet* i (1990): 969–970.
Manuci, P.; et al. "KS Without HIV in Hemophiliacs." *ANN Intern Med.* (1986): 105–466.
Jansen, R.; et al. "Neurological Complications of HIV in Patients with Lymphadenopathy Syndrome." *ANN. Neurol.* 23 (1988): 49–55.
Pankhurst, C.; et al. "Reduced CD4 T Cells and Severe Oral Candidiasis in Absence of HIV." *The Lancet* (Mar 25, 1989) (8639): 672.
Jacobs, J.; et al. "A Cluster of PCP in Adults Without Predisposing Illnesses." *New England Journal of Medicine* (Jan 24, 1991) 324 (4).
15 Mannucci, P.; et al. "Kaposi's Sarcoma Without HIV Antibody in Hemophiliacs." *Annals of Internal Medicine* 105: 466, (1986).
Jacobs, J.; et al. "A Cluster of PCP in Adults Aithout Predisposing Illness." *New England Journal of Medicine* (Jan 24, 1991) 324 (4).
16 Root-Bernstein, R. *Rethinking AIDS.* New York: Macmillan Free Press, 1992.
17 CDC. July, 1991. HIV/AIDS Surveillance Report, 1–18.
18 Duesberg, P. H. "AIDS Acquired by Drug Consumption and Other Noncontagious Risk Factors. "*Pharmac. Ther.* vol. 55 (1992): 201–277.
19 World Health Organization. International Classification of Diseases, 10th Edition. Geneva: World Health Organization, 1992.
20 Farber, C. "Fatal Distraction." *SPIN Magazine* 8 no. 3 (May, 1992): 36.
21 Farber, C. "Fatal Distraction." *SPIN Magazine* 8 no. 3 (May, 1992): 36.
22 Farber, C. "Fatal Distraction." *SPIN Magazine* 8 no. 3 (May, 1992): 36.
23 Farber, C. "Fatal Distraction." *SPIN Magazine* 8 no. 3 (May, 1992): 36.
24 Reported by Doctors Jorge Eichberg and Krishna Murthy, of the Southwest Foundation for Biomedical Research.
25 Reviewed in Descotes. *Immunotoxicology* (1988): 107–111.
26 Farber, C., Liversidge, A. "Words From The Front." *SPIN Magazine* (Sept, 1990): 71.
27 Farber, C., Liversidge, A. "Words From

The Front." *SPIN Magazine* (Sept, 1990): 71.
28 *Science,* vol. 260 (May 28, 1993).
29 Callen, M. *Surviving AIDS.* New York: HarperCollins, 1990, 5.
30 Haverkos, H. W.; et al. (eds.). "Health Hazards of Nitrite Inhalants." 1988, National Institute on Drug Abuse Monograph 83, ff.
31 Learmont, J.; et al. "Long-Term Symptomless HIV-1 Infection in Recipients of Blood Products From a Single Donor." *The Lancet* (Oct 10, 1992) 340(8824): 863–7.
32 Health and Human Services Press Release, August 17, 1989.
33 Mosley, J. W. "Idiopathic CD4+ Lymphocytopenia: Other Lymphocyte Subset Changes" as presented at IX International Conference on AIDS, Berlin, June 6–11, 1993.
34 Koszinowski; et al. "The Role of CD4 and CD8 T Cells in Viral Infections." *Current Opinion in Immunology* (Aug 3, 1991) (4):471–5
Goldberg, B. *International Journal of Alternative and Complimentary Medicine* (Dec, 1993): 2.
Bird, A. Graham (ed.). "Immunology of HIV Infection." *Kluwer Academic Publishers* (1992):59.
35 Goldberg, B. *International Journal of Alternative and Complimentary Medicine* (Dec, 1993): 2.
36 Farber, Celia. "Fatal Distraction." *SPIN Magazine* 8 no. 3 (May, 1992): 36.
Kolata, G. "Doctors Stretch Rules on AIDS Drug: Some Give Possibly Toxic AZT Before Symptoms Develop." *New York Times* 137 (Dec 21, 1987): A1. Dr. Douglas Dietrich, of the New York Medical Center, told *Times* reporter Gina Kolata, "I've followed patients who've had T-cell counts of less then 10 for a year, and nothing happened to them."
37 Farber, C. "Sins of Omission." *SPIN Magazine* (Nov, 1989).
38 Farber, C. "Words From The Front." *SPIN Magazine* (Oct, 1993).
39 *Immunotoxicology* (1988) (107–111).
40 Root-Bernstein, R. *Rethinking AIDS.* New York: Macmillan Free Press, 1992, 133.
41 Editorial. *Continuum Magazine* (Oct/Nov 1993).
42 Farber, C. "Sins of Omission." *SPIN Magazine* (Nov, 1989).
43 Farber, C. "Word from the Front." *SPIN Magazine* (May, 1991).
Farber, C. "Sins of Omission." *SPIN Magazine* (Nov, 1989)·
44 Concorde Coordinating Committee. "Concorde: MRC/ANRS Randomized Double-blind Controlled Trial of Immediate and Deferred Zidovudine in Symptom-free HIV Infection." *The Lancet* (April 8, 1994) 343: 871–880.
45 "ARC," a term not officially recognized by the CDC, refers to patients with some HIV-related symptoms such as recurrent fevers, unexplained weight loss, swollen lymph nodes, and/or fungus infection of the mouth and throat, but with no AIDS-defining diagnosis.
46 Standish, L.; et al. "One Year Open Trial

of Naturopathic Treatment of HIV Infection Class IV-A in Men." *Journal of Naturopathic Medicine* 3(1) (1992): 42–64.

Chapter Two
1 See Chapter 10, "Malnutrition AIDS," in *AIDS Inc.*, by Jon Rappoport, for medical studies linking malnutrition, T-cell depletion, and immune-collapse. (Listed under BOOKS.)
2 Seligman, Maxime. "AIDS—An Immunologic Reevaluation." *New England Journal of Medicine* (Nov, 1984).
3 Dowd, P.; et al. "Influence of Undernutrition on Immunity." *Clinical Science* 66: 241–248, 1984.
4 Reviewed in Descotes. *Immunotoxicology* (1988): 107–111.
5 Root-Bernstein, R., *Rethinking AIDS* . New York: Macmillan Free Press, 1992, 305.
6 See chapter, "Parasitic Infections" in *Alternative Medicine: The Definitive Guide.* Puyallup, WA: Future Medicine Publishing, Inc., 1993.
7 Root-Bernstein, R. *Rethinking AIDS.* New York: Macmillan Free Press, 1992, 224.
8 See *When Antibiotics Fail,* by Marc Lappe, North Atlantic Books, 1986. It describes problems with overuse of these drugs, and also discusses the most toxic antibiotics.
9 Root-Bernstein, R. *Rethinking AIDS.* New York: Macmillan Free Press, 1992, 228.
10 Some researchers also state that ingestion or other reception of sperm, especially from many partners, is immunosuppressive.
11 See the CDC description in its "Morbidity and Mortality Report" of June 5, 1981. Reprinted as Appendix 2 in *AIDS Inc.*
12 Haverkos, H. W.; et al. (eds.). "Health Hazards of Nitrite Inhalants." 1988, National Institute on Drug Abuse Monograph 83, ff.
13 To say nothing of other immunosuppressive drugs such as heroin, cocaine, crack, qualudes, Ecstasy, ethyl chloride, amphetamines, psychiatric tranquilizers, etc.
14 Stoneburner, R., et al. "A Large Spectrum of Severe HIV-1 Related Disease in Intravenous Drug Users in New York City." *Science* (Nov 11, 1988) 242(4880): 916–9.
15 Root-Bernstein, R. *Rethinking AIDS.* New York: Macmillan Free Press, 1992, 234.
16 McDonough, R. J.; et al. (1980) *J. Immunol* 125: 2539.
17 Root-Bernstein, R. *Rethinking AIDS.* New York: Macmillan Free Press, 1992, 244.
18 Ward J. W., Bush T. J., Perkins H. A., et al. "The Natural History of Transfusion-associated Infection With Human Immunodeficiency Virus." *New England Journal of Medicine* (Oct 5, 1989) 321(4): 947–52.
19 Root-Bernstein, R. *Rethinking AIDS.* New York: Macmillan Free Press, 1992, 242.
20 Ward J. W., Bush T. J., Perkins H. A., et al. "The Natural History of Transfusion-associated Infection With Human Immunodeficiency Virus." *New England Journal of Medicine* (Oct 5, 1989) 321(4): 947–52.
21 Root-Bernstein, R. *Rethinking AIDS.* New York: Macmillan Free Press, 1992, 244.

22 CDC. July, 1991. HIV/AIDS Surveillance Report, 1–18.
23 Root-Bernstein, R. *Rethinking AIDS.* New York: Macmillan Free Press, 1992, 239.
24 Root-Bernstein, R. *Rethinking AIDS.* New York: Macmillan Free Press, 1992, 239.
Cummings, P.; et al. *New England Journal of Medicine* 321:941–946.
25 Ward; et al. "Serum Erythropoitin Levels After Renal Transplant." *New England Journal of Medicine* 321(14): 947–52.
26 Aronson, D. L. (1988) *Am. J. Haematol* 27: 7—12.
27 Root-Bernstein, R. *Rethinking AIDS.* New York: Macmillan Free Press, 1992, 246–247.
28 Tsoukas, C.; et al. "Association of HTLV-III Antibodies and Cellular Immune States of Hemophiliacs." *New England Journal of Medicine* (Dec 6, 1984) 311(23): 1514–5.
29 Hilgartner, M. W.; Aledort, C. M. "AIDS in Hemophilia." *Annals of the New York Academy of Science* (1984) 437: 466–71.
30 Root-Bernstein, R. *Rethinking AIDS,* New York: Macmillan Free Press, 1992, 55.
31 Goedert, J. J., Kessler, C. M., Aledort, L.M.; et al. "A Prospective Study of HIV Type 1 Infection and the Development of AIDS in Subjects With Hemophilia." *New England Journal of Medicine* (Oct 26, 1989) 321 (17): 1141–8
32 Hodgkinson, Neville. "Factor 8 Hope in HIV Battle." Report in *London Sunday Times* (Feb 21, 1993).
33 Ibid.

Chapter Three

1 Newman, Turner R. *Naturopathic Medicine.* London: Thorsons, 1990.
2 Siegel, B. *Love, Medicine, & Miracles.* New York: Harper & Row, 1987.
Chaitow, L., Martin, S. *A World Without AIDS.* London: Thorsons/HarperCollins, 1989.
3 Selye, H. *The Stress of Life.* New York: McGraw Hill, 1978.
Naylor, V. *Emotional Problems of Cancer Patients.* Kershaw Press, 1977.
Simonton, C. "Role of the Mind in Cancer Therapy." Lecture UCLA, 1972.
4 *AIDS 1990: A Physicians Manual.* Laurel, MD: Life Science Universal Inc.
5 Suskind, R. (ed.). *Malnutrition and the Immune Response.* New York: Raven Press, 1977.
6 Jerrels, T.; et al. "Ethanol-associated Immunosuppression." and Donahue, R.; et al. "Neuroimmunomodulation by Opiates and Other Drugs." Both in Bridge, T.; et al. (eds.). *Psychological, Neuropsychiatric, and Substance Abuse Aspects of AIDS.* New York: Raven Press, 1988.
7 Ibid.
Standish, L. "One Year Open Trial of Naturopathic Treatment of HIV Infection." (HARP study) *Journal of Naturopathic Medicine* 3(1)42–64 (1992).
8 Guyton, Arthur C. *Basic Physiology.* Philadelphia: Saunders, 1941.

9 Werbach, M. *Nutritional Influences on Illness.* Third Line Press, 1992.
Davies, S. *Nutritional Medicine.* London: Pan Books, 1989.
Report by McKauliffe, K. in *Omni* (Nov, 1987).
10 Goedert, J. "Recreational Drugs: Relationship to AIDS." *Annals of New York Academy of Sciences* (437) (1984).
Brown, R. *AIDS, Cancer, and the Medical Establishment.* New York: Robert Speller, 1986.
Culbert, M. *AIDS—Terror, Truth, and Triumph.* Bradford Foundation, 1986.
Chaitow, L., Martin, S. *A World Without AIDS.* London: Thorsons/HarperCollins, 1989.
11 Briggs, J.; et al. "Severe Systemic Infections Complicating Heroin Addiction." *The Lancet* (Dec 9, 1967) 2 (528): 1227–31.
Brown, S.; et al. "Immunological Dysfunction in Heroin Addicts." *Archives of Internal Medicine* 134 (1974): 1001.
Harris, P.; et al. "Susceptibility of Addicts to Infection and Neoplasia." *New England Journal of Medicine* (Aug. 10, 1972) 287(6): 310.
Selwyn, P.; et al. "Impact of AIDS on Morbidity and Mortality Among Intravenous Drug Users." *America Journal of Public Health* (79) (1989): 1358.
12 Ostrow, D.; et al. "Multicentre AIDS Cohort Study (MACS) Recreational Drug Use and Sexual Behavior in Homosexual Men." *AIDS* (4) (1990): 759.
13 Ibid.
14 Duesberg, P. "Role of Drugs in Origin of AIDS." *Biomedical and Pharmacotherapy* (46) (1992): 3–15.
15 Descotes, J. *Immunotoxicology of Drugs and Chemicals.* Amsterdam: Elsevier, 1988.
16 Lerner, W. "Cocaine Abuse and AIDS." *American Journal of Medicine* (8) (1989): 661.
Ettinger, N., Albin, R. J., "Respiratory Effects of Smoking Cocaine." *American Journal of Medicine* (Dec, 1989) 87, (6): 664–8.
17 Haverkos, H.; et al. "Health Hazards of Nitrite Inhalants." National Institutes for Drug Abuse Monograph 83, 1988.
18 San Francisco Department of Health Substance Abuse Assessment. August, 1991.
19 Neuman, H. "Use of Steroid Creams as Possible Cause of Immunosuppression in Homosexuals." *New England Journal of Medicine* (April 15, 1982). 306(15): 935.
20 Descotes, J. *Immunotoxicology of Drugs and Chemicals.* Amsterdam: Elsevier, 1988.
21 *AIDS 1990: A Physicians Manual.* Laurel, MD: Life Science Universal Inc.
22 "A Little Fever is Good for You." *Science.* (Nov, 1984).
23 Cohen, S. "Antiretroviral Treatment for AIDS." *New England Journal of Medicine* (Sept 3, 1987) 317(10): 629–30.
Dournon, E.; et al. "Effects of AZT in 365 Consecutive Patients with AIDS and ARC." *The Lancet* Dec 3, 1988. 2(8632): 1297–302.
Duesberg, P. "AIDS Epidemiology." *PNAS* 88 (1991): 1575.

Gill, P.; et al. "Azydomythmidine Associated with Bone Marrow Failure in AIDS." *Annals of Internal Medicine* (Oct, 1987) 107(4): 502–5.

Institute of Medicine. *Confronting AIDS*, updates 1986, 1988.

Richman, D.; et al. "Toxicity of AZT in Treating AIDS and ARC." The AZT Working Group. *New England Journal of Medicine* (July 23, 1987) 317(4): 192–7.

Smothers, K. "Pharmacology and Toxicology of AIDS Therapies." *The AIDS Reader* 1, 29 1991.

Volberding, P. "Zidovudine in Asymptomatic Human Immunodeficiency Virus Infection." *New England Journal of Medicine* (April 5, 1990) 322(14): 941–9.

Yarchoan, R., Broder, S. "Development of Antiretroviral Therapy for AIDS and Related Disorders. A Progress Report." *New England Journal of Medicine* (Feb 26, 1987) 316(9): 557–64.

24 Cohen, S. "Antiretroviral Treatment for AIDS." *New England Journal of Medicine*. (Sept 3, 1987) 317(10): 629–30.

Dournon, E.; et al. "Effects of AZT in 365 Consecutive Patients With AIDS and ARC." *The Lancet* (Dec 3, 1988) 2(8632): 1297–302.

Duesberg, P. "AIDS Epidemiology." *PNAS* 88: 1575, (1991).

Gill, P.; et al. "Azydomythmidine Associated With Bone Marrow Failure in AIDS." *Annals of Internal Medicine* (Oct, 1987) 107(4): 502–5.

Institute of Medicine. *Confronting AIDS*, updates 1986, 1988.

Richman, D.; et al. "Toxicity of AZT in Treating AIDS and ARC." The AZT Working Group. *New England Journal of Medicine* (July 23, 1987) 317(4): 192–7.

25 Groopman, J. "Clinical Spectrum of HTLV-III in Humans." *Cancer Research* (supplement) 45(4649s–4654s) (1985).

26 Brown, R.; et al. "IgA Mediated Elimination of Antigens by Hepatobiliary Route." *Fed. Proc.* 42 (1985) 3218–3221.

Brown, R. *AIDS—The Third Pivot*. Unpublished manuscript, 1992.

27 Chaitow, L., Martin, S. *A World Without AIDS*. London: Thorsons/HarperCollins, 1989.

28 Null, G. "The AIDS Cover-up." *Penthouse* (1985).

Chapter Four

1 Monitovo, J., Menitove, J. E. "Status of Recipients of Blood from Donors Subsequently Found to Have Antibodies to HIV." *New England Journal of Medicine* (Oct. 23, 1986) 315(17): 1095–6.

Tabor, E. "Review of Transmission of Hepatitis by Clotting Factor Concentrates." *Scan. J. Haematol. Supplement* 40 33: 23–328 (1984).

2 Duffort, G.; et al. "No Clinical Signs Fourteen Years After HIV-2 Transmission Via Blood Transfusion." *The Lancet* (Aug 27, 1988) 2(8069): 510.

Aiuti, F.; et al. "Delayed Appearance of HIV Infection in Children." *The Lancet* (Oct 10, 1987) 2(8563): 510.

3 Lemaitre, P., Montagnier, L., et al. "Protective Activity of Analogs of Tetracycline Against Cytopathic Effects of HIV." *Res. Virol.* 141: 5 (1990).

4 Root-Bernstein, R. "HIV and Immuno-suppressive Factors in AIDS/EOS." *Revista Immunologica Ed Immunofarmacolgica* 12(4) (1992).

5 Barnes, D. "Losing AIDS Antibodies." *Science* (June 10, 1988) 240 (4858): 1407.

Imagawa, D.; et al. "HIV-1 in Seronegative Homosexual Men." *New England Journal of Medicine* (Oct 24, 1991) 325(17): 1250–1.

6 Lindhoe, C.; et al. "Autopsy Findings in Family Members With Presumed Acquired Immunodeficiency Syndrome of Unknown Etiology." *Acta. Pathol. Microbiol. Immunol. Scand.* A 94: 17–123 (1986).

Montagnier, L. and others. Statements at International AIDS Conference, Amsterdam, July, 1992.

7 Callen, M. *Surviving AIDS*. New York: HarperCollins, 1990.

8 Root-Bernstein, R. *Rethinking AIDS*. New York: Macmillan Free Press, 1992, 68.

9 Garry, R.; et al. "Documentation of an AIDS Virus Infection in the USA in 1968." *Journal of the American Medical Association* 260: 2085–2087 (1988).

Huminer, D.; et al. "AIDS in the Pre-AIDS Era." *Review Infect. Dis.* 9: 1102–1108 (1987).

10 Culbert, M. *Townsend Letter for Doctors*. Aug/Sept 1993, 984–992.

11 Ludlam, C. "Letters." *The Lancet* (June 20, 1992): 1547–1548.

12 "Risk of Developing AIDS in Hemophiliac and Homosexual Men." *Journal of the American Medical Association* 262: 3129–3130.

13 "Report." *General Practitioner* 7 (June, 1987).

14 "Letter." *British Medical Journal* (Aug 8, 1987).

15 Learmont, J.; et al. "Long Term Symptomless HIV-1 Infection in Recipients of Blood Products from a Single Donor." *The Lancet* (Oct, 1992) 340: 863–867.

16 "Report." *General Practitioner* 7 (Sept, 1987).

17 Duffort, G.; et al. "No Clinical Signs 14 Years after HIV Transmission via Blood Transfusion." *The Lancet* (Aug 27, 1988) 2(8609): 510.

18 Root-Bernstein, R. *Rethinking AIDS*. New York: Macmillan Free Press, 1992, 52.

19 Root-Bernstein, R. *Rethinking AIDS*. New York: Macmillan Free Press, 1992, 52.

20 Wells, Jody; and McTaggert, Lynn. "HIV Infection: Tested to Death." *What Doctors Don't Tell You*. Vol. 5, No. 4: 1–3.

21 Abstracts. VII International Conference on AIDS. Florence, Italy, 1991; Vol. 1:326.

22 Ward, J.; et al. "Laboratory and Epidemiological Evaluation of an Enzyme Immunoassay for Antibodies to HTLV-III." *Journal of the American Medical Association* 256: 357–361 (1986).

Burke, D.; et al. "Measurement of the False Positive Range in a Screening Program for HIV Infections." *New England Journal of Medicine* Oct 13, 1988. 319(15): 961–4.
23 *Biotechnology* June, 1993. Reported in Root-Bernstein, R. *Rethinking AIDS*. New York: McMillan Free Press, 1992, 51.
24 *Biotechnology* June, 1993. Reported in Root-Bernstein, R. *Rethinking AIDS*. New York: Macmillan Free Press, 1992, 51.
25 Hodgkinson, Neville. *Sunday Times*. 22 May, 1994.
26 *New England Journal of Medicine*, 1986; 314:647.
27 Wells, Jody; and McTaggert, Lynn. "HIV Infection: Tested to Death." *What Doctors Don't Tell You.* Vol 5, No. 4: 1–3.
28 *Nature*, 1985; 317:395–403.
Lancet, 1989; 11:1023–25.
29 Root-Bernstein, R. "Research in Immunology," 141:321–329, Pasteur Institute, 1992.
Peters, R. "Is AIDS an Autoimmune Disease?" *Townsend Letter for Doctors* (April, 1992): 272–280.
30 Root-Bernstein, R. "Research in Immunology," 141:321–339, Pasteur Institute, 1992.
31 Peters, R. "Is AIDS an Auto-immune Disease?" *Townsend Letter for Doctors* (April, 1992) 278–280.
32 Root-Bernstein, R. *Rethinking AIDS*. New York: Macmillan Free Press, 1992, 52.
33 Suitable reference from *World Without AIDS*.
Campbell, D. "Living Positively." *New Statesman* 29 (Jan, 1989).
34 Campbell, D. "AIDS: The Race Against Time." *New Statesman* 6 (Jan, 1989).
Gavrzer, B. "Why Do Some People Survive AIDS?" *Daily Breeze* (Sept 18, 1988).
Elliott, Michael Verney. "AIDS, the Unheard Voices." Channel Four Television, November, 1987 (Meditel Productions).
35 Standish, L.; et al. "One Year Open Trial of Naturopathic Treatment of HIV Infection in Class IV-A in Men." *Journal of Naturopathic Medicine* 3 no. 1 (1992): 42–64.

PART TWO: ALTERNATIVE TREATMENTS FOR AIDS

Introduction

1 Chaitow, L., Martin, S. *A World Without AIDS*. London: Thorsons/HarperCollins, 1989, 91.
Campbell, D. "Living Positively." *New Statesman* 29 (Jan, 1989).

Chapter Five

1 Williams, R. *Biochemical Individuality*. Austin, TX: University of Texas Press, 1982.
2 Standish, L.; et al. "One Year Open Trial of Naturopathic Treatment of HIV Infection." *Journal of Naturopathic Medicine* 3 no. 1 (1992): 42–64.

3 Sanchez, A.; et al. "Role of Sugars in Human Neutrophilic Phagocytosis." *American Journal of Clinical Nutrition* 26 no. 11 (1973): 1180–1184.
4 Mertin, J. "Essential Fatty Acid and Cell-Mediated Immunity." *Prog. Lipid Research* 20 (1981): 851–856.
Johnston, D.; et al. "Dietary Fat, Prostaglandins and the Immune Response." *Prog. Food Nutr. Science* 8 no. 1–2 (1984): 3–25.
5 Brayton, R.; et al. "Effects of Alcohol on Leucocyte Mobilization, Etc." *New England Journal of Medicine* 282 (3): 123–8.
Saxena, A.; et al. "Immunomodulating Effect of Caffeine." *Indian Journal of Experimental Biology* 22 no. 6 (1984): 293–301.
6 McGovern Senate Committee on Nutrition: Guidelines.
NACNE Dietary Recommendations UK, 1986.
7 Standish, L.; et al. "One Year Open Trial of Naturopathic Treatment of HIV Infection Class IV-A in Men." *Journal of Naturopathic Medicine* 3 no. 1 (1992): 42–64.
8 Brayton, R.; et al. "Effects of Alcohol on Leucocyte Mobilization, Etc." *New England Journal of Medicine* 282 (3): 123–8.
Saxena, A.; et al. "Immunomodulating Effects of Caffeine in Rodents." *Indian Journal of Experimental Biology* 22 no. 6 (1984): 293–301.
9 Huang, C.; et al. "Nutritional Status of Patients with AIDS." *Clinical Chemistry* 34 no. 10 (1988): 1957–1959.
10 Mantera-Tienza, E.; et al. "Low Vitamin B6 in HIV Infection." *Fifth International Conference on AIDS*. Montreal, (June, 1989): 468.
11 Herbert, V. "Vitamin B12, Folate and Lithium in AIDS."
12 Harriman, G.; et al. "Vitamin B12 Malabsorption in AIDS." *Archives Internal Medicine* 149 no. 9 (1989): 2039–2041.
13 Dworkin, B.; et al. "Selenium Deficiency in AIDS." *Journal of Parenteral and Enteral Nutrition* 10 no. 4 (1986): 405–407.
14 Fabris, N.; et al. "AIDS, Zinc Deficiency, and Thymic Hormone Failure." *Journal of the American Medical Association* 259 (1988): 839–840.
15 Pulse, T.; et al. "A Significant Improvement in a Clinical Pilot Study Utilizing Nutritional Supplements, Essential Fatty Acids, and Stabilized Aloe Vera Juice in 29 HIV Seropositive, ARC and AIDS Patients." *Journal for the Advancement of Medicine* 3 no. 4 (1990): 209–230.
16 Guitierrez, P. "Influence of Ascorbic Acid on Free Radical Metabolism of Xenobiotics." *Drug Metabolism Review* 18 nos. 3 and 4 (1989): 319–343.
Blakeslee, J.; et al. "Human T-Cell Leukaemia Virus: Inhibition by Retinoids, Ascorbic Acid and Vitamin E." *Cancer Research* 45 (1985): 3471–3476.
Bouras, P.; et al. "Monocyte Locomotion—In Vivo Effect of Ascorbic Acid." *Immuno-pharmocology and Immunotoxicity* 11 no. 1 (1989): 119–129.

17 Cathcart, R., M.D. "Vitamin C in the Treatment of AIDS." *Medical Hypotheses* 14 (1984): 432–433.

18 To preserve privacy, no names of doctor's patients or people with AIDS are mentioned in this book. Unless full names are given, the names used are fictitious.

19 *Medical Tribune.* (Feb 25, 1993).

20 Rheinhardt, A.; et al. "Mechanisms of Viricidal Activity of Retinoids Antimicrobial Agents Chemotherapy." 17(6) (1980): 1034–1037.

Dolbeare, F.; et al. "Beta Carotene—an Unusual Type of Lipid Antioxidant." *Science* 224 (1984): 569–573.

21 Guitierrez, P. "Influence of Ascorbic Acid on Free Radical Metabolism of Xenobiotics." *Drug Metabolism Review* 18 (3&4) (1989): 319–343.

Blakeslee, J.; et al. "Human T-cell Leukemia Virus Inhibition by Retinoids, Ascorbic Acid, and Vitamin E." *Cancer Research* 45 (1985): 3471–3476.

Bouras, P.; et al. "Monocyte Locomotion - in Vivo Effect of Ascorbic Acid." *Immunopharmacology and Immunotoxicology* 11(1) (1989): 119–129.

22 Chaitow, L., Martin, S. *World Without AIDS* London: Thorsons/HarperCollins, 1989.

23 Mann, C. "Vitamin C KOs HIV" in *QQQ* (UK) 1991.

24 Harakeh, S.; et al. "Suppression of HIV Replication by Ascorbate in Chronically and Acutely Infected Cells." *Proceedings of National Academy of Sciences* (Sept, 1990): 7245–7249.

25 Weiner, M. *Maximum Immunity* (UK): Gateway Books, 1986.

26 Davies, S. Stewart. *A Nutritional Medicine.* London: Pan Books, 1987.

27 *AIDS 1990: A Physicians Manual.* Laurel, MD: Life Science Universal Inc.

28 *AIDS 1990: A Physicians Manual.* Laurel, MD: Life Science Universal Inc.

29 *AIDS 1990: A Physicians Manual.* Laurel, MD Life Science Universal Inc.

30 Chaitow, L. *Candida Albicans* Healing Arts Press: Vermont, 1989.

31 *AIDS 1990: A Physicians Manual.* Laurel, MD: Life Science Universal Inc.

32 Truss, C. Orion. *The Missing Diagnosis.* Published by the author: 1986.

33 *AIDS 1990: A Physicians Manual.* Laurel, MD: Life Science Universal Inc.

Chaitow, L. Martin, S. *World Without AIDS.* Thorsons/HarperCollins, 1989.

34 *AIDS 1990: A Physicians Manual.* Laurel, MD: Life Science Universal Inc.

Chaitow, L., Martin, S. *World Without AIDS.* Thorsons/HarperCollins, 1989.

Falutz, J. et al. "Zinc as co-factor in HIV induced immunosuppression" *Journal of American Medical Association* 259(19) 1881–2 1989.

35 *Nutrition Almanac (3rd edition)* New York: McGraw-Hill, 1990.

36 Staal, F., et al. "Glutathione Deficiency and HIV Infection." *The Lancet* (April 11, 1992): 909–912.

37 Robinson, M.; et al. "Glutathione Deficiency in HIV Infection." *The Lancet* (June 27, 1992): 1603–1604.

38 Standish, L.; et al. "One Year Open Trial of Naturopathic Treatment of HIV Infection." *J. Naturopathic Medicine* 3(1) (1992): 42–64.

39 Pulse, T.; et al. "A Significant Improvement in a Clinical Pilot Study Utilizing Nutritional Supplements, Essential Fatty Acids, and Stabilized Aloe Vera Juice in 29 HIV-seropositive, ARC and AIDS Patients." *Journal for the Advancement of Medicine* 3(4)209–230 (1990).

40 Erdmann, R. Ph.D. "AIDS Re-examined." *Felmore Newsletter* UK (1987).

41 Chaitow, L., Trenev, N. *Probiotics* London: Thorsons/HarperCollins, 1990.

42 Standish, L.; et al. "One Year Open Trial of Naturopathic Treatment of HIV Infection" *J. Naturopathic Medicine* 3(1) (1992): 42–64.

Chapter Six

1 Dharmananda, S., Ph.D. "Chinese Herbal Therapies for the Treatment of Immuno-deficiency Syndromes." *Oriental Healing Arts International Bulletin* 12(1) (Jan, 1987): 24–38.

Dharmananda, S., Ph.D. *Chinese Herbal Therapies for Immune Disorders.* Institute for Traditional Medicine, 1993.

2 Dharmananda, S., Ph.D. "Chinese Herbal Therapies for the Treatment of Immuno-deficiency Syndromes." *Oriental Healing Arts International Bulletin* 12(1) (Jan, 1987): 24–38.

3 Lien, Dr. "Analysis of Natural Products Against HIV." *International Journal of Oriental Medicine* 17(1) (1992).

4 Standish, L. "One Year Open Study of Naturopathic Treatment of HIV Infection." *Journal of Naturopathic Medicine* 3(1) (1992) 42–64.

5 Sun, Y.; et al. "Preliminary Observation on the Effects of Chinese Herbs." *Journal of Biological Response Modifiers* 2 (1983): 227–237.

6 Walker, M. "Carnivora Therapy for Cancer and AIDS." *Explore* 3 no. 5 (1992): 10–15.

Walker, M. "Carnivora and AIDS." *Townsend Letter for Doctors* (May, 1992): 351–359.

7 Stimpel, M.; et al. "Macrophage Activation and Induction of Cytotoxicity by Purified Polysaccharide Fractions from Echinacea Purpurea." *Infection and Immunity* 46 (1984): 845–849.

Wacker, A.; et al. "Virus Inhibition by Echinacea Purpurea." *Planta Medica.*

8 Abe, N.; et al. "Interferon Induction by Glycyrrhizin." *Microbiology and Immunology* 26 no. 6 (1982): 535–539.

9 Sharma, R.; et al. "Berberine Tannate in Acute Diarrhea." *Indian Pediatrics Journal* 7 (1978): 496–502.

Choudray, V.; et al. "Berberine in Giardiasis." *Indian Pediatrics Journal* 9 (1979): 143–146.

Sack, R.; et al. "Berberine Inhibits Intestinal Secretory Response in Vibrio Cholerae, E. Coli Enterotoxins." *Infection and Immunity* 35 no. 2 (1982): 471–475.

10 Adetumbi, M.; et al. "Allium Sativum: a Natural Antibiotic." *Medical Hypotheses* 12 (1983): 227–237.

Vahora, S.; et al. "Medicinal Use of Indian Vegetables." *Planta Medica* 23 (1973): 381–393.

"Garlic in Cryptococcal Meningitis." *Chinese Medical Journal* 93 (1980): 123–126.

11 Sharma, R.; et al. "Berberine Tannate in Acute Diarrhea." *Indian Pediatrics Journal* 7 (1978): 89–102.

12 Brekhmann, E. *Man and Biologically Active Substances.* London: Pergamon Press, 1980.

Takada, A.; et al. "Restoration of Radiation Injury by Ginseng." *Journal of Radiation* 22 (1981): 323–325.

13 Meruelo, D.; et al. "Therapeutic Agents with Dramatic Retroviral Activity." *Proceedings of National Academy of Sciences* 85 (1988): 5230–5234.

Someya, H. "Effect of a Constituent of Hypericum on Infection and Multiplication of Epstein Barr Virus." *Journal of Tokyo Medical College* 43 no. 5 (1985): 815–826.

Barbagallo, C.; et al. "Antimicrobial Activity of Three Hypericum Species." *Fitoteripia* LVIII no. 3 (1987): 175–177.

14 Zhang, Q. C. "Preliminary Report on the Use of Momordica Charantia Extract by HIV Patients." *Journal of Naturopathic Medicine* 3 no. 1 (1992): 65–90.

Baker, R. "MAP30: Momordica Anti-HIV Protein Research Notes." *BETA* (1991): 14.

Hierholzer, J.; et al. "In Vitro Effects of Monolaurin Compounds on Enveloped RNA and DNA Viruses." *Journal of Food Safety* 4 no. 1 (1982).

Sands, J.; et al. "Extreme Sensitivity of Enveloped Viruses to Long Chained Unsaturated Monoglycerides and Alcohols." *Antimicrobial Agents and Chemotherapy* 15 no. 1 (1979): 67–73.

Aoki, T.; et al. "Antibodies to HTLV-1 and HTLV-III in Sera from Two Japanese Patients." *The Lancet* 20 (Oct, 1984): 936–937.

15 *Immunopharm and Immunotox*, vol. 14, (1992): 63–77.

16 Dharmananda, S. with Fruehauf, H. *The Key Link: A Detailed Analysis of an Epidemic Disease.* Portland, OR: Institute of Traditional Medicine, 1994.

17 Poster, 6th Int. Conf. on AIDS, "HIV-1 Infected Patients Respond Favorably to Oral Acemannan," McDaniel et al.

18 Sun, Y.; et al. "Preliminary Observation on the Effects of Chinese Herbs." *Journal of Biological Response Modifiers* 2 (1983): 227–237.

19 Sun, Y.; et al. "Immune Restoration and/or Augmentation of Local Versus Host Reaction by Traditional Chinese Herbs." *Cancer* 52(1) (1983): 70–73.

20 Walker, M. "Carnivora Therapy in Cancer and AIDS." *Explore* 3(5) (1992): 10–15.

Walker, M. "Carnivora and AIDS." *Townsend Letter for Doctors* (May, 1992).

Walker, M. "Carnivora Therapy." *Raum & Zeit* 4(2) (1991).

21 McGrath, M.; et al. "GLQ223: Inhibitor of HIV Replication in Acutely and Chronically Infected Cells of Lymphocytes and Mononuclear Phagocyte Lineage." *Proc. Nat. Acad. Sci.* (1989): 862844–48.

McGrath, M.; et al. "Effect of GLQ223 on HIV Replication in Human Monocyte/Macrophages Chronically Infected in Vitro with HIV." *AIDS Res. Retrovir.* (1990); 6(8): 1039–43.

Baker, R.A. "MAP 30: Momordica Anti-HIV Protein, Research Notes." *BETA* (1991): 14.

22 Stimpel, M.; et al. "Macrophage Activation and Induction of Cytotoxicity by Purified Polysaccharide Fractions from Echinacea Purpurea." *Infection and Immunity* 46: (1984): 845–849.

23 Adetumbi, M.; et al. "Allium Sativum: A Natural Antibiotic." *Medical Hypothesis* 12 (1983): 227–237.

24 Sharma, R.; et al. "Berberine Tannate in Acute Diarrhea." *Indian Pediatric Journal* 7 (1973): 496–502.

25 Information on Medical Science and Technology, Guangdong Institute of Medicine and Health 8–9 (1973): 33.

26 Abe, N.; et al. "Interferon Induction by Glycyrrhizin." *Microbiology and Immunology* 26(6) (1982): 535–539.

27 Ponpei, R.; et al. "Glycyrrhizic Acid Inhibits Virus Growth and Inactivates Virus Particles." *Nature* 281 (1979): 689–690.

28 Nakashima, H.; et al. "New Anti-HIV Substance-Glycyrrhizin Sulfate." *Japanese Journal of Cancer Research* 78 (1987): 767–771.

29 Mischer, L.; et al. "Antimicrobial Agents from Higher Plants." *Journal of Natural Products* 43(2): (1980): 259–269.

30 Kiso, Y.; et al. "Mechanism of Anti-hepatotoxic Activity of Glycyrrhizin." *Planta Medica* 50(4) (1984): 298–302.

31 Juroyanagi, T.; et al. "Effect of Prednisone and Glycyrrhizin on Passive Transfer of Experimental Ellergic Encephalomyitis." *Allergy* 15 (1966): 67075.

32 Kumazai, A.; et al. "Effects of Glycyrrhizin on Thymolytic and Immunosuppressive Action of Cortisone." *Endocrinology* Japan 14(1) (1967): 39–42.

33 Brekhmann, E. *Man and Biologically Active Substances.* London: Pergamon Press, 1980.

34 Meruelo, D.; et al. "Therapeutic Agents With Dramatic Retroviral Activity." *Proceedings of National Academy of Sciences* 85 (1988): 5230–5234.

35 *Foundations of Chinese Herb Prescribing*, Oriental Healing Arts Institute, Long Beach.

Chapter Seven
1 Sidhu, G., El-Sadr, W. "Some Thoughts on AIDS." *Nutrition Research* Vl.3 (1985): 7.

2 Sohn, N.; et al. "Gay Bowel Syndrome." *American Journal of Gastroenterology* 67 (1977): 478–484.

3 Chaitow, L. *Beat Fatigue Workbook*. London: Thorsons, 1986.

4 Alexander, M.; et al. "Oral Beta-carotene Can Increase Number of OKT4+ Cells in Human Blood." *Immunology* (letters) 9(4) (1985): 221–224.

5 Harakeh, S.; et al. "Suppression of HIV Replication by Ascorbate." *Proceedings of National Academy of Sciences* vol.87 (1990): 7245–7249.

Blakeslee, J.; et al. "Human T-cell Leukemia Virus Induction Inhibited by Retinoids, L-ascorbic Acid, and DL-alpha Tocopherol." *Cancer Research* 45 (1985): 3471–3476.

Schwerdt, P., Schwerdt, C. "Effect of Ascorbic Acid on Rhinovirus Replication." *Proc. Soc. Exp. Biol. Med* 148(4) (1975): 1237–1243.

Beisel, W.; et al. "Single Nutrient Effects on Immunological Functions." *Journal of the American Medical Association* 245(1) (1981): 53–58.

6 Cathcart, R. "Vitamin C: Titrating to Bowel Tolerance." *Medical Hypotheses* 7 (1981): 1359–1376.

7 Hierholzer, J.; et al. "In Vitro Effects of Monolaurin Compounds on Enveloped RNA and DNA Viruses." *Journal of Food Safety* 4:1 (1982).

8 Sun, Y.; et al. "Immune Restoration by Traditional Chinese Medical Herbs." *Cancer* 52(1) (1983): 70–73.

9 Yunde, H.; et al. "Effects of Radix Astragalis on Interferon System." *Chinese Medical Journal* 94 (1980): 35–40.

10 Walker, M. "Carnivora Therapy for Cancer and AIDS." *Explore* 3(5) (1992): 10–15.

11 Zhang, Q. C. "Preliminary Report on Use of Momordica Charantia Extract by HIV Patients." *Journal of Naturopathic Medicine* 3(1) (1992): 65–69.

12 Pizzorno, J., Murray, M. *Textbook of Natural Medicine*. Seattle, WA: Bastyr Publications, 1989.

13 *Information on Medical Science and Technology*. Guangdong Institute of Medicine and Health 9–9:33, 1973.

Encyclopedia of Chinese Materia Medica. Shanghai People's Publishing House 1:126, 1975.

14 Abe, N.; et al. "Interferon Induction by Glycyrrhizen in Mice." *Microbiology and Immunology* 26(6) (1982): 535–539.

15 Aoki, T.; et al. "Antibodies to HTLV-1 and HTLV-III in Sera from Two Japanese Patients." *The Lancet* 20 (Oct, 1984): 936–937.

16 Truss, C. O. *The Missing Diagnosis*. Birmingham, Alabama, 1982.

17 Stretch, E. "Clinical Manifestations of HIV Infection in Women." *Journal of Naturopathic Medicine* 3(1) (1992): 12–19.

18 Carlson, E. "Enhancement by Candida of S. aureus, S. marcescens, S. faecalis in the Establishment of Infection." *Infection and Immunity* 39(1) (1983): 193–197.

19 Chaitow, L., Trenev, N. *Probiotics* New York: HarperCollins, 1989.

20 Chaitow, L., Trenev, N. *Probiotics* New York: HarperCollins, 1989.

21 Crook, W. *The Yeast Connection*. Jackson, TN: Professional Books, 1984.

22 Anthony, M.; et al. "Infectious Diarrhea in Patients with AIDS." *Digestive Disease* 33 (1988): 1141–1146.

23 Bihari, B. "Ambulatory Management of HIV." *Journal of Naturopathic Medicine* 3(1) (1992): 20–30.

24 Bihari, B. "Ambulatory Management of HIV." *Journal of Naturopathic Medicine* 3(1) (1992): 20–30.

25 Sharma, R.; et al. "Berberine Tannate in Acute Diarrhea." *Indian Pediatric Journal* 7 (1970): 496–501.

26 Shehani, K.; et al. "Nutritional and Therapeutic Aspects of Cultured Dairy Products." *Prox XIX International Dairy Congress* vol.1e (1974): 569–570.

27 Gibson, R., Gibson, S. *Homoeopathy for Everyone*. New York: Penguin, 1987.

28 Data from the Allergy Research Group, San Leandro, CA. 1-800-545-9960.

29 "Garlic in Cryptococcal Meningitis: A Preliminary Report of Twenty-one Cases." *Chinese Medical Journal* 93 (1980): 123–6.

30 Bihari, B. "Ambulatory Management of HIV." *Journal of Naturopathic Medicine* 3(1) (1992): 20–30.

31 Nahmias, A.; et al. *New England Journal of Medicine* 289: 781–789.

Nahmias, A.; et al. *Journal of Infectious Diseases* Supplement 69:19–36, 1990.

32 Brown, R. *AIDS—The Third Pivot*. To be published shortly. 1992.

33 Root-Bernstein, R. *Rethinking AIDS*, New York: Macmillian Free Press, 1992.

34 Kagan, C. "Lysine Therapy for Herpes Simplex." *The Lancet* 1(137) (Jan 26, 1974).

35 Pompei, R.; et al. "Antiviral Activity of Glycyrrhizic Acid." *Experientia* 36(3) (1980): 304.

36 Ibid.

37 Sofroniou, P. "AIDS and Nutrition." *Journal of Alternative and Complementary Medicine* (April, 1993).

Adetumbi, M. "Allium Sativum (Garlic): a Natural Antibiotic." *Medical Hypothesis* 12 (1983): 227–237.

38 Sands, J.; et al. "Extreme Sensitivity of Enveloped Viruses Including Herpes Simplex to Long Chained Unsaturated Monoglycerides and Alcohols." *Antimicrobial Agents and Chemotherapy* 15(1) (1979): 67–73.

39 Chaitow, L., Martin, S. *A World Without AIDS*. London: Thorsons/HarperCollins, 1989.

40 Taylor-Papadimitriou. "Effects of Interferon on Cell Growth and Function." *Interferon* Edited by I. Gresser. New York: Academic Press, 1982.

41 Bihari, B. "Ambulator Management of HIV." *Journal of Naturopathic Medicine* 3(1) (1992): 20–30.

42 Pizzorno, J., Murray, M. *Textbook of Natural Medicine* Seattle, WA: Bastyr Publications, 1989.

43 Field, D. "Adverse Reactions and Side Effects of HIV Treatment." *Journal of Naturopathic Medicine* 3(1) (1992):74–76.

44 Stimpel, M.; et al. "Macrophage Activation and Induction of Cytotoxicity from the Plant Echinacea Purpurea." *Infect. Immun.* 46: (1984): 845–849.
45 Standish, L. "One Year Open Trial of Naturopathic Treatment of HIV Infection." *Journal of Naturopathic Medicine* 3(1) (1992): 42–64.
46 Chaitow, L. *Thorsons Guide to Amino Acids.* New York: HarperCollins, 1990.
47 Bihari, B. "Ambulatory Management of HIV." *Journal of Naturopathic Med.* 3(1) 20–30 (1992) and report *London Daily Telegraph* (Dec 30, 1992).

Chapter Eight
1 Cracium, T.; et al. "Neurohumoural Modification After Acupuncture." *American Journal of Acupuncture* 21 (1973): 67.
Tykochinskaia, E. "Acupuncture as a Method of Reflex Therapy." *Veprosy Psikhatrii I Nerripathologii* 7 (1960): 249–260.
Yang, C. Clinical Report, Sansi Acupuncture Symposium reported in *Acupuncture in Medical Practice* by Louise Wensall, M.D. Reston Publishing, 1980.
2 Misha Cohen, O.M.D., L.Ac. (415) 861–1101.
3 Adetumbi, M.; et al. "Allium Sativum: a Natural Antibiotic." *Medical Hypotheses* 12 (1983): 227–237.
Vahora, S.; et al. "Medicinal Use of Indian Vegetables." *Planta Medica* 23 (1973): 381–393.
"Garlic in Cryptococcal Meningitis." *Chinese Medical Journal* 93 (1980): 123–126.
4 Sharma, R.; et al. "Berberine Tannate in Acute Diarrhea." *Indian Pediatrics Journal* 7 (1978): 89–102.
5 Ponpei, R. et al. "Glycyrrhizic Acid Inhibits Virus Growth and Inactivates Virus Particles." *Nature* 281 (1979): 689–690.
Nakashima, H.; et al. "New Anti-HIV Substance—Glycyrrhizin Sulfate." *Japanese Journal of Cancer Research* 78 (1987): 767–771.
6 Zhang, Q. C. "Preliminary Report on the Use of Momordica Charantia Extract by HIV Patients." *Journal of Naturopathic Medicine* 3 no. 1 (1992): 65–69.
Baker, R. "MAP30: Momordica Anti-HIV Protein Research Notes." *BETA* (1991): 14.
Hierholzer, J.; et al. "In Vitro Effects of Monolaurin Compounds on Enveloped RNA and DNA Viruses." *Journal of Food Safety* 4 no. 1 (1982).
Sands, J.; et al. "Extreme Sensitivity of Enveloped Viruses to Long Chained Unsaturated Monoglycerides and Alcohols." *Antimicrobial Agents and Chemotherapy* 15 no. 1 (1979): 67–73.
Aoki, T.; et al. "Antibodies to HTLV-1 and HTLV-III in Sera from Two Japanese Patients." *The Lancet* 20 (Oct, 1984): 936–937.
7 Meruelo, D.; et al. "Therapeutic Agents with Dramatic Retroviral Activity." *Proceedings of National Academy of Sciences* 85 (1988): 5230–5234.
Someya, H. "Effect of a Constituent of Hypericum on Infection and Multiplication of Epstein Barr Virus." *Journal of Tokyo Medical College* 43 no. 5 (1985): 815–826.
Barbagallo, C.; et al. "Antimicrobial Activity of Three Hypericum Species." *Fitoteripia* LVIII no. 3 (1987): 175–177.
8 Zhang, Q. "Chinese Medicine and AIDS." Qingcai Zhang, M.D., 8789 5th Avenue, Suite 604, New York, NY 10003.
9 Orman, D., Margetis, D. "Effectiveness of Acupuncture and Chinese Phytomedicinals in the Treatment of HIV and AIDS." *Journal of Naturopathic Medicine* 3 no. 1 (1992): 80–82.
10 Smith, M., Rabinowitz, N. "Acupuncture Treatment of AIDS." Lincoln Hospital Acupuncture Clinic, March, 1985.
11 Smith, M., Rabinowitz, N. "Acupuncture Treatment of AIDS." Lincoln Hospital Acupuncture Clinic, March, 1985.
Smith, M. "Research in Use of Acupuncture with AIDS." *American Journal of Acupuncture* 16 no. 2 (April–June, 1988).
12 Chaitow, L., Martin, S. *A World Without AIDS.* London: Thorsons/HarperCollins, 1989, 131.

Chapter Nine
1 Steven Bailey, N.D. Northwest Naturopathic Clinic, 2606 NW Vaughn, Portland, OR 97210. (503) 224-8083
2 Standish, L.; et al. "One Year Open Trial of Naturopathic Treatment of HIV Infection Class IV-A in Men." *Journal of Naturopathic Medicine* 3 no. 1 (1992): 42–64.
3 Brayton, R.; et al. "Effect of Alcohol and Various Diseases on Leucocyte Mobilization, Phagocytosis, and Intracellular Bacterial Killing." *New England Journal of Medicine* 2 no. 3 (1970): 123–128.
Saxena, A.; et al. "Immunomodulating Effects of Caffeine in Rodents." *Indian Journal of Experimental Biology* 22 no. 6 (1984): 293–301.
4 Standish, L.; et al. "One Year Open Trial of Naturopathic Treatment of HIV Infection Class IV-A in Men." *Journal of Naturopathic Medicine* 3 no. 1 (1992): 42–64.

Chapter Ten
1 Solomon, G. "The Emerging Field of Psychoneuroimmunology." *Advances* 2(1) (1985): 6–19.
2 Callen, M. *Surviving AIDS.* New York: HarperCollins, 1990.
3 Solomon, G. *Brain/Mind Bulletin* (May, 1988).
4 Healey, D.L.; et al. "The Thymus-Adrenal Connection: Thymosin Has Corticotropin-Releasing Activity in Primates." *Science* 222 no, 4630 (1983): 1353–1355.
5 Solomon, G. "The Emerging Field of Psychoneuroimmunology." *Institutes for the Advancement of Health* 2 no.1 (1985): 6–19.

6 "Depression, Stress, and Immunity." *The Lancet* (June 27, 1987): 1487–1488.
7 Quoted in Chaitow, L., Martin, S. *A World Without AIDS*. London: Thorsons/Harper-Collins, 1989.
8 Eric Peper, Ph.D., Associate Director, Institute for Holistic Healing Studies, San Francisco State University, 1600 Holloway Avenue, San Francisco, CA 94132. (415) 338-7683.
9 Chaitow, L. *The Stress Protection Plan*. London: Thorsons/HarperCollins, 1991.
10 Patricia Norris, Ph.D., Director, Biofeedback and Psychophysiology Clinic, Menninger Clinic, Box 829, Topeka, Kansas 66601. (913) 273-7500.
11 Janet Konefal, Ph.D., Associate Professor of Psychiatry, University of Miami School of Medicine, 1425 NW 10th Avenue, Suite T-1, Miami, FL 33136. (305) 548-4751.
12 Cohen, S. I. "Voodoo Death, the Stress Response, and AIDS." In Peter Bridge, et al. (eds.) *Psychological, Neuropsychiatric, and Substance Abuse Aspects of AIDS*. New York: Raven Press, 1988.
13 Antoni, M., Baggett, L, Ironson, G.; et al. "Cognitive-behavorial Stress Management Intervention Buffers Distress Responses and Immunologic Changes Following Notification of HIV-1 Seropositivity." *Journal of Consulting and Clinical Psychology* 59(6): 906–915.
Ironson, G., LaPerriere, A., Antoni, M.; et al. "Changes in Immune and Psychological Measures as a Function of Anticipation and Reaction to News of HIV-1 Antibody Status." *Psychosomatic Medicine* 52(3): 247–270.

Chapter Eleven
1 Nault, K. "AIDS, Cancer - An Answer (Ozone Therapy)." Report in *Crosswinds*. Santa Fe, NM, December, 1988, based on Associated Press wires services report, October 28, 1988.
2 Warburg, O. "The Prime Cause and Prevention of Cancer." Revised lecture at the meeting of the Nobel-laureates on June 30, 1966. National Cancer Institute, Bethesda, MD, 1967.
3 Farr, C. H. Presented at the Fourth International Conference on Bio-Oxidative Medicine. Reston, VA, April 1–4, 1993.
4 Farr, C. H. "Workbook on Free Radical Chemistry and Hydrogen Peroxide Metabolism Including Protocol for the Intravenous Administration of Hydrogen Peroxide." Contains thirty-two citations with references in the workbook, and 123 in the Protocol. Available from the International Bio-Oxidative Medicine Foundation, P.O. Box 13205, Oklahoma City, OK 73113, 1992.
5 Based on literature provided by Life Sciences Universal Inc., P.O. Box 2890, Laurel, MD 20709. (301) 567-3484.
6 Wells, K., Latinok J., Gavalchin, J., Poiesz, P. "Inactivation of Human Immunodeficiency Virus Type I By Ozone in Vitro." *Blood* 78(7) 1882–90, (1991).

7 Sweet, F., Ka, M., Lee, S. "Ozone Selectively Inhibits Growth of Human Cancer Cells." *Science* 2009(72)931 (1990).
8 Wells, K.; et al. "Inactivation of Human Immunodeficiency Virus Type 1 by Ozone in Vitro." *Blood* 78 (1991): 1882–1890.
9 Vallancien, B., Winkler, J. M. "Immunomodulating Effect of Ozone Among Patients with AIDS." *Conference Report* New York (1989).
10 Forest, W. "AIDS, Cancer Cured by Hyperbaric Oxygenation." *Townsend Letter for Doctors* 105 (April, 1992): 231–238.
11 The off-the-record source states that, "When medical ozone use is discontinued, T-cell counts can drop quickly and steeply." "Therefore," he continues, "a person should have another way of supporting T-cell levels before he stops ozone."
12 Farr, C. H. *The Therapeutic Use of Intravenous Hydrogen Peroxide*, Genesis Medical Center, Oklahoma City, OK 73120, 1987.
13 Farr, C. H. "Workbook on Free Radical Chemistry and Hydrogen Peroxide Metabolism Including Protocol for the Intravenous Administration of Hydrogen Peroxide." Contains thirty-two citations with references in the workbook, and 123 in the Protocol. Available from the International Bio-Oxidative Medicine Foundation, P.O. Box 13205, Oklahoma City, OK 73113, 1992.
14 Farr, C. H. "The Use of Dilute Hydrogen Peroxide to Inject Trigger Points, Soft Tissue Injuries, and Inflamed Joints." International Bio-Oxidative Medicine Foundation, P.O. Box 13205, Oklahoma City, OK 73113, 1992.
15 Farr, C. H. "Rapid Recovery from Type A/Shanghai Influenza Treated with Intravenous Hydrogen Peroxide." Geneses Medical Center, Oklahoma City, OK 73120.
16 Farr, C. H. "Rapid Recovery from Type A/Shanghai Influenza Treated with Intravenous Hydrogen Peroxide." Geneses Medical Center, Oklahoma City, OK 73120.

Chapter Twelve
1 Pizzorno, J., Murray, M. *Textbook of Natural Medicine*. Seattle, WA: Bastyr College Publications, 1989.
2 Neville, A.; et al. "Whole Body Hyperthermia (41*–42*C) Induces Interleukin-1 in Vivo." *Lymphokine Research* 7(3) (1988): 201–205.
Park, M., et al. "Effect of Whole Body Hyperthermia on Immune Cell Activity of Cancer Patients." *Lymphokine Research* 9(2) (1990): 213–221.
3 Tyrrell, D., Barrow, I., Arthur, J. "Local Hyperthermia Benefits Natural and Experimental Common Colds." *British Medical Journal* 298 (1989): 1280–1283.
4 Spire, B.; et al. "Inactivation of Lymphadenopathy-Associated Virus by Heat, Gamma Rays, and Ultraviolet Light." *The Lancet* 1 no. 8422 (Jan 26, 1985): 188–189.
5 Thrash, A., M.D., Thrash, C. L. Jr., M.D. *Home Remedies: Hydrotherapy, Massage,*

Charcoal, and Other Simple Treatments. Groveland, CA: New Life Books, 1981.

6 Weatherburn, H. "Hyperthermia and AIDS Treatment." *British Journal of Radiology* 61, no. 729 (Sept, 1988): 862–863.

7 Standish, L.; et al. "One Year Open Trial of Naturopathic Treatment of HIV Infection Class IV-A in Men." *Journal of Naturopathic Medicine* 3 no. 1 (1992): 42–64.

8 DeMarco, C. "To Those Interested in Hyperthermia as a Treatment for AIDS." Monograph, HEAT INFO, 1994. (Copies available from HEAT INFO, (201) 865–4483.)

9 "Summary of Findings: Site Visit Report - Clinical Use of Hyperthermia in AIDS." Backgrounder. National Institute of Allergy and Infectious Diseases. August 30, 1990.

10 "Summary of Findings: Site Visit Report - Clinical Use of Hyperthermia in AIDS." Backgrounder. National Institute of Allergy and Infectious Diseases. August 30, 1990.

Stanley, S. K., Bressler, P. B., Poll, G., and Fauci, A. S. "Heat Shock Induction of HIV Production from Chronically Infected Promonocytic and T Cell Lines." *The Journal of Immunology* 145, no. 4 (Aug 15, 1990): 1120–1126.

11 Yatvin, M. B., Stowell, M. H., Steinhart, C.R. "Shedding Light on the Use of Heat to Treat HIV Infection." *Oncology* 50 (1993): 380–389.

Yatvin, M. B. "An Approach to AIDS Therapy Using Hyperthermia and Membrane Modification." *Medical Hypotheses* 27 (1998): 163–165.

Alonso, K., Pontiggia, P., DeBartolomei, E., Curto, F. C., Calvi, G., Nardi, C. "Systemic Hyperthermia in the Treatment of HIV-Related Kaposi's Sarcoma (KS) Confers a Survival Advantage: Long Term Results of a Phase I Study." *AIDS Weekly* (Sept 27, 1993).

Alonso, K., Pontiggia, P., Nardi, C., Sabato, A., Curto, F. C. "Systemic Hyperthermia in the Treatment of HIV-Related Kaposi's Sarcoma—A Phase I Study." *Biomed & Pharmacother* 46 (1992): 21–24.

12 DeMarco, C. "To Those Interested in Hyperthermia as a Treatment for AIDS." Monograph, HEAT INFO, 1994.

13 DeMarco, C. "To Those Interested in Hyperthermia as a Treatment for AIDS." Monograph, HEAT INFO, 1994.

[14] DeMarco, C. "To Those Interested in Hyperthermia as a Treatment for AIDS." Monograph, HEAT INFO, 1994.

15 Yatvin, M. B., Stowell, M.H., Steinhart, C. R. "Shedding Light on the Use of Heat to Treat HIV Infection." *Oncology* 50 (1993): 380–389.

Yatvin, M. B. "An Approach to AIDS Therapy Using Hyperthermia and Membrane Modification." *Medical Hypotheses* 27 (1998): 163–165.

Alonso, K., Pontiggia, P., DeBartolomei, E., Curto, F. C., Calvi, G., Nardi, C. "Systemic Hyperthermia in the Treatment of HIV-Related Kaposi's Sarcoma (KS) Confers a Survival Advantage: Long Term Results of a Phase I Study." *AIDS Weekly* (Sept 27, 1993).

Alonso, K., Pontiggia, P., Nardi, C., Sabato, A., Curto, F. C. "Systemic Hyperthermia in the Treatment of HIV-Related Kaposi's Sarcoma—A Phase I Study." *Biomed & Pharmacother* 46 (1992): 21–24.

16 DeMarco, C. "To Those Interested in Hyperthermia as a Treatment for AIDS." Monograph, HEAT INFO, 1994.

17 Sawtell, N. M., Thompson, R. L. "Rapid in Vivo Reactivation of Herpes Simplex Virus in Latently Infected Murine Ganglionic Neurons after Transient Hyperthermia." *Journal of Virology* 66 no. 4 (April, 1992): 2150–2156.

18 Skibba, J. L.; et al. "Oxidative Stress as a Precursor to the Irreversible Hepatocellular Injury Caused by Hyperthermia." *International Journal Hyperthermia* 7 no. 5 (Sept/Oct 1991): 749–761.

Chapter Thirteen

1 Chaitow, L. *Soft Tissue Manipulation.* Rochester, VT: Healing Arts Press, 1989.

2 Ironson, G., M.D., Ph.D.; Field, T., Ph.D.; Kumar, A., Ph.D.; Price, A., B.A.; Kumar, M., Ph.D.; Hansen, K., R.N.; Burman, I., B.A. "Relaxation Through Massage Therapy is Associated with Decreased Distress and Increased Serotonin Levels." Touch Research Institute, University of Miami School of Medicine. Reported in *Journal of Alternative and Complementary Medicine* (UK), (Dec, 1992).

3 Robert King, Director, Chicago School of Massage Therapy, 2918 N. Lincoln, Chicago, IL 60657. (312) 477-7256.

PART THREE: LONG TERM SURVIVORS

Chapter Fourteen

1 Solomon, George, M.D. *Brain/Mind Bulletin* (May, 1988).

2 *Resist* is available from Pacific BioLogic Inc., 5337 College Avenue, Oakland, CA 94618. (800) 869-8783.

3 Information available by calling Health First, (415) 922-5147.

4 Laurence Badgley, M.D., 1020 Foster City Boulevard, Suite 205, Foster City, CA 94404-2345. (415) 349-0646.

5 Orth, G. *Raum & Ziet* (German) 56: (1992). Orth, G. *Journal of Alternative and Complementary Medicine* (tr. Derek Wolfe), (April, 1993).

6 "Alkala-N" powder and "Multiplasen H33" are available from Sanum-Kehlbeck Gmbh, Arzneimittelherstellung, Bahnfostr.2, pf1355, W2812 Hoya, Germany.

7 "Pefrkehl," "D5" drops, "D4" capsules. and "D3" suppositories are available from Sanum-Kehlbeck Gmbh, Arzneimittelherstellung, Bahnfostr.2, pf1355, W2812 Hoya, Germany.

8 "Multiplasen GL17" is available from Planta-trakt Gmbh., Postfach 20, W8974 Oberstaufen Steibis, Germany.

9 Clark, Hulda R., *The Cure for HIV and AIDS*. San Diego, CA: ProMotion Publishing, 1993. (Available through Future Medicine Publishing, Inc. (800) 249-8500.)

10 Burzynski Research Institute, Inc., 12000 Richmond Avenue, Suite 260, Houston, TX 77082-2431. (713) 597-0111.

11 Dr. Burzynski states that three patients out of those who began the three studies died. In each situation, this was from an opportunistic infection. These three people had full-blown AIDS before entering the studies, and had not done well on previous antiviral therapy.

12 Robert Cathcart, III, M.D., 127 2nd Street, Suite 4, Los Altos, CA 94022. (415) 949-2822.

13 Cathcart, Robert, III, M.D. "Vitamin C in the Treatment of AIDS." (1984).

14 To determine the availability of L-51, inquire at Dr. Coronel's office, in Mexico City: 011-525-549-2281.

15 Bird, C. *The Persecution and Trial of Gaston Naessens*. Tiburon, CA: H.J. Kramer, 1991.

16 Pleomorphic theory states that microorganisms can change and take on multiple forms during a single life cycle. Accordingly, viruses, bacteria, and fungi are seen as actual interchangeable forms of a single, fundamental unit of life. The theory holds that when there is a state of health and balance, these microorganisms live in harmony with the body. However, when that balance is lost due to illness or other immunosuppressive factors, these same microorganisms change form and fight against their host.

17 For more information regarding 714-X, call Writers and Research Inc. at (716) 266-4630. There is also a number in Canada where information can be obtained: (819) 564-7883.

18 Qingcai Zhang, M.D. (China), Lic.Ac., 383 5th Avenue, 4th Floor, New York, NY 10016. (212) 889-0633.

19 McGrath, M.; et al. "GLQ223: Inhibitor of HIV Replication in Acutely and Chronically Infected Cells of Lymphocytes and Mononuclear Phagocyte Lineage." *Proc. Nat. Acad. Sci.* (1989) 862844–48.

McGrath, M.; et al. "Effect of GLQ223 on HIV Replication in Human Monocyte/Macrophages Chronically Infected in Vitro with HIV." *AIDS Res. Retrovir.* (1990) 6(8): 1039–43.

Baker, R. A. "MAP 30: Momordica Anti-HIV Protein, Research Notes." *BETA* 1991, 14.

20 Baker, R. A. "MAP 30: Momordica Anti-HIV Protein, Research Notes." *BETA* 1991, 14.

21 Zhang, Q. "Preliminary Report on the Use of Momordica Charantia Extract by HIV Patients."*The Journal of Naturopathic Medicine* vol. 3, no. 1: 65–69.

22 *Jiangsu New Medical College Great Dictionary of Chinese Materia Medica*. Shanghia Science and Technology Publishers, 1985, 12,801.

23 Lee-Huang (1990): 13.

24 Zhang (1992): Abs. 7597.

Chapter 15
1 Sharon Lund, c/o Mary McDonald, 155 West 72nd Street, 7th floor, New York, NY 10023 (212)580-4128.

APPENDIX

Scientific Appendix: Human Immunondeficiency Virus

1 *AIDS Weekly*. (Jan 4, 1993).

2 "Asia May Become New Leader in HIV Infections." *AIDS Weekly* (Jan 4, 1993).

3 Greene-Warner, C. "Review Article: Mechanisms of Disease - The Molecular Biology of Human Immunodeficiency Virus Type 1 Infection." *The New England Journal of Medicine* (Jan 31, 1991) 324 (5): 308–317.

4 Greene-Warner, C. "Review Article: Mechanisms of Disease—The Molecular Biology of Human Immunodeficiency Virus Type 1 Infection." *The New England Journal of Medicine* (Jan 31, 1991) 324 (5): 308–317.

5 Greene-Warner, C. "Review Article: Mechanisms of Disease—The Molecular Biology of Human Immunodeficiency Virus Type 1 Infection." *The New England Journal of Medicine* (Jan 31, 1991) 324 (5): 308–317.

Weiss, R. A. "Retroviruses and Human Disease." *Journal of Clinical Pathology* (Sept, 1987) 40(9): 1064–1069.

6 Greene-Warner, C. "Review Article: Mechanisms of Disease—The Molecular Biology of Human Immunodeficiency Virus Type 1 Infection." *The New England Journal of Medicine* (Jan 31, 1991) 324 (5): 308–317.

7 Greene-Warner, C. "Review Article: Mechanisms of Disease—The Molecular Biology of Human Immunodeficiency Virus Type 1 Infection." *The New England Journal of Medicine* (Jan 31, 1991) 324 (5): 308–317.

8 *AIDS Weekly*. (Nov 2, 1992). "Crosslinking CD4 by Human Immunodeficiency Virus gp120 Primes T Cells for Activation-Induced Apoptosis." *Journal of Experimental Medicine* (Oct, 1992) 176(10): 1099–1106.

VIII International Conference on AIDS, "AIDS Onset Associated With Loss of Active, Anti-HIV CD8+ Cells." *AIDS Weekly* (July 27, 1992).

9 Greene-Warner, C. "Review Article: Mechanisms of Disease—The Molecular Biology of Human Immunodeficiency Virus Type 1 Infection." *The New England Journal of Medicine* (Jan 31, 1991) 324 (5): 308–317.

10 Greene-Warner, C. "Review Article: Mechanisms of Disease—The Molecular Biology of Human Immunodeficiency Virus Type 1 Infection." *The New England Journal of Medicine* (Jan 31, 1991) 324 (5): 308–317.

11 "NIH Conference: Immunopathogenic Mechanisms in Human Immunodeficiency Virus HIV Infection." *Annals of Internal Medicine* (April 15, 1992) 114(8): 678–93.

12 "NIH Conference: Immunopathogenic Mechanisms in Human Immunodeficiency Virus HIV Infection. "*Annals of Internal*

Medicine (April 15, 1992) 114(8): 678–93.
Clark, Stephen J., Saag, Michael S., Decker, W. Don., Campbell-Hill, Sherri, Roberson, Joseph L., Veldkamp, Peter J., Kappes, John C., Hahn, Beatrice H., Shaw, George M. Original Articles: "High Titres of Cytopathic Virus in Plasma of Patients with Symptomatic Primary HIV-1 Infection." *The New England Journal of Medicine* (April 4, 1991) 324 (14): 954–960.
Baltimore, David, Feinberg, Mark B. Editorials: "HIV Revealed: Toward a Natural History of the Infection." *The New England Journal of Medicine* (Dec 14, 1989) 321 (24): 1673–1675.
13 "Rockefeller University Study Suggests HIV Hitchhikes on Blood Cell." *AIDS Weekly* (Aug 3, 1992).
"Programmed Death of T Cells in HIV-1 Infection." *AIDS Weekly* (Aug 3, 1992) *Science* (July 10, 1992) 257(5067): 217–219.
"Superantigen-presenting Dendritic Cells Carrying HIV Virions Cause an Explosive Cytopathic Infection in CD4+ T Cells." *AIDS Weekly, Science* (July 17, 1992): 383–387.
Editorials: "AIDS: How Can a Pussy Cat Kill?" *The Lancet* (April 4, 1992) 339(8797): 839–840.
14 Baltimore, David; Feinberg, Mark B. Editorials: "HIV Revealed - Toward a Natural History of the Infection." *The New England Journal of Medicine* (Dec 14, 1989) 321 (24): 1673–1675.
Schnittman, Steven M., M.D. "NIH Conference: Immunopathogenic Mechanisms in Human Immunodeficiency Virus HIV Infection." "Viral Burden in Human Immunodeficiency Virus Type 1 (HIV-1) Infection." *Annals of Internal Medicine* (April 15, 1992) 114(8): 678–693.
15 Editorials: "AIDS: How Can a Pussy Cat Kill?" *The Lancet* (April 4, 1992) 339(8797): 839–840.
16 Guido Poli, M.D. "The Role of Mononuclear Phagocytes in the Pathogenesis of HIV Infection." *Annals of Internal Medicine* (April 15, 1992) 114(8): 678–93.
"NIH Conference: Immunopathogenic Mechanisms in Human Immunodeficiency Virus HIV Infection."
17 Tersmette, M., Lange, J. M. A., de-Goede, R. E. Y., de Wolf, F., Eeftink-Schattenkerk, J. K. M., Schellekens, P. Th. A., Coutinho, R. A., Huisman, J. G., Goudsmit, J., Miedema, F. Original Article: "Association Between Biological Properties of Human Immunodeficiency Virus Variants and Risk for AIDS and AIDS Mortality." *The Lancet* May 6, 1989. 1(8645): 983–985.
18 Montagnier, Luc. "VIII International Conference on AIDS. HIV, Mycoplasmal Superantigens Program T Cells for Death." *AIDS Weekly* (Aug 17, 1992).
19 Montagnier, Luc. "VIII International Conference on AIDS. HIV, Mycoplasmal Superantigens Program T Cells for Death." *AIDS Weekly* (Aug 17, 1992).

20 Pantaleo, Giuseppe, M.D. "Mechanisms of CD8+ Cell Dysfunction in HIV Infection. "*Annals of Internal Medicine.* (April 15, 1992) 114(8): 678–93.
"NIH Conference: Immunopathogenic Mechanisms in Human Immunodeficiency Virus HIV Infection."
21 VIII International Conference on AIDS. "Study Links Depression to More Rapid Decline in Those With HIV Infection." *AIDS Weekly* (July 27,1992).
22 VIII International Conference on AIDS. "GP160 Vaccine Immunotherapy Showing Promise." *AIDS Weekly* (July 27, 1992).
Koenig, Scott, M.D. "HIV-specific Immunity and the Pathogenesis of AIDS." *Annals of Internal Medicine* (April 15, 1992) 114(8): 678–93.
NIH Conference. "Immunopathogenic Mechanisms in Human Immunodeficiency Virus HIV Infection."
23 VIII International Conference on AIDS. "Vaccine Pioneer Jonas Salk Questions Strategy of AIDS Researchers." *AIDS Weekly* (Aug 3,1992).
24 Concorde Coordinating Committee. "Concorde: MRC/ANRS Randomized Double-blind Controlled Trial of Immediate and Deferred Zidovudine in Symptom-free HIV Infection." *The Lancet* (April 8, 1994) 343: 871–880.
25 VIII International Conference on AIDS. "Aggressive HIV Strain May Cause AIDS Progression." *AIDS Weekly* (July 27, 1992).
26 "Reports of Immunodeficiency in Patients Without HIV Create Furor." *AIDS Weekly* (July 27, 1992).
Editorials: " 'AIDS' Without HIV: Fire Without Smoke." *The British Medical Journal* (Aug 8, 1992) 3305(6849): 325–326.
"Clinically Diagnosed AIDS Cases Without Evident Association With HIV Type 1 and 2 Infections in Ghana." *AIDS Weekly* (Nov 2, 1992).
27 VIII International Conference of AIDS. "Physician Association for AIDS Care Launches Nutrition Program for HIV Patients." *AIDS Weekly* (Aug 3, 1992).
28 "Glutathione Depletion in HIV-Infected Patients: Role of Cysteine Deficiency and Effect of Oral N-Acetylcysteine." *AIDS Weekly, AIDS* (Aug, 1992) 6(8): 815–819.
VIII International Conference on AIDS. "Evidence Suggests Nutritional Supplements Can Decrease Malnutrition in AIDS Patients and Improve Quality of Life." *AIDS Weekly* (Aug 3, 1992).

Index

A

Absorption, nutrient, 63, 70
Acemannan, treatment with, 91
Acupressure, 189
    recommended reading, 192
    resources, 190–91
Acupuncture
    American Association of Acupuncture and Oriental Medicine, 119
    herbal medicine in conjunction with, 86–87
    naturopathic medicine and, 125
    practitioners of, 119–20
    recommended reading, 120–22
    resources, 119–20
    treatment of AIDS-related illnesses, 114, 116, 118
Acyclovir, herpes treatment with, 107
Adrenaline level, 38
Aerobic exercise, patient-physician partnership and, 201
Africa
    gender distribution of AIDS cases, 12
    HIV test results and, 51
    incidence of AIDS, 4–5
AIDS
    alternative treatment approaches, overview of, 59–60
    autoimmune features, 13, 52–53
    definitions, 6
    HIV exposure and, questions concerning, 48–50
    HIV-negative patients with, 9–10, 275–76
    myths surrounding, 3–4
    positive actions for patients, 55–56
    prevention of infections associated with, 54–55
    prognosis for future, 45–47, 56
    recommended reading, 23–24, 260–62

    regaining health after illness, 54–55
    worldwide differences, 4–6
AIDS organizations, 255–59
AIDS Project Los Angeles, 248, 255–56
Alcohol
    avoidance of, 64
    effects of, 37–38
Allergen elimination, 218
Allergy testing, resources, 80
Aloe vera, treatment with, 91
Alonso, Kenneth, M.D. 173–75, 177
Alternative healing program, patient-physician partnership in, 205–11
Alternative health professionals, selection of, 263–65
    acupuncture, practitioners of, 119–20
    biofeedback, practitioners of, 149
    hypnotherapy, practitioners of, 149–50
    massage therapy, practitioners of, 190
    mind/body medicine, practitioners of, 148–49
    neuro-linguistic programming (NLP), practitioners of, 150
    physicians. *See* Physicians, selection of
    Therapeutic Touch, practitioners of, 191
    Traditional Chinese Medicine (TCM), practitioners of, 119–20
American Association of Acupuncture and Oriental Medicine, 119
American Association of Naturopathic Physicians, 95
Amino acids, dietary supplements, 65, 76–77, 110
Amphetamines, effects of, 39–40
Amyl nitrite, AIDS and, 14, 28, 39–40
Anal intercourse, 28, 52
Anal intercourse, AIDS and, 28, 42–43
ANA-10 treatment, 231
Anemia, 207

intravenous drug users and, 29
Antibiotics
  AIDS-related illnesses, treatment
    with, 41
  AIDS risks associated with use of, 14
  Bifidobacteria supplement use, 41
  intravenous drug users and, 29
  Lactobaccillus acidophilus supple-
    ment use, 41
  overuse as risk factor in homosexual
    men, 27–28
  Pneumocystis carinii pneumonia
    (PCP), treatment with, 109
Antibodies
  HIV, 8, 52
  hyperthermia and, 170
Antimalarial drug use, AIDS and, 26
Antineoplastin AS2-1 treatment, 221–24
Antiviral therapies, patient-physician
  partnership and, 202
Apoptosis, HIV mechanism of, 10
Ascorbic acid. *See* Vitamin C
Aspirin, treatment of AIDS-related ill-
  nesses with, 41
Astragalus *(Astragalus membranaceus)*,
  treatment with, 91–92, 102
Astragalus *(Radix astragalus)*, treatment
  with, 102
Astra Isatis, treatment with, 88, 132
Attitude, patient-physician partnership
  and, 201–2, 208
Autoimmune disease, AIDS as, 13, 52–53
Ayurvedic medicine, 89–90
AZT
  adverse effects, 19–20, 207
  characteristics of, 41–42
  natural methods compared with,
    21–22
  questionable benefits of, 20–21
  resistance to, 207
  side effects, 41–42
  toxicity, 42

B

Bacteria, friendly. *See* Probiotics
Badgley, Laurence, M.D., 62, 197,
  211–16

Bailey, Steven, N.D., 27, 29, 38,
  123–30, 140
Bastyr University, 179. *See also* Healing
  AIDS Research Project (HARP)
Baths, hot, hyperthermia and, 169–70,
  172, 178
B cells, definition, 17
Benzene, AIDS and, 220–21
Beta-carotene, 72–73, 101
Bialy, Harvey, Ph.D., 10–11
Bifidobacteria
  antibiotics supplemented with, 41
  candidiasis treatment with, 104
  diarrhea treatment with, 106
  dietary supplements, 78
Bihari, Bernard, 105
Biochemical Defense System (BDS),
  221–22
Biofeedback, practitioners of, 149
Biotin, 75
Birk, Thomas J., Ph.D., 185
Bitter melon. *See* Chinese bitter melon
Blood acidity level, alteration of, 217
Blood cell counts, diagnosis and, 207
Blood transfusion recipients
  amount of blood transfused as factor,
    31
  hemophiliacs, 14, 31–32
  HIV test results in, 52
  immunosuppressive effects of trans-
    fusion, 30
  risk of AIDS in, 29–30
  study results, 49
Bowel disorders, AIDS-related illnesses
  and, 100
Bowel flora, normalization of, 218
Breathing, massage therapy and, 185
Brown, Raymond Keith, M.D., 107
Burzynski, Stanislaw, M.D., Ph.D., 197,
  221–24, 244
Buyer's clubs, 259

C

Caffeine
  avoidance of, 64
  effects of, 38
Callen, Michael, 137

Canada, somatidian orthobiology in, 226–34

Candidiasis, 103–4
  herbal treatment, 104
  nutritional therapy, 105
  treatment, alternative, 104–5
  treatment, conventional, 104

Carbohydrates, refined, 64

Cargile, William Michael, B.S., D.C., 114-115

Carlson, Eunice, 104

Carnivora *(Dionaea muscipula)*, treatment with, 92, 102

Carpendale, Michael, M.D., 155

Case histories
  Badgley, Laurence, M. D., 213–16
  Bailey, Steven, Ph.D., 127-130
  Burzynski, Stanislaw, M.D., Ph.D., 222–24
  Cathcart, Robert, III, M. D., 224–25
  Chinese bitter melon, treatment with, 236–37
  hyperthermia, 173–77
  Kaiser, Jon, M.D., 203–5
  massage therapy, 186
  naturopathic medicine, 127–30
  nutrition, 72
  Orth, Gerhard, Dr., 219
  ozone therapy, 161–62
  Priestley, Joan, M.D., 209–11
  714-X treatment, 231–34
  vitamin C treatment, 224–25
  woman as long-term survivor, 241–52

Cathcart, Robert, III, M.D., 71, 108, 197, 224–25

Causes of AIDS, 5. *See also* Co-factors; Lifestyle factors; Risk groups
  multifactorial, 13, 46–47
  treatment method and, 25

CBC test, 207

CD4 cells. *See* T4 cells

CD8 cells. *See* T8 cells

Centers for Disease Control (CDC)
  blood transfusion study, 30
  conditions associated with AIDS, recognition by, 99
  diagnostic criteria for AIDS, 4, 9–10

HIV test guidelines, 51

Chinese bitter melon *(Momordica charantia)*, treatment with, 92–93, 102, 116
  anti-HIV effects, 235
  patient-physician partnership, 235–37

Chinese herbal medicine, 86, 113–14, 116

Chinese Medicine, Traditional. *See* Traditional Chinese Medicine (TCM)

Chocolate, effects of, 38

Chronic Fatigue Syndrome (CFS), 47

Clark, Hulda R., N.D., Ph.D., 26, 220–21

Cocaine, effects of, 39–40

Co-factor illnesses. *See* Illnesses, AIDS-related

Co-factors, 14–15. *See also* Antibiotics; Drug use; Homosexual men; Malnutrition
  hemophiliacs, 14, 31–32
  mycoplasma, 13
  parasites, 26, 105–6, 220–21
  psychoimmunoneurological factors, 14, 35, 138–39
  requirement for AIDS development, 10, 13, 45, 277
  sexually transmitted diseases, 14, 27–29

Coffee, effects of, 38

Cohen, Misha, O.M.D., L.Ac., 115

Composition-A, treatment with, 86–87

Concorde study, AZT findings, 21

Condoms, 43

Coronel, Ignacio, M.D., 197, 225–26

Counseling, naturopathic medicine and, 124, 132–33

Curran, James, Dr., 13, 30

Cytomegalovirus
  herbal medicine and, 108
  HIV test results and, 51–52

D

ddC, 22, 207
  problems associated with, 19

side effects, 22
ddI, 22, 207
    problems associated with, 19
    side effects, 22
Definitions of AIDS, history of, 6
Detoxification, acupuncture and, 125
Dharmananda, Subhuti, Ph.D., 86–88,
        91, 114–15, 184
Diagnosis
    African AIDS patients, 12
    blood cell counts, 207
    CBC test, 207
    Centers for Disease Control (CDC)
        criteria, 4, 9–10
    criteria, 4, 9–10
    difficulties encountered, 5
    ELISA (Enzyme Linked Immuno-
        sorrbent Assay) test, 50–51
    HIV, 50–51, 275
    T cell count, 15, 18, 207
    Traditional Chinese Medicine
        (TCM) methods, 117
    Western Blot HIV tests, 50–51
Diarrhea, 105–6, 209, 218
Diathermy, 170
Diet. *See also* Nutrition
    alcohol, avoidance of, 64
    alkaline, 217
    balanced, 63, 65
    caffeine, avoidance of, 64
    case history, 72
    cooked foods, 64
    cooking methods to avoid, 64
    emotional considerations, 63
    fats, avoidance of, 64
    foods to avoid, 63–64
    fungal treatment and, 217
    guidelines, 63–70
    Healing AIDS Research Project
        (HARP), 66, 70, 130–31
    naturopathic study, 130–31
    patient-physician partnership and,
        199, 206, 212, 217–18
    protein intake, 64–65
    raw foods, 64
    recommended reading, 82–83
    refined carbohydrates, avoidance of,
        64

resources, 80–82
    sample daily diet, 67–69
    saturated fats, avoidance of, 64
    supplements. *See* Dietary
        supplements
    vegetarian, 65
    whole foods, 63
Dietary supplements
    amino acids, 65, 76–77
    benefits of, 70
    digestive enzymes, 65, 110
    dosage recommendations, 72–78
    essential fatty acids, 77
    folic acid, 109
    friendly bacteria, 77–78
    future of, 78
    Healing AIDS Research Project
        (HARP), 131-132
    herpes infections, treatment of, 107–8
    intravenous nutrition, 71
    minerals. *See* Minerals
    monolaurin, 102
    multivitamin supplements, 78
    N-acetyl-cysteine (NAC), 76
    naturopathic study, 131–32
    patient-physician partnership,
        199–200
    PCP infections, 109
    probiotics, 77–78
    protein, 76–77
    quercetin, 206
    recommended reading, 83–84
    skin rashes, treatment of, 109
    types of, 70–71
    vitamins. *See* Vitamins
Digestion, 63, 66, 70
    enzymes as dietary supplements, 65,
        110
Diseases associated with AIDS. *See*
        Illnesses, AIDS-related
Drug resistance, 207
Drug treatment, 14
    antibiotics. *See* Antibiotics
    antineoplastin AS2-1, 221–24
    aspirin, 41
    AZT. *See* AZT
    co-factor illnesses, 40–41
    ddC, 19, 22, 207

ddI, 19, 22, 207
diarrhea, 105–6
drug resistance, 207
HIV, 274–75
Investigational New Drug classification, 222
natural compounds in conjunction with, 206
non-steroidal anti-inflammatory drugs, 41
Pneumocystis carinii pneumonia (PCP), 109
problems associated with, 19–20
prophylactic, 276–77
side effects, 19–20
steroid drugs, 40–41
toxicity, 19–20
Drug use
antimalarial drug use as risk factor, 26
intravenous drug use, 14, 28–29
pharmaceutical drug use, 14
recreational drug use, 14
risk of AIDS and, 5, 14
Duesberg, Peter, Ph.D., 8–12, 39

E

Echinacea *(Echinacea angustifolia)*, treatment with, 93
ELISA (Enzyme Linked Immunosorrbent Assay) test, 50–51
Emotional states
mind/body medicine and, 140, 142–45
psychoimmunoneurology and, 138–39
shiatsu and, 189
Endorphins, psychoimmunoneurology and, 138
Environmental risk factors, 5, 35–36
Epstein, Gerald, M.D., 140
Essential fatty acids, dietary supplements, 77
Essex, Max, Dr., 51
Exercise, patient-physician partnership and, 201

F

False positive HIV test results, 50–51
Farr, Charles H.,M.D., Ph.D., 157, 162–63
Fat, dietary, 64
Fatty acids
dietary supplements, 77
monolaurin, 102
Female long-term survivor, case history of, 241–52
Fever, induced. *See* Hyperthermia
Fields, Tiffany, Ph.D., 185
Folic acid, 74, 109
Food. *See* Diet; Nutrition
Foot reflexology, 189
Friendly bacteria. *See* Probiotics
Fungal treatment, 217–18

G

Gallo, Robert, M.D., 7–8
Garlic *(Allium sativum)*, treatment with, 93, 102
herpes infections, 108
immune enhancement, 116
Gay men. *See* Homosexual men
Gay Related Immune Deficiency, 14
Gender, AIDS distribution by, 12
Germany, naturopathic methods in, 216–21
Ginseng, Siberian *(Eleutherococcus sentiocosus)*, treatment with, 94
Glandular extracts, Healing AIDS Research Project (HARP) study, 131–32
Glandular fever, 52
Goldenseal *(Hydrastis canadensis)*, treatment with, 93
Gonorrhea, AIDS in homosexual men and, 27–28
Gordon, Garry F., M.D., 140, 263–65

H

Haas, Elson, M.D., 264–65
Hamilton, John, Dr., 20

HARP study. *See* Healing AIDS
    Research Project
Haverkos, Harry, Dr., 28
HBOT. *See* Hyperbaric oxygen therapy
Healing AIDS Research Project
    (HARP), 130-133
    dietary guidelines, 66, 70, 130–31
    dietary supplements, 131–32
    glandular extracts, 131–32
    herbal medicine, 88, 131–32
    hyperthermia, 132, 171–72
    natural treatment methods, 21–22
    naturopathic study, 130–33
    psychological counseling, 132–33
    results, 133
Health professionals, selection of. *See*
    Alternative health professionals,
    selection of
Health workers, accidental exposure to
    HIV, 11–12
Heat, treatment with. *See* Hyperthermia
Helper cells. *See* T4 cells
Hemophiliacs, 14, 31–32
Hepatitis, Minor Bupleurum
    Combination treatment for, 88
Hepatitis B virus, 52
Hepatitis C virus, 52
Herbal medicine, 85–86, 125
    acemannan, 91
    acupuncture in conjunction with,
        86–87
    aloe vera, 91
    astragalus *(Astragalus mem-
        branaceus)*, 91–92, 102
    astragalus *(Radix astragalus)*, 102
    Astra Isatis, 88, 132
    Ayurvedic medicine, 89–90
    candidiasis, treatment of, 104
    carnivora *(Dionaea muscipula)*, 92,
        102
    Chinese, 86, 113–14, 116
    Chinese bitter melon. *See* Chinese
        bitter melon (Momordica
        charantia)
    combination formulas, 86–88
    Composition-A, 86–87
    diarrhea, treatment of, 106

Echinacea *(Echinacea angustifolia)*,
    93
garlic *(Allium sativum)*. *See* Garlic
goldenseal *(Hydrastis canadensis)*,
    93
HARP study, 131–32
herpes infections, treatment of, 107–8
immune enhancement with, 100–3
immune function supported by, 70
isatis *(Isatis tinctoria)*, 94, 102
licorice *(Glycyrrhiza glabra)*, 94,
    103
liver dysfunction, treatment of, 108
Minor Bupleurum Combination, 88
patient-physician partnership in,
    200–201, 208, 217
physicians specializing in, 95
recommended reading, 96–97
resources, 95–96
role of, 88, 90–91
safety considerations, 95
St. John's Wort *(Hypericum perfora-
    tum)*, 94, 103
Shiitake mushroom extract
    (Lentinan), 103
Siberian ginseng *(Eleutherococcus
    sentiocosus)*, 94
side effects, 95
symptoms treated, 87
Traditional Chinese Medicine
    (TCM). *See* Traditional Chinese
    Medicine (TCM)
types of herbology, 89–90
Venus Fly Trap, 92
Western medicine, 90
Heroin use, risk of AIDS and, 28–29
Herpes infections, 106–8
Hiatt, Alice, R.N., 141, 143, 188–89
HIV, 3
    accidental exposure in medical per-
        sonnel, 11–12
    accuracy of test results, 50–51
    AIDS in HIV-negative patients,
        275–76
    AIDS relationship to, controversy
        regarding, 6, 12–14
    antibodies, 8, 52

causative agent of AIDS, recognition as, 7
characteristics of, 8, 45–46
co-factors for disease progression, 15, 45, 277
drug treatment, 274–75
drug treatment, prophylactic, 276–77
ELISA (Enzyme Linked Immuno-Sorbent Assay) test, 50–51
exposure leading to AIDS, questions concerning, 48–50
false positive test results, 51–52
hyperthermia and, 171
incidence, 267
infection without AIDS, 50
infectivity of, 48–49
latency period, 48
lifestyle factors, 276
natural therapy, 277–78
negative test results in immune suppressed patients, 9–10
pathogenesis, 267–73
positive test results without AIDS, 50
prevention of infections associated with, 54–55
prognosis for future, 45–47
testing, 50–52, 275
vaccines, 273
Western Blot tests, 50–51
Holder, Jay, M.D., D.C., Ph.D., 118, 264
Homeopathy, 106, 125–26
diarrhea treatment, 106
Healing AIDS Research Project (HARP) study, 132
Homosexual men
antibiotic overuse as risk factor for AIDS in, 27–28
autoimmunity in, 53
bowel disorders and, 100
Gay Related Immune Deficiency, 14
international differences, 4
mind/body medicine and, 140
nutritional problems, 100
recreational drug use as risk factor, 14, 28, 39–40
risk factors, 27–28
sexual activity and, 42–43

sexually transmitted diseases and, 27–28
Hughes, David, D.Sc., 164–65
Human immunodeficiency virus. *See* HIV
Humatin, diarrhea treatment with, 105–6
Hydrogen peroxide therapy, 162–63
side effects, 163
Hydrotherapy, 126
Hyperbaric oxygen therapy (HBOT), 163–65
physicians specializing in, 165
Hyperthermia, 169–70
case histories, 173–77
HARP study, 132, 171–72
HEAT INFO, 177–78, 180
HIV virus and, 171
home treatment, 178
induction methods, 170
local, 178
recommended reading, 180–81
resources, 179–80
risks associated with, 178–79
viral infection, treatment of, 172
Hypnotherapy
practitioners of, 149–50
recommended reading, 151

I

Idiopathic CD-4 lymphocytopenia (ICL), 10
Illnesses, AIDS-related
acupuncture as treatment for, 114, 116, 118
candidiasis. *See* Candidiasis
cytomegalovirus, 108
diarrhea, 105–6, 209, 218
drug treatment for, 40–41
herbal medicine, 102–3
herpes infection, 106–8
international differences, 4
Kaposi's sarcoma. *See* Kaposi's sarcoma
liver dysfunction, 108
nutrition, 101–2

Pneumocystis carinii pneumonia. *See*
    Pneumocystis carinii pneumonia
    (PCP)
  prevention of infection, 54–55
  skin rashes, 109–10
  Traditional Chinese Medicine
    (TCM), treatment with, 113–14,
    116, 118
  treatment methods, overview of,
    99–101
  weight loss, 110
Immune collapse, 18
Immune enhancement, 100–101
  acupuncture and, 114
  massage therapy and, 183
  Traditional Chinese Medicine
    (TCM) and, 114–15
Immune function
  foods shown to impair, 63–64
  mind/body medicine and, 142
  nutritional support for, 70–72
Immune suppression
  blood transfusion recipients and,
    30–31
  HIV-negative patients and, 9
Immune system, 15–19
Interferon, hyperthermia and, 170
Intestinal parasites, AIDS and, 26,
    105–6, 220–21
Intravenous drug use, 14, 28–29
Iron, 76
Ironson, Gail, M.D., Ph.D., 185
Isatis *(Isatis tinctoria)*, treatment with,
    94, 102

J

Joiner-Bey, Herb, N.D., 141
*Journal of American Medical
    Association*, HIV tests and, 51

K

Kabat-Zinn, Jon, Ph.D., 146
Kaiser, Jon, M.D., 141, 197–205
Kaposi's sarcoma, 99
  acupuncture and, 118

  inhalant nitrite use associated with,
    28
  Therapeutic Touch and, 190
  treatment, 108
King, Robert, L.M.T., 183–86
Kleinman, Steven, M.D., 155
Koch, Robert, 8–11
Konefal, Janet, Ph.D., M.P.H., C.A.,
    145, 147
Krieger, Dolores, R.N., Ph.D., 189–90
Kunz, Dora, 189

L

Lactobacillus acidophilus, 78
  antibiotics supplemented with, 41
  candidiasis treatment with, 104–5
  diarrhea treatment with, 106
  sources of, 105
Lange, Michael, 15
Latency period, HIV, 48
Lautenberg, Frank, 177
Lee, John R., M.D., 264
Lee-Huang, Sylvia, 236
Leprosy, 52
Levy, Jay, 13
Lewis, Douglas, N.D., 171–72
Licorice (Glycyrrhiza glabra), treatment
    with, 94, 103
Life Sciences Institute of Mind-Body
    Health, 143–45
Lifestyle factors, 35, 37, 44
  alcohol, 37–38
  AZT. *See* AZT
  caffeine, 38
  drugs for treatment of co-factor ill-
    nesses, 40–41
  environmental considerations, 35–36
  HIV and, 276
  patient-physician partnership in
    changing, 206, 219
  pharmaceutical drugs, 40–41
  recreational drugs. *See* Recreational
    drug use
  responsibility, acceptance of, 36
  sexual considerations, 42–44
  stress, 36
  tobacco, 38

Liver dysfunction, treatment, 108
Logan, William D., M.D., 173–74
Long-term survivors
    female, case history of, 241–52
    patient-physician partnership and.
        See Patient-physician partnership
Ludlum, C., Dr., 48
Lund, Sharon, 241–52, 263–64
Lymphocytes. *See* B cells; T cells

M

Macrophage, definition, 17
Magnesium, 76
Malaria
    HIV test results and, 51–52
    treatment, AIDS and, 26
Malnutrition, 70
    AIDS and, 14, 63
    AIDS-related illnesses and, 99–100
    intravenous drug users and, 29
    third world poor and, 26
Manganese, 76
Manipulation, treatment with, 126
Marijuana, effects of, 39
Massage therapy, 126, 183–86
    AIDS patients, 186–88
    case history, 186
    practitioners, 190
    precautions for AIDS patients,
        187–88
    psychoneurological benefits, 186
    recommended reading, 191–92
    resources, 190
McKenna, Joan, 28
Medical personnel, accidental exposure
    to HIV, 11–12
Meditation
    mind/body medicine and, 146
    recommended reading, 152
Methylxanthines, effects of, 38
Mexico, L-51 treatment in, 225–26
Mind/body medicine, 137
    immune system and, 139–40
    individual responsibility and, 140–41
    Life Sciences Institute of Mind-Body
        Health, 143–45
    meditation, 146

    mindfulness, development of, 142
    neuro-linguistic programming
        (NLP), 145–47
    patient-physician partnership, 198–99
    practitioners of, 148–49
    psychoimmunoneurology, 14, 35,
        138–39
    psychological support, 140–41
    recommended reading, 151–54
    resources, 148–49
    stress reduction, 141–43
Minerals
    deficiencies, 75–76
    dietary supplements, 70–71, 75–76,
        78, 206
    iron, 76
    magnesium, 76
    manganese, 76
    potassium, 75
    selenium, 75
    zinc, 75
Minor Bupleurum Combination, treat-
    ment with, 88
Monocyte, definition, 17
Monolaurin, diet supplemented with, 102
Montagnier, Luc, 7, 12–13, 45
Mullis, Kary, Ph.D., 8
Multifactorial causes of AIDS, 13, 46–47
Mushrooms, Shiitake, treatment with
    extract from, 103
Mycoplasma, 13, 52

N

N-acetyl-cysteine (NAC), dietary sup-
    plements, 76, 110, 200
Naessens, Gaston, 198, 226–34
Nardi, Christian Dr., 175, 177
National Institutes of Health (NIH), AZT
    recommendations, 20
Natural killer cells
    definition, 17
    massage therapy and, 185
Natural therapy
    HIV, 277–78
    patient-physician partnership in. *See*
        Patient-physician partnership
Naturopathic medicine, 123

acupuncture and, 125
American Association of
    Naturopathic Physicians, 95, 133
case histories, 127–30
counseling and, 124
dietary guidelines, 130–31
dietary supplements, 131–32
directories of physicians specializing
    in, 95, 133, 135
Healing AIDS Research Project
    (HARP) study, 130–33
herbal medicine. *See* Herbal
    medicine
homeopathy, 125–26
hydrotherapy, 126
hyperthermia. *See* Hyperthermia
manipulation, 126
massage, 126
nutrition. *See* Nutrition
physicians specializing in, 95, 133,
    135
physiotherapy, 126
power blend recipe, 126
protocol recommendations, 124
psychological counseling, 132–33
recommended reading, 135–36
resources, 133–35
Traditional Chinese Medicine
    (TCM) and, 125
Needlestick wounds, accidental exposure
    to HIV via, 11–12
Needle-transmitted infections, in intra-
    venous drug users, 29
Neuro-linguistic programming (NLP),
    145–47
    practitioners of, 150
    recommended reading, 152
New England Journal of Medicines, HIV
    tests and, 51
Newsletters, 262
Non-steroidal anti-inflammatory drugs,
    treatment of co-factor illnesses
    with, 41
Norris, Patricia, Ph.D., 143–45
Null, Gary, 43
Nutrition, 35, 61. *See also* Malnutrition
    absorption, 63, 70
    AIDS-related illnesses and, 99
    benefits of healthy diet, 61–62

candidiasis, treatment of, 105
case history, 72
deficiencies, 62, 70, 199, 212
dietary guidelines. *See* Diet
digestion, 63, 66, 70
herbal medicine. *See* Herbal medi-
    cine
herpes infections, treatment of,
    107–8
immune enhancement with, 100–101
immune function supported by,
    70–72
individual requirements, 62–63
minerals. *See* Minerals
naturopathic medicine and, 125
patient-physician partnership and,
    212
PCP infections, 109
physicians specializing in, 79
professional advice, recommendation
    for, 63
recommended reading, 82–84
supplements. *See* Dietary supple-
    ments
vitamins. *See* Vitamins

O

Olson, Melodie A., Ph.D., 189
Opiodes, effects of, 39
Oral sex, AIDS and, 43
Organic foods, resources for, 80–82
Orth, Gerhard, Dr., 197, 216–19
Orthobiology, somatidian, 226–34
Oxygen therapy, 155–56
    hydrogen peroxide, 162–63
    hyperbaric oxygen therapy (HBOT),
        163–65
    oxidation, 155–57
    oxygenation, 155–56
    ozone therapy, 155, 157–62
    recommended reading, 167–68
    resources, 165–66
    side effects, 162–63
    vitamin C and, 157, 160
Ozone therapy, 155, 157–61
    case histories, 161–62
    side effects, 162

P

p24 antigen
  hyperthermia and, 176
  level in HIV test, 176
Pantothenic acid (vitamin B6), 74
Papadopulos-Elepulos, Eleni 51
Papillomavirus warts, 52
Parasites
  AIDS and, 26, 220–21
  treatment for, 105–6
Patient-physician partnership, 198–99,
    236–37
  alkaline diet, 217–18
  allergen elimination, 218
  antineoplastin AS2-1 and, 221–24
  attitude adjustment and, 201–2, 208
  Badgley, Laurence, M. D., 211–16
  blood acidity level, alteration of, 217
  bowel flora, normalization of, 218
  Burzynski, Stanislaw, M.D., Ph.D.,
    221–24
  case histories. *See* Case histories
  Cathcart, Robert, III, M. D., 224–25
  Chinese bitter melon, treatment with,
    235–37
  Clark, Hulda R., N.D., Ph.D.,
    220–21
  Coronel, Ignacio, M. D., 225–26
  diet, 199, 206, 212, 217–18
  dietary supplements, 199–200
  exercise, 201
  fungal treatment, 217–18
  herbal medicine, 200–201, 208, 217
  Kaiser, Jon, M.D., 198–205
  lifestyle changes, 206, 219
  L-51 treatment, 225–26
  medical therapies, 202
  medication limitations, 219
  mind/body medicine, 198–99
  Naessens, Gaston, 226–34
  Orth, Gerhard, Dr., 216–19
  parasites, treatment of, 220–21
  positive attitude, 201–2, 208
  Priestley, Joan, M. D., 205–11
  recommended reading, 239–40
  selection of health care professional,
    263–65
    714-X treatment, 226–34
    somatidian orthobiology, 226–34
    stress reduction, 201–2
    tissue acidity level, alteration of, 217
    vitamin C, treatment with, 224–25
    Zhang, Qingcai, M.D., 235–37
PCP *See* Pneumocystis carinii pneumonia
PCR (Polymerase Chain Reaction), 8, 275
Peper, Erik, Ph.D., 141–43
Peptide-T, treatment with, 208
Pert, Candace, Ph.D., 138–39, 208
Pharmaceutical drug treatment. *See* Drug
    treatment
Physician-patient partnership. *See*
    Patient-physician partnership
Physicians, selection of, 263–65
  American Association of
    Naturopathic Physicians, 95
  herbal medicine, 95
  hyperbaric oxygen therapy (HBOT),
    specialists in, 165
  naturopathic medicine, 95, 133–135
  nutrition, specialists in, 79
Physiotherapy, 126
Pittman, John, M.D., 160
Pneumocystis carinii pneumonia (PCP),
    99
  acupressure and, 189
  Therapeutic Touch and, 189
  treatment, 109
Pontiggia, Paolo, M.D., 174
Poppers, AIDS and, 14, 28, 39–40
Potassium, 75
Poverty, third world, AIDS and, 25–26
Preuss, ALexander, M.D., 159
Priestley, Joan, M.D., 71, 116, 197,
    205–11, 244
Probiotics
  candidiasis, treatment with, 104
  dietary supplements, 77–78
Prostitution, intravenous drug users and,
    29
Protein
  dietary guidelines, 64–65
  dietary supplements, 76–77
  malnutrition in third world poor and,
    26
  recommendations, 206

Protein p24, HIV test results and, 52
Pro-vitamin A. *See* Beta-carotene
Psychoimmunoneurology, 14, 35, 138–39
Psychological counseling, naturopathic medicine and, 132–33
Psychological support, mind/body medicine and, 140–41
Pyridoxine (vitamin B6), 74

Q

Quercetin, 206

R

Rarick, Mark, M.D., 155
Rashes, treatment of, 109–10
Rebultan, Stanley, 236–37
Recreational drug use
    amyl nitrite, 14, 28, 39–40
    marijuana, 39
    opiodes, 39
    risks associated with, 14, 28, 38–39
Rectal retention enema, bitter melon used with, 93
Rectum, sexual activity effects on, 42–44
Reflexology, 189
    recommended reading, 192–93
    resources, 191
Relaxation techniques, immune function and, 142
Resist, herbal formula, 200
Retroviruses, 8, 52
Riboflavin (vitamin B2), 74
Risk groups, 25, 33
    blood transfusion recipients, 29–31, 49
    hemophiliacs, 14, 31–33
    homosexual men. *See* Homosexual men
    international differences, 4
    intravenous drug users, 14, 28–29
    third world poor, 25–26
Root-Bernstein, Robert, PhD., 9, 20, 28–30, 46, 50, 52–54
Russia, AIDS education in, 251–52

Ryan, Mary Kay, N.C.C.A., Dipl. Ac., 113–14

S

Safe sex, 43
St. John's Wort *(Hypericum perforatum)*, treatment with, 94, 103
Saunas, hyperthermia and, 170
Scafidi, Frank, Ph.D., 185
Selenium, 75
Seligmann, Maxime, 25–26
Selye, Hans, 36
VII International Conference on AIDS, 51
714-X treatment, 226–34
Sex, AIDS distribution by, 12
Sexual activity, AIDS and, 42–44
Sexually transmitted diseases (STDs)
    AIDS and, 14
    gonorrhea, 27–28
    homosexual men and, 27–28
    intravenous drug users and, 29
    syphilis, 27–28
Shiatsu, 189
    recommended reading, 192
Shiitake mushroom extract *(Lentinan)*, treatment with, 103
Siberian ginseng *(Eleutherococcus sentiocosus)*, treatment with, 94
Side effects
    antibiotics for PCP, 109
    AZT, 41–42
    drug treatment, 19–20, 22
    herbal medicine, 95
    hydrogen peroxide therapy, 163
    ozone therapy, 162
Skin rashes, treatment of, 109–10
Smith, Michael, M.D., 118
Smoking, effects of, 38
Socially disadvantaged groups, AIDS in, 5
Social Security Disability Benefits, women as recipients of, 248
Solomon, George, Dr., 137, 197
Somatidian orthobiology, 226–34
Sonnabend, Joseph, M.D., 13, 53

Spirituality, patient-physician partnership and, 209
Standish, Leanna, N.D., Ph.D., 132
Steam treatment, 170
Steroid drugs, treatment of AIDS-related illnesses with, 40–41
Stewart, Gordon, Professor, 6, 32
Stimulant drugs, effects of, 39
Stress
  acupuncture and, 115
  cumulative effects of, 36
  massage therapy and, 183
  mind/body medicine and, 141–43
  reduction, patient-physician partnership and, 201–2
Sunnen, Gerard, M.D., 158–59
Suppressor cells. *See* T8 cells
Survivors, long-term
  female, case history of, 241–52
  patient-physician partnership and.
    See Patient-physician partnership
Symptoms
  AIDS-related illnesses, 99–100
  HIV-negative cases, 9
Syphilis
  HIV test results and, 27–28
  homosexual men and, 27–28

T

T cell counts
  antineoplastin AS2-1 and, 221
  case histories, 203–5
  diagnosis and, 15, 18, 207
  L-51 treatment and, 225–26
  naturopathic medicine and, 127
  T4 cells, 15, 18, 116, 236–37
  T8 cells, 18, 207
  Traditional Chinese Medicine effects on, 116
  vitamin C and, 224
T cells. *See also* Natural killer cells
  aupuncture and, 115
  definition, 16
T4 cells, 15
  Chinese bitter melon effects on count, 116, 236–37
  count, 15, 18, 116, 236–37

definition, 16
  immune system role of, 17–19
  massage therapy and, 185
T8 cells
  count, 18, 207
  definition, 16
  immune system role of, 17–19
  significance of, 207
Tea, effects of, 38
Temperature, treatment and. *See* Hyperthermia
T-helper lymphocytes. *See* T4 cells
Theobromine, effects of, 38
Theophyllin, effects of, 38
Therapeutic Touch, 189–90
  practitioners, 191
  recommended reading, 193
  resources, 191
Thiamine (vitamin B1), 74
Third world poor, AIDS and, 25–26
Tissue acidity level, alteration of, 217
Tobacco, effects of, 38
Total parenteral nutrition (TPN), treatment with, 209–10
Touch therapy, 188–90. *See also* Massage therapy
  acupressure, 189
  recommended reading, 191–93
  reflexology, 189
  resources, 190–91
  shiatsu, 189
  Therapeutic Touch, 189
Toxicity
  AZT, 41–42
  pharmaceutical drugs, 19–20
Traditional Chinese Medicine (TCM), 89, 113–14, 125
  acupuncture. *See* Acupuncture
  diagnosis in, 117
  herbs, 86, 113–14, 116
  practitioners of, 119–20
  recommended reading, 120–22
  resources, 119–20
  treatment of AIDS-related illnesses, 116, 118
Treatment
  acupuncture. *See* Acupuncture
  alternative approaches, 59–60

antineoplastin AS2-1, 221–24
blood acidity level, alteration of, 217
candidiasis, 104–5
diarrhea, 105–6
diet. *See* Diet
drug treatment. *See* Drug treatment
fungal, 217
herbal medicine. *See* Herbal medicine
herpes infections, 107–8
hyperthermia. *See* Hyperthermia
illnesses associated with AIDS,
    99–111
Kaposi's sarcoma, 108
liver dysfunction, 108
L-51 treatment, 225–26
massage therapy, 183–88
mind/body medicine. *See* Mind/body
    medicine
naturopathic medicine. *See*
    Naturopathic medicine
nutrition. *See* Nutrition
oxygen therapy. *See* Oxygen therapy
Pneumocystis carinii pneumonia
    (PCP), 109
714-X treatment, 226–34
skin rashes, 109–10
somatidian orthobiology, 226–34
tissue acidity level, alteration of, 217
touch therapy, 188–90
Traditional Chinese Medicine
    (TCM). *See* Traditional Chinese
    Medicine
vaccine, development of, 53
vitamin C. *See* Vitamin C
weight loss, 110
Trimethoprim-sulfamethoxazole, PCP
    treatment with, 109
T-suppressor lymphocytes. *See* T8 cells
Tuberculosis, 52

U

Ultrasound therapy, 170
Universal Reactor Syndrome, 47

V

Vaccines, development of, 53, 273

Vaginal yeast infections. *See* Candidiasis
Vallancien, Bertrand, 159
Vegetarian diets, 65
    protein guidelines, 65
    recommended reading, 83
    resources, 81
Venezeula, HIV test results and, 51
Venus Fly Trap, treatment with, 92
Veterans Administration, AZT study, 20
Viral infections, hyperthermia treatment
    of, 151
Vitamin A, 73. *See also* Beta-carotene
Vitamin B-complex, 73–75
    biotin, 75
    folic acid, 74
    pantothenic acid (B5), 74
    pyridoxine (B6), 74
    riboflavin (B2), 74
    thiamine (B1), 74
    vitamin B12, 74
Vitamin C
    bowel tolerance, 101
    dietary supplements, 71
    dosage, 71, 73
    immune enhancing effects, 71
    Kaposi's sarcoma treatment, 108
    megadose treatment, 224–25
    oxygen therapy and, 157, 160
Vitamin E, 73
    selenium and, 75
Vitamins
    ascorbic acid. *See* Vitamin C
    beta-carotene, 72–73, 101
    deficiencies, 70, 199
    dietary supplements, 70–71, 200,
        206
    dosage recommendations, 72–75
    multivitamin supplements, 78
    pro-vitamin A, 72–73, 101

W

Wagner, Kenneth, M.D., 155
Water testing, resources, 81
Weight loss, treatment of, 110
Western Blot HIV tests, 50–51
Western medicine, herbal, 90
Whole foods, 63

Winkler, Jean-Marie, 159
Winson, Beth, 186–87
Women
    case history of long-term survivor,
      241–52
    special challenges for AIDS patients,
      247–52
    vaginal yeast infections in. *See*
      Candidiasis
World Health Organization, diagnostic
    criteria for AIDS, 9–10
Wright, Jonathan, M.D., 160

Y

Yeast infections. *See* Candidiasis
Yogurt, *Lactobacillus acidophilus* in,
    105

Z

Zablow, Andrew, M.D., 175
Zhang, Qingcai, M.D., 113, 116, 235–37
Zidovudine. *See* AZT
Zinc, 75

What Experts are Saying about *You Don't Have to Die: Unraveling the AIDS Myth*

"This book is a godsend and will be a lifesaver for many. It also clearly shows the danger and futility of our conventional belief that AIDS is simply an infectious viral disease and offers reasonable and hopeful alternatives. Conventional treatment for AIDS with toxic immunotherapy drugs stems from the same mind set that, for over a century, has used the same futile approach with cancer. Having read this book and many others, it seems that the conventional beliefs of 'modern medicine' are far more inaccurate and thus dangerous than the beliefs of the past.

"For those who have AIDS, I strongly suggest that you steer your own ship, educate yourself with this and other books, and take an active part in all decisions concerning your treatment. This book will help you enormously."

—Julian Whitaker, M.D., President,
American Preventive Medical Association

"An honest and well written presentation of material that is an excellent resource for anyone who is HIV positive or at risk. I highly recommend it."

—Dr. Bernie Siegel, Author,
Love, Medicine & Miracles

"As the Chief Executive Officer and founder of Project AIDS, International, I take the endorsement of literature very seriously, as it may mean the difference between life and death. As for this book, we can only state that it is mandatory for the survival of persons with AIDS."

—Jeremy Selvey, Founder,
Project AIDS, International

"Highly recommended! At last, clear thinking and clear writing about AIDS and its treatment. A wealth of invaluable information."

—Bernard Rimland, Ph.D.,
Author and Lecturer

"This volume demonstrates the variety of treatment and prevention regimens that are available NOW, once one is liberated from the 'HIV causes AIDS' mythology."

—Charles A. Thomas, Jr., Ph.D.,
Secretary, The Group for the Scientific
Reappraisal of the HIV/AIDS Hypothesis,
Former professor of Molecular Biology, Harvard University

"This book offers the precious gift of life to two groups of people: those who suffer from AIDS (the syndrome), and those who test HIV-positive—which are quite different. You Don't have to Die: Unraveling the AIDS Myth *has clearly been researched in unusual depth by a team of dedicated experts in every aspect of the central subject, and should be of significant interest to anyone concerned with immunosuppressive diseases."*

—Charles Wallach, Ph.D., Director,
AIDS Policy Research Center

"Congratulations on another success! You Don't Have to Die: Unraveling the AIDS Myth *fills a long-standing void in the education and treatment options for HIV infection. This exceptional book will become required reading for all my AIDS patients and should be a 'must read' for anyone interested in HIV, AIDS, and immune depression."*

—Steven Bailey, N.D., Assistant Professor of
Pharmacognosy and Nutrition,
National College of Naturopathic Medicine

"*To be empowered with choices and information is a great gift. To have so much life-affirming options is a BLESSING. Thank you.*"

— Gregg Cassin, Founder and President,
San Francisco Center for Living

"*This sober, dispassionate, and informative survey of what is called the 'AIDS epidemic' goes a long way to unraveling the tangle of premature medical judgments which have brought this monster into being. And it offers a plethora of therapeutic suggestions for those who do not want to shorten their lives with AZT.*"

— Harris L. Coulter, Ph.D., Author,
*Divided Legacy: A History of
the Schism in Medical Thought*

Author Bios

Leon Chaitow, N.D., D.O., is a practicing naturopath, osteopath, and acupuncturist in the United Kingdom, with over thirty years clinical experience. He is a prolific writer (40+ books) and edits the *International Journal of Alternative and Complementary Medicine*. He regularly lectures in the United States as well as Europe and has recently been appointed as a senior lecturer by London's University of Westminster. In 1993, he became the first naturopath/osteopath to be appointed as consultant to a Government-funded conventional medical practice.

James Strohecker is an author, consultant, and authority in the field of natural health. Executive Editor of the highly acclaimed *Alternative Medicine: The Definitive Guide*, he has co-authored three books and collaborated on numerous titles in the fields of natural health, yoga, and human potential. A Phi Beta Kappa graduate of the University of Tennessee, James is Vice-President and Executive Editor of Future Medicine Publishing, and is a member of the Advisory Boards for the Institute of Naturopathic Medicine and the College of Homeopathy. James and his wife Nancy reside in Santa Monica, California.

If you are an AIDS patient and are unable to afford *You Don't Have to Die: Unraveling the AIDS Myth*, please call us with the name, address, and phone number of your local public library. We will send a copy to the library free of cost, providing the AIDS patients in your community with access to this valuable resource.

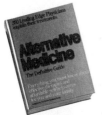

Alternative Medicine: The Definitive Guide

Spanning a global effort of 4 years and input from nearly 400 health professionals, this one-stop reference offers in-depth explanations to 43 of the leading alternative therapies. In addition to covering over 200 of the most common health problems, a wide range of choices to maintaining and regaining your health are highlighted with graphic illustrations. This is truly the "Voice of Alternative Medicine."   ISBN# 0-9636334-3-0 $59.95

Alternative Medicine Yellow Pages

The perfect companion to *Alternative Medicine: The Definitive Guide*, this publication is the most comprehensive directory of health care practitioners of alternative medicine in the United States and Canada. Practitioners of over 70 therapies can be located by state and city. Patients can now instantly find the most appropriate practitioner in their geographical region.   ISBN# 0-9636334-2-2 $12.95

Alternative Medicine Digest

This monthly update reports on leading-edge research and advances in the field of alternative medicine. The information is simply, easily, and quickly accessed through our bottom-line format. Where the book *Alternative Medicine: The Definitive Guide* began, the Digest continues with information on the politics of healthcare and the future of medicine today. $36.00/12 issues

Natural Home Remedies

A concise, easy-to-use handbook which lists remarkable yet simple and natural remedies to help you get relief from common health conditions such as colds and flus, headaches, allergies and much more. With this book, you can build your 'natural medicine chest' with products found in health food stores everywhere.   ISBN# 0-9636334-8-1 $4.95

Alternative Medicine Natural Home Remedies Video

Make natural, safe remedies in your home. Host, Jay Gordon, M.D., gives hands-on demonstrations in this instructional video. *Natural Home Remedies* handbook also included.

ISBN# 0-9636334-7-3 $29.95

You Don't Have to Die - Unraveling the AIDS Myth

A cutting-edge publication that redefines AIDS by shattering the myths surrounding this controversial and sometimes deadly disease. Alternative therapies from around the world coupled with case histories and the latest research make this one of the most promising and compelling books on coping with AIDS today.   ISBN# 0-9636334-4-9 $14.95